CONTENTS

PREFACE

The study of human sexuality has been accepted as a scientific discipline for several decades, as has sexuality education as part of the formal education of children in kindergarten through 12th grade. Although in some educational settings it stands as a separate and distinct discipline, comprehensive sexuality education most frequently occurs as one of the subcontent areas subsumed under health education. Hence, it is for the preparation of preservice as well as professional health education students that this book is intended. We envision it to be used as the primary text in a sexuality education course for prospective health educators, bridging the gap between the content and pedagogy specific to this subcontent area. It may also be used as a supplemental text in a K–12 methods course and as a resource for K–12 teachers already in service.

The book considers specific areas associated with sexuality education deemed appropriate for young people to learn about, the basic information necessary for the prospective teacher to feel comfortable with the knowledge base, as well as comments and segments about the age/developmental appropriateness of the content. Also included are examples of learning experiences designed for prospective teachers to experience themselves, and then to adapt or apply in their future classrooms. In addition, each chapter directs the reader to several websites and additional resources where additional information and activities can be found.

One can teach about human sexuality taking a content-based approach, a skills-based approach, or a combination of both skills and content. We believe that the combination of skills and content is most effective in contributing to student achievement of the National Standards for Health Education established by the professional community. Moreover, we believe that using a combination approach of skills and content will better prepare prospective teachers to help their future students to develop living styles that are consistent with their own personal value system, with concerns for their family, religious, and social community. The book provides opportunities to reflect on the diversity of thoughts, beliefs, preferences, and behaviors associated with sexual issues. Such an approach also considers the sometimes controversial issues related to gender equity, sexual orientation, family planning, adolescent pregnancy, parenting styles, sexual violence, and media portrayals of sexuality. This approach attempts to further develop prospective students' skills as communicators, problem solvers, decision makers, stress managers, and goal setters as each role applies to their sexuality.

We recognize that teaching about human sexuality to all grade levels frequently presents academic and political problems. Some school districts do not permit teaching sexuality education at all; others allow an abstinence-only curriculum; still others restrict the amount and type of information provided; and finally, there are those who support a comprehensive approach including an "abstinence-plus" curriculum. It is our opinion, supported by research, that information, delivered appropriately with due consideration for the developmental stages of the students being taught, will not interfere with students' healthy sexual development or support their early involvement in sexual intercourse or other "promiscuous" behaviors. Knowing does *not* mean doing! Knowing makes one smarter rather than more stupid. The more information and skills students have, the better equipped they are to deal with their sexual thoughts and make wise and critical decisions about their sexual behaviors, less influenced by peer pressure. The more knowledgeable and skilled they are, the more they can reflect on their lives as sexual beings (since they are sexual beings from the moment that they are born); the better they can evaluate their sexual behaviors relative to others such as friends, peers, family, and community; and the more likely they will make decisions that will enhance their lives. Hence, the text provides opportunities for prospective teachers to help their students to develop both skills and knowledge.

Each of the chapters discussed here introduces a critical subcontent area included in a comprehensive sexuality education curriculum.

Chapter 1, "Introduction," presents an overview of the discipline and a history of sexuality research as it applies to sexuality education. This chapter reinforces the need for sexuality education to be taught as a component of health education. It identifies, explains, and outlines the skills that prospective students need to develop in order to be effective in their adult lives. Also presented are the rationale for developmental appropriateness, the format for teaching methodologies, and an explanation of the components that constitute effective learning experiences and lesson plans.

Chapter 2, "Male and Female Sexuality Development through the Life Cycle: Birth to Aging," describes the anatomy and physiology of the reproductive systems in males and females and the characteristics and behaviors involved in sexual growth and maturation. This chapter discusses some of the theories of psychosexual development especially as they pertain to the complexities of puberty and adolescence.

Chapter 3, "Sexual Behaviors," focuses on those behaviors directly associated with sexual arousal and sexual attraction such as the human sexual response cycle, sexual variations, and dysfunctions. The chapter explains the processes involved in self-pleasuring, noncoital, and coital behaviors. It also deals with other sexual expressions such as fetishes and provides an overview of prostitution and its impact on culture.

Chapter 4, "Gender Issues in Sexuality Education," begins with the way gender is assigned at birth and how social scripting and socializing affect the development of gender roles and masculinity and femininity. By the time children enter school, gender differences can impact their learning potential, thus limiting their development as males and females. The chapter emphasizes the position that learning should not be limited by gender. It goes on to develop the notion of gender equity in education and the issues that teachers need to be sensitized to. Thus, the teaching of life skills must not have a gender bias. The chapter also describes the ways that families, peers, and communities influence gender.

Chapter 5, "Sexual Orientation: Gay, Lesbian, Bisexual, and Transgender People," indicates that these areas are the most misunderstood and undertaught components in sexuality education curricula. It uses a developmental model to describe the various sexual orientations as a part of normal human sexual development. It emphasizes that orientation should not be seen as a dichotomous model (straight or gay) but as a continuum between the two extremes, that behaviors cannot be predicted by applying a stereotype and the coming out process can be better understood. By describing the variability of GLBT people, a safer academic environment can be created.

Chapter 6, "Relationships," describes the components of a healthy relationship. It begins with the various forms of relationships and how they differ in attachments, boundaries, and styles—family, friends, dates, and mates and how they are chosen. The necessary skills required for their selection are discussed. Some will involve forms of intimacy; others will not. Also important are recognizing when relationships are unhealthy and identifying the resources in the community that can help.

Chapter 7, "Parenting," helps students to explore the roles, attitudes, and expectations that they will have should they become parents. It explains the gender differences between mothers and fathers and the stresses that adolescents may face if they become parents prematurely. Along with their economic challenges, teenage parents face a myriad of informational and emotional problems in their parenting roles. By exploring these issues, teenagers can develop the skills needed in order to defer becoming parents prematurely. Also described are the essential skills, such as conflict resolution and stress management, required for effective parenting. Talking about the different types of families helps children to identify the preferential and cultural diversity that exists. Also essential to effective parenting is developing students' knowledge about infant and child development and the social support systems that are available.

Chapter 8, "Pregnancy and Childbirth," extends the information on parenting to include the processes of conception, pregnancy, and childbirth so that much of the misinformation can be rooted out, allowing students to be informed about these natural processes. Concerns about fertility and developmental abnormalities are also discussed. To improve the chances of fertility, stress management and fertility awareness are presented, as are options in cases of infertility. Included is a review of the postpartum experience and how it can influence family dynamics.

Chapter 9, "Contraception and Abortion," extends parenting skills to include pregnancy prevention. After presenting the history of the methods applied to contraception and abortion, including religious and cultural issues, the chapter describes each contraceptive and abortion method, along with their advantages and disadvantages. This information is meant to enable people to make the best decisions about these matters for themselves.

Chapter 10, "Sexually Transmitted Infections and HIV/AIDS," provides students with the information necessary to remain sexually healthy, to prevent illness resulting from STIs, and to understand the risk-taking process when making a decision to become sexually active. Inherent in this discussion is an understanding of the functioning of the human immune system and the differences between infections from bacterial, viral, and parasitic organisms. The various diseases and their symptoms, diagnoses, and treatments are presented. In addition, there is a full discussion of acquired immune deficiency syndrome (AIDS) and its prevention. Finally, because much concern persists on giving STI and AIDS information to students, there is a brief discussion of the information from a developmentally appropriate perspective.

Chapter 11, "Sexual Violence," introduces the topics of sexual abuse, sexual assault, forcible rape, and date rape without frightening students, faculty, and parents. The data clearly show that students who are exposed to these topics will more readily disclose instances of victimization. The antivictimization material is presented using a clearly defined developmental approach and reinforces the need to identify persons available in the school and community whom students can speak with about abuse and assault. The chapter emphasizes effective communication that can enhance personal safety and alerts educators to symptoms of victimization.

The text concludes with Chapter 12, "Sexuality in Society and Culture," which addresses the way that society and culture heavily influence who we are as sexual beings. Legal institutions and religious traditions are examined as to their impact on people's sexuality. The chapter recognizes the ethnic and racial diversity in the United States and the resulting wide variety of views, traditions, and expectations related to human sexuality. It also considers works of art and their impact on people's sexuality, as well as the influences of the media (books, TV, movies, newspapers, the Internet, and so forth). Hence, censorship and the ongoing struggle it elicits, especially as it relates to youth, are also discussed.

CONTRIBUTORS

Estelle Weinstein, Ph.D., is a full Professor in the School of Education and Allied Human Services at Hofstra University. She served as the chairperson of the Department of Health Professions and Family Studies for more than 6 years and as the director of Graduate Programs in Health (Health Education and Health Administration) for more than 18 years. She has co-authored, with Efrem Rosen, *Critical Issues in Sexuality: Implications for Psychotherapy* (American Press, 2003); and coedited, also with Rosen, *Teaching Children about Health: A Multidisciplinary Approach* (Wadsworth/Thomson Learning, 2003). She has published chapters in edited texts, research collections, and workbooks and journal articles on various topics in human sexuality, adolescence, chronic illness, obesity, and other health-related topics. She regularly presents workshops and seminars at national and regional professional association conferences and has a private practice in Sex and Family Therapy.

Efrem Rosen, Ph.D., earned a Bachelor of Science Degree at Brooklyn College in biology. He received his Master of Science Degree at Long Island University in biology and his Ph.D. at Rutgers University in zoology. He is a Professor Emeritus of biology and the coordinator of the Natural Sciences and Master of Arts in Human Sexuality programs at New College of Hofstra University, Hempstead, New York. Since 1966, he has taught courses in biology, ecology, animal behavior, and human sexuality. He is certified in sex education and counseling by the American Association of Sex Educators, Counselors and Therapists (AASECT). He is a member of the Medical Advisory Committee of Planned Parenthood of Nassau County and a consultant for education and training in human sexuality. He has co-authored, with Estelle Weinstein, *Sexuality Counseling: Issues and Implications* (Brooks/Cole, 1988); and coedited, also with Weinstein, *Teaching Children about Health K-6: A Multidisciplinary Approach* (Wadsworth/Thomson Learning, 2003). He also authored several articles on adolescent sexuality and AIDS, which have been presented at several national and state conferences.

Patricia Cathers, M.S.W., a Burghardt Turner Fellow, received her M.S.W. from the State University of New York at Stony Brook. With over 18 years of experience in the field of child welfare, she specializes in staff development and training. She currently is the director of Program and Volunteer Services at Child Abuse Prevention Services, Roslyn, New York, where she develops child abuse prevention curricula and child safety workshops. She frequently gives presentations and provides training to school personnel on violence prevention, sexual harassment prevention, bully prevention, and other child safety issues.

Jenine DeMarzo, Ed.D., received her Master's and Doctorate Degrees from Teacher's College, Columbia University, in community health. She holds a B.S. in Health Administration from State University of New York at Cortland. She is an Assistant Professor at Adelphi University in the Health and Physical Education Department. Her research focuses on adolescent and young adult sexual behaviors and their relationship to selected socio-cultural variables. She has presented her work at several professional meetings and conferences and has contributed to edited collections. Prior to university teaching, she spent her early career teaching Health and Physical Education for the New York City Board of Education.

Alane Fagin, M.S., is a Child Development Specialist with a Master's Degree in Child Development from the University of Pittsburgh. She has been the executive director of Child Abuse Prevention Services (CAPS) since its inception in 1982. She is an Adjunct Assistant Professor at Hofstra University, where she teaches courses on child abuse and violence prevention. She has published several articles on child abuse and neglect, has written a chapter in a health education textbook, and has presented workshops at state and national conferences. She is an active board member and participant on Long Island Coalition's task forces, and advisory committees on youth violence, child abuse, teen pregnancy, and family violence.

Rhona Feigenbaum, M.A.; A.C.E., is currently an Associate Professor in the Department of Health, Physical Education, and Recreation at Nassau Community College, New York, where she teaches human sexuality and women's studies courses. She has served as a consultant in sex education curriculum and staff development for local public schools and community agencies. She was the Coordinator of Counseling at Planned Parenthood of Nassau County, New York. She has published several journal articles, coauthored chapters in textbooks, and presented seminars at national and regional conferences.

Jean L. Harris, Ph.D., is an Assistant Professor in Health Studies in the Department of Health Studies, Physical Education, and Human Performance Science at Adelphi University. She received both her Ph.D. and M.S. in Health Education from Pennsylvania State University. She has a B.S. in Health and Physical Education from East Stroudsburg University. She received a national Public Health Award from the Department of Health and Human Services for her Trading Cards program, a peer education drug prevention program. She has published in peer-reviewed journals and is a frequent presenter at local, state, and national conferences. She also has an extensive background in K–12 education, having taught in the Billings Public School System for 12 years.

Mary Grenz Jalloh is the founder and Executive Director of the New York State (NYS) Center for School Safety, New Paltz, New York. The center is a government-coordinating agency for school violence prevention, funded by the New York State Education Department, Office of the Governor,

Office of the NYS Attorney General, and the NYS Department of Health. She has served as a Health Education Consultant for organizations such as the Department of Health, American Cancer Society, Carolina Hospitals, Girl Scouts, and University of North Carolina. Previously, she was an administrator at a county health department in North Carolina and a member of the faculty at the University of Missouri School of Medicine. She is the author of a textbook in rural sociology, coauthor with Kathleen Schmalz of a book chapter on health education and violence prevention for elementary school teachers, and creator of curricula on safe school planning and violence prevention for educators. She holds graduate degrees in Public Health (M.P.H.) and Rural Sociology (M.S.) and is a Certified Health Education Specialist (CHES); she is board certified in school crisis response from the American Academy of Experts in Traumatic Stress (B.C.S.C.R.).

David Kilmnick is a cofounder and the Executive Director of Long Island Gay and Lesbian Youth, Inc., and a Professor of human sexuality, social welfare, and health and diversity. He teaches courses at Adelphi University, Nassau Community College, and State University of New York, Empire State College. He has been widely recognized for his work with GLBT youth.

Janice Koch, Ph.D., is a Professor of Science Education for the Department of Curriculum and Teaching at Hofstra University on Long Island, New York. She teaches courses in elementary and middle school science methods, gender issues in the classroom, and techniques of classroom research. She has written several chapters in edited texts on issues relating to the lives of girls and women in schools and has most recently coedited, with Beverly Irby, *Defining and Redefining Gender Equity in Education* (Infoage, 2002). She is the author of *Gender Issues in the Classroom,* Volume 7 for the *Handbook of Psychology* (Wiley, 2002). Her elementary science methods text, *Science Stories: A Science Methods Book for Elementary School Teachers* (Houghton Mifflin, 2002), is in its third edition as an elementary and middle school text. She consults broadly to schools all over the United States and in Australia addressing issues in science education as they connect to other academic disciplines.

Michael Ludwig, Ph.D., is an Assistant Professor in the Department of Health Professions and Family Studies at Hofstra University. He received his Ph.D. from Pennsylvania State University in Health Education. He also holds an M.S. and B.S. in Health Education from the State University of New York at Cortland. His research focuses on the social, political, and cultural aspects of education and health. He has published in peer-reviewed journals and has presented his work at local and national conventions. He serves as a reviewer for the *American Journal of Health Behavior* and for the research consortium of the American Association for Health Education (AAHE).

Nancy O'Keefe, M.S.W., received a Bachelor of Social Work Degree at Penn State University and a Master's of Social Work from Fordham University. In 1987, she began her social work career in women's reproductive health care, working in a storefront clinic in Brooklyn, New York. She then moved to Planned Parenthood of Nassau County as the Director of Counseling, later advancing to the position of Vice President for Health Services.

Kathleen Schmalz, Ed.D., is an Associate Professor with over 30 years of experience in teaching, leadership, and management roles within public school, college, corporate, clinical pharmaceutical research, and hospital settings. She is the associate chair of a unique, interdisciplinary Department of Health & Human Services at the College of Mount Saint Vincent in Riverdale, New York, which encompasses seven different degree programs, including a Master's in Allied Health and two five-year B.S./M.S. programs in Community Health and Allied Health. She serves as a consultant to schools, businesses, government agencies, nonprofits, and private sectors and as a nongovernmental representative to the United Nations (associated with the Department of Public Information of the UN) for three health promotion and education organizations. She is the author of more than 30 publications on current health issues and topics. She has coauthored, with Mary Grenz Jalloh, a book chapter on Health Education and Violence Prevention for elementary school teachers. She also cowrote, with Jalloh, a technical assistance guide for the National Resource Center for Safe Schools titled *Acquiring and Utilizing Resources to Enhance and Sustain a Safe Learning Environment.* She is a registered nurse, holds graduate degrees in Health Education (Ed.D., M.S., M.A.), and is a Certified Health Education Specialist (CHES).

Andrina Veit, C.S.W, received a Master of Arts Degree in Health Education and a Master of Social Work Degree from Adelphi University. She is currently a Full Professor of Health Education at Nassau Community College, Garden City, New York. She specializes in health, mental health, and chemical dependency. She is the recipient of the New York State Chancellor's Award for Excellence in Teaching. She has presented several workshops at professional conferences and community organizations and coauthored chapters in two health textbooks. She has a private practice in Great Neck, New York.

Shannon Whalen, Ed.D., is an Associate Professor in the Health Studies Division of the Department of Health Studies, Physical Education, and Human Performance Science at Adelphi University. She received her Baccalaureate Degree in Health and Physical Education from the University of Delaware, her first Master's Degree in Health Education from New York University, and her second Master's and Doctorate of Education Degrees in Health Education from Columbia University, Teachers College. Prior to joining the faculty at Adelphi University, she taught Health, Physical Education, and Athletic Training courses at the College of Mount Saint Vincent and John Jay College, City University of New York. She has also worked as a health teacher in the Clarkstown Central School District and the Yonkers Public School System. In addition to her responsibilities at Adelphi University, she has served as an Adjunct Assistant Professor and Director of Student Teaching in the Department of Health and Behavior Studies at Columbia University, Teachers College. She serves as a consultant for many private and public health organizations. She is currently working as an advocate for health education on state and national committees. Whalen served on the New York State Goals 2000 Higher Education committee and is a member of the National Board of Professional Teaching Health Standards Committee. She presents health education workshops at many conferences each year and has begun publishing some of her teaching techniques and research efforts in health education journals. Her areas of expertise are school health, technology integration, women's health, HIV/AIDS, and human sexuality education. Her current research efforts are focused on advocacy for health education, both on collegiate campuses and in the public schools.

ACKNOWLEDGMENTS

To that which defines my life and gives it meaning: To Mel, my love and inspiration. To my children Tammy, Scott, and Adam and their life partners Gregg, Ilene, and Dawn, who by their inclusiveness, thoughtfulness, and generosity validate all that is important to me. And to each of the eight grandchildren they brought to me as my footprints to the future.

—Estelle Weinstein

To my wife, Sherry, whose unconditional support, companionship, and love has made this task possible. To my children and grandchildren who continue to give my life meaning. And to my new family of children and grandchildren whose total acceptance of me has given me a new happiness and continued productivity.

—Efrem Rosen

INTRODUCTION

ESTELLE WEINSTEIN

"Education is never neutral; it is either for freedom or for domination."
(FREIRE, 1972)

OBJECTIVES

After reading this chapter, students will be able to

1. Describe the study of human sexuality from a historical perspective.
2. Explain what constitutes comprehensive sexuality education and why it is important in a school curriculum.
3. Identify the data on sexual behavior among school-age children.
4. Describe the national health education standards and the scope and sequences suggested in the professional literature.
5. Explain a personal life skills approach to sexuality education, and identify the various skills.
6. Create a learning environment.
7. Develop all of the components necessary for effective lessons.

REFLECTIVE QUESTIONS

Reflective questions such as these may be discussed at the beginning of a session or at the conclusion of a session depending on the previous knowledge and academic experiences of the students.

1. How might you respond to a parent who says that sexuality education belongs in the home or in religious institutions and not in the schools?
2. What are the advantages of a skills-based approach versus a content-based approach to sexuality education?
3. What skills are important to develop?
4. What would you (the prospective teacher) need to be an effective sexuality educator?
5. What are some of the outcomes you would strive for in a K–12 sexuality education curriculum?
6. What are the advantages or disadvantages of an "abstinence-only" versus and abstinence-plus curriculum?

─────────── **SCENARIO** ───────────

Ms. Jordan Jones has been the director of health programs in The East Magical Middle and Senior High School for more than 5 years. She and her faculty have been asked to develop and implement a sexuality education curriculum. They have worked diligently on the curriculum and have had several meetings with the district's Health Advisory Council. Ms. Jones has been asked to present the program next week to the local parents' group. Knowing this to be a somewhat conservative school district, she must impress them with the importance and relevance of what the faculty hope to include in the curriculum.

What are some of the key points Ms. Jones must include in her presentation?
What skills and content will be included in the sexuality curriculum? Why?
How can the curriculum be adjusted to accommodate for the several developmental levels of the students?
Who will teach the subject matter, and what will be that individual's expertise?
What do you anticipate will be the problems Ms. Jones will encounter?
What will parents be concerned about?
How will Ms. Jones deal with controversial issues?

INTRODUCTION

As the globe becomes smaller, travel becomes easier and life becomes more complicated for families to negotiate, schools are more frequently called upon to take the role of parent and caregiver. Teachers are often expected to recognize, understand, and teach children with different cultural, intellectual, and physical characteristics. Increasingly, they are asked to comfort, mentor, and meet students' emotional needs, believing that meeting these needs would result in a greater ability for the students to learn about and lead more healthful and productive lives. Hence, the subject matter includes traditional math, the natural sciences, the social sciences, language arts, as well as content and skills associated with physical, social, emotional, and spiritual health. In this latter context, the subjects of human sexuality and sexual health have been incorporated.

A Historical Perspective

People's interest in sexuality issues are evidenced in art, theological papers, and religious testaments by the ancient Egyptians, Hebrews, Greeks, and Romans. Much of the early literature explains sexuality in terms of morality and religious doctrine in a framework of what might be considered "acceptable" behaviors in a particular society. Folklore, religious influences, and eventually the social controls espoused by an early and relatively unscientific medical community about human sexuality, particularly concerning the "dreadful" things that might emerge from participating in masturbation and contracting a "venereal disease," can be traced to early European history. These influences set the stage for the sexually restrictive and repressive characteristics of the European Victorian era of the 1800s. Embedded within this repressive Victorian culture was an embracing of a traditional philosophy where male dominance was the accepted way and where the inequalities between men and women were considered appropriate (Reiss & Reiss, 1997). Limitations in sexual behavior, especially those related to gender and gender identity, were apparent within marital and other heterosexual relationships (little information was available about homosexual relationships). Yet, moral restraints and gender disparities were not shared across all social classes. The working class adopted them, but the aristocracy was considerably permissive in their sexual attitudes and behaviors. Class differences regarding sexual and gender behaviors can be traced across cultures.

Westheimer and Lopater (2004) chronicle the work of several historical researchers on human sexuality. What emerges is a picture of the profound influences of the sexual fears, restrictive attitudes, and gender disparities that reflect the European Victorian era. Moreover, social class differences were also evident in American society. According to Reiss and Reiss (1997), the oldest related research on sexual practices in the United States conducted by Clelia Mosher during her years as a student (and left unpublished in the archives of student monographs at Stanford University) supported the notion of class differences. Although much of society was sexually Victorian, especially toward women, Mosher's sample of highly educated married women in 1892 indicated that they participated in sexual intercourse approximately five times per week, and more than 40 percent reported usually or always experiencing orgasm.

As the 19th century drew to an end, a more intellectual and academic climate regarding sexuality research began to emerge. For example, through 1939, the work of Havelock Ellis probably had the most profound effect on present thinking about masturbation. His work counteracted previous medical and religious teachings of serious health problems emerging from masturbation and instead proclaimed that masturbation was a way of releasing tension. Yet, while asserting his belief that one is born with a homosexual orientation, it was his classification of homosexuality as a psychopathology that influenced psychological classifications and the treatment of homosexuals for many decades.

Sigmund Freud's research introduced the concept of libido as a "natural" and lustful drive from within the individual that expresses itself in sexual ways. Through understanding this force, one could understand the drives and actions of human beings. Freud also introduced the notion that sexual and sensual pleasure is derived from erogenous zones throughout the body and not just genitally focused (Westheimer & Lopater, 2004).

Much of what Freud theorized about the development of personality was associated with sexual development and sexual experiences (see Chapter 2).

Many believe that Alfred Kinsey was, in recent history, the most influential researcher about American sexuality. His large-scale sociological research initially legitimized the study of human sexuality in the United States. Although his famous Kinsey Studies were published in 1948 (*Sexual Behavior in the Human Male*) and 1953 (*Sexual Behavior in the Human Female*), respectively, his earlier data had indicated an emergence from "Victorian" culture and gender disparate behaviors. Kinsey's research indicated that 50 percent of women and 80 percent of men, born between 1900 and 1909, experienced sexual intercourse before marriage. While the change was not so pronounced for men, it did represent a doubling of premarital sexual experience for women from 25 to 50 percent. His data, three decades later, revealed continuing changes. Kinsey reported that most males participated in sexual activities by 15 years of age, and extramarital sexual activity existed among 50 percent of married men (Kinsey, Pomeroy, & Martin, 1948). Among females, more variability in sexual behaviors was reported, particularly among more educated women; extramarital relationships were not uncommon, and 50 percent still reported sexual intercourse before marriage (Kinsey, Pomeroy, Martin, & Gebhard, 1953). Yet, little was learned about the sexual practices of gay and lesbian people in relationships. But the Kinsey research did provide a dearth of information about sexual practices including the experience of orgasm, the frequency of participation in various sexual activities, the frequency of homosexuality in the population, and support for the changing notion that homosexuality is not caused by early negative psychological influences. This research opened the door to continued scientific scrutiny of what was always considered a "private" topic, sexuality.

It must be noted that, although Kinsey used a very large sample size, the data's ability to be generalized to the greater American society was compromised. The research neglected to include sufficient representation from diverse ethnic groups, and since the culture at the time impeded the ability to ask very young children, adolescents, or the elderly about their sexual practices, they were largely omitted. (See the cited Kinsey publications for a more in-depth review.)

One cannot discuss human sexual research without including the famous works of William Masters and Virginia Johnson (1966, 1970). Masters, a gynecologist, and Johnson, a sociologist, contributed a great deal to our understanding of human sexual response and human sexual dysfunction. Their initial research concerned itself with the physiology of human sexual response. By monitoring sexual behavior in the laboratory by observation, they chronicled the physical changes in the male and female body resulting from sexual stimulation. Out of their research came a description of the phases of the human sexual response cycle, a classification of a variety of specific sexual dysfunctions (which had both physiological and psychological components), and behavioral treatment modalities (all discussed in Chapter 3) that continue to be practiced today. Their research expanded to include a range of sexual behaviors and sexual orientations, and although they are recently deceased, their work continues to provide information through the many sexologists at the institute they founded in St. Louis. Hence, it was Masters and Johnson's research that provided a significant contribution to our understanding of the physical phenomenon of human sexual behavior and the sex therapy approaches to treatment.

Although the Masters and Johnson behavioral models of treatment became the accepted practice, it was others, especially Helen Singer Kaplan (1979), who added additional dimensions to our understanding of the more psychological influences on sexual dysfunction and treatment. Kaplan's explanation of inhibited sexual desire and her combination of insight therapy with behavioral sex therapy in a more dynamic orientation also recognized the more intrapsychic conflicts that may be contributing to people's sexual problems.

In the 1980s, Laumann, Gagnon, Michael, and Michaels undertook an extensive social research survey about human sexual behavior in relationships. They attempted to explain sexual behavior by applying three social theories: scripting theory, choice theory, and network theory (Laumann et al., 1994). "Scripting Theory explained sexual conduct, Choice Theory explained sexual decision-making and Network Theory was used to explain the sexual dyad" (Laumann et al., 1994, p. 44). These theoretical concepts also made a significant contribution to our understanding of the social phenomenon surrounding human sexual behavior.

After the middle of the 20th century, it became apparent that sexual behavior, attitudes, and values in American society were continuing to change. The activities of the feminist movement resulted in increasing unrest between the genders as women became more overt about their sexuality and sexual rights. More young people of both genders were participating in sexually intimate activities outside permanently committed relationships more openly, and the activities and interests of the gay, lesbian, and bisexual community became more evident to the larger population. Moreover, the popular literature was replete with social research findings translated into public information. Shere Hite (1976), in her report on the sexual behavior of 100,000 American women, indicated such things as 70 percent of her population was having extramarital relationships during the first 5 years of marriage, and most women did not experience an orgasm during sexual intercourse. Information about the famous "G-spot" was being disseminated to the lay public (Ladas, Whipple, & Perry, 1983). Still, little was available about sexual behaviors in childhood. Over time, the information and resources about human sexual behavior expanded to include a broader range of subgroups.

The validity of sex research established by these early researchers continues today. Scholars in universities, institutes, and national and international professional associations participate in research that crosses the related disciplines (psychological, social, physiological, and spiritual) as we continue to move toward a better understanding of human sexuality. Fairly recently the pharmacological community joined the so-called sexual revolution by developing drugs that effectively intervene in certain sexual dysfunctions (although most drugs are geared to male dysfunction) and are making that information readily available through the mass media. Physicians and other practitioners are more frequently considering the sexual problems associated with chronic diseases and their treatments. What is important to this text is that the research is being translated into the development of comprehensive sexuality education curricula based on the scientific literature at all levels of education, from preschool through graduate school, and there is an ongoing evaluation of their effectiveness.

Why Sexuality Education?

How does one begin to explain the conflict surrounding the topic of human sexuality, let alone the virtual "war of words" that sexuality education in the public schools precipitates? Society is replete with sexual innuendos in the mass media, oftentimes portraying sexuality with unrealistic images of attractiveness, bizarre behaviors, and unhealthy circumstances under which sexual behaviors occur, including abuse and coercion. Sex is mostly presented as exciting and enticing, on the one hand, and dirty and dangerous, on the other (Kelly, 2004). From the sheer number of these messages available in easily accessible newspapers, popular magazines, and television programs, one would think America is an open society, comfortable with diversity in sexual expression and, more important, knowledgeable about ourselves as sexual beings. Yet, although we are intrigued and titillated by the overt sexual stimuli provided, we find very little communication is available about sexual information that can positively enhance our lives. Moreover, young people often claim that they have had little if any discussion with their parents or other trusted caretakers about sex to counteract mass media influences. Schools, restricted by public pressure, are most often left to offer the very barest of physiological information, if any at all. So that leaves young people to become sexually educated consumers from their peers (who often know little more than they do) or from experimentation. Children will learn about sexuality from any source available. Although they represent the sometimes silent but vast majority, parents want their children to learn. So here lies the problem: How do we balance the sexuality learning of young people so that it more effectively represents the values and attitudes of their family, community, or chosen adult lifestyle?

What Is Sexuality Education?

Before we can explain what constitutes effective sexuality education, we will discuss what education is in a democratic society. Furthermore, we will discuss how education is or is not administered in the United States so that it can embrace the controversial nature of sexuality education. Education is the primary institution charged with preparing young people to take their full place as democratic citizens. Moreover, education occurs in concert with the philosophical views of a society.

Robert Silverstone (2000) explains that societies are organized "autocratically" or "democratically." In an *autocratic* society, the leadership is the determining force by which the society operates, and the community is rarely approached for input. In a *democratic* society, the leadership represents the views of the community. Silverstone goes on to explain that while American society embraces the ideals of democracy and individual rights, autocratic power threads throughout U.S. history. Autocracy minimizes critical thinking, reflection, personal decision making, and problem solving. Autocratic thinking and restrictive practice in education limits the development of personal skills and the ability of individuals to assume responsibility for their behaviors and outcomes. It supports the notion that there is one right way. Democracy supports the development of autonomous moral reasoning (Kohlberg, 1964) and the expression of one's values and morals despite their difference from society's accepted postures. Moreover, democracy acknowledges and respects difference, open discourse, and the sharing of opposing points of view. It is this battle between autocracy and democracy that drives the themes underlying the U.S. educational system and that adds support to the limitations and controversy surrounding sexuality education.

One of the primary controversies surrounding sexuality education is based on the notion that there exists some finite set of "appropriate" values, attitudes, and behaviors to learn and accept. Thus, "inappropriate" ones also exist. Also, there is a clash between restrictive and permissive ideologies. A *restrictive* ideology limits sexuality education to reproductive anatomy and physiology and an "abstinence-only" until marriage philosophy. A *permissive* ideology extends teaching to include the biological, psychological, spiritual, and other aspects of a wide range of topics (McKay, 1999). It is not a question of which of these ideologies should be implemented but rather the acceptance of one being "right" and the other being "wrong" that compromises democratic sexuality education. Furthermore, a position by the educator to one ideology or the other will ultimately be reflected in the curriculum and the classroom, representing compromises of democratic ideals. According to McKay, the notion of which is best for students to assure their development into sexually healthy democratic citizens and the "democratic ideals of justice, equality, critical deliberation, debate, representation, pluralism, individual rights and responsibilities" (p. 11) should determine sexuality curricula.

According to the National Guidelines Task Force (Sexuality Information and Education Council of the United States [SIECUS], 1996),

> Sexuality education is a lifelong process of acquiring information and forming attitudes, beliefs, and values about identity, relationships and intimacy. It encompasses sexual development, reproductive health, interpersonal relationships, affection, intimacy, body image, and gender roles. Comprehensive Sexuality Education (CSE) addresses the biological, sociocultural, psychological, and spiritual dimensions of sexuality from the cognitive, affective, and the behavioral domains. Among the primary goals of comprehensive sexuality education is the promotion of sexual health. It seeks to assist people in understanding a more positive view of sexuality,

to provide them with information and skills about taking care of their sexual health, and to assist them in acquiring skills to make decisions now and in the future. (p. 6)

Hence, one would expect decreases in the incidence of sexually transmitted infections (STIs) and unintended pregnancies as an outcome of effective comprehensive sexuality education.

THE STATUS OF SCHOOL SEXUALITY EDUCATION

It often takes a crisis to create change. It is what society defines as the crisis of early adolescent sexual activity, adolescent pregnancy, and STIs, especially HIV, that enhanced opportunities for more sexuality education, especially in schools across this country where it had previously been restricted. Although the door seems more open at this time, education continues to emphasize preventing social problems and their related negative outcomes through teaching restrictive practices rather than highlighting the benefits of developing a healthy and enjoyable sexuality. Furthermore, the present political environment encourages and primarily funds an "abstinence-only" sex education perspective rather than a comprehensive positive approach. The result is the implementation of courses or discussions that do not resonate with the sexual activities and decisions of the majority of students. Hence, formal sexuality education takes place primarily in the higher grades, often after students have already become sexually active.

The Data

Various studies have looked at what is actually happening in the schools. According to an extensive poll by National Public Radio, the Henry J. Kaiser Family Foundation, and the Harvard University Kennedy School of Government Representatives (2003), only 7 percent of Americans are against sexuality education in the public schools. Only 15 percent believe that it should address abstinence-only and not include information about contraception. However, 46 percent believe sexuality education should be an abstinence-plus curriculum, and another 36 percent believe that the focus should be on responsible decision making about sexuality. Yet, of the school principals surveyed in this study, 30 percent reported that their school taught abstinence-only, 47 percent taught abstinence-plus, and 20 percent taught responsible decision making.

According to the Alan Guttmacher Institute's *State Policies Brief* (AGI, 2003), 22 states and Washington, DC, require HIV/STI and sexuality education, and 17 more require only HIV/STI education. A policy to teach sexuality education exists at the district level in more than two of every three public schools; of those remaining districts, approximately one-third leave the policy of whether it will be taught to the individual school or teachers. Yet, most of the districts that have a public policy to teach sexuality education require that abstinence only be promoted (86 percent). Of these, only half permit discussion of contraception as an effective method of preventing pregnancy and STIs, and less than 15 percent permit the teaching of abstinence as one of the other options, not the only option, in preparing young people to be sexually healthy.

Various sources continue to collect data about adolescent sexual behavior. The Henry J. Kaiser Family Foundation (2000), for example, notes a decline in the number of those students who reported ever having sexual intercourse and an increase in those who use condoms. The Youth Risk Behavior Surveillance System (Centers for Disease Control and Prevention [CDC], 2004) report indicates that 46 percent of 9th to12th graders have ever had sexual intercourse (slightly more boys than girls); by 12th grade, 61 percent have had sexual intercourse; and 37.3 percent of males and 27.9 percent of females have had sex by 9th grade. Moreover, 7.4 percent of teens had sexual intercourse before age 13. The survey also indicates that 14.4 percent of teens had more than four sex partners in their short lifetime. Of the teens who were sexually active during the last 3 months prior to the survey (34 percent or one-third of all students), 63 percent had used a condom during their last sexual intercourse (thus, 37 percent had not), and 25 percent had used alcohol or other drugs during their last sexual experience. Of note, the survey indicated that 9 percent of students reported having been forced to have sexual intercourse when they did not want to and 4.2 percent had been pregnant or partnered a pregnancy.

The data on behaviors other than sexual intercourse are somewhat scanty in the literature. Data collected in 1995 reported that 53 percent of males, age 15 to19, had been masturbated by a female, 49 percent had received oral sex, 39 percent had given oral sex, and 11 percent had engaged in anal sex (CDC, 2002a, 2002b). The *Morbidity and Mortality Weekly Report* (*MMWR;* CDC, 1998) reported that 29 percent of teens who hadn't had vaginal intercourse had masturbated, 31 percent had been genitally stimulated by a partner, 9 percent had performed oral sex on a male, and 10 percent had performed oral sex on a female. Almost 1 million teens will become pregnant each year, or one-fifth of all sexually active teenagers between 15 and 19 years of age (Terry & Manlove, 2000; Henshaw, 1998).

The data on teen sexual behavior patterns generally do not provide information that differentiates among heterosexual, homosexual, bisexual, or transgender youth. Furthermore, in a society where cultural diversity abounds, sexual orientations, other than heterosexual and gender- and age-related inequities, clearly exist. Yet, at best sexuality education curricula are usually biased toward young to midlife, white, middle-class, heterosexual experiences.

Trained teachers of sexuality education believe in a more comprehensive approach to sexuality education presented in a developmentally appropriate sequence, occurring long before the conclusion of the 12th grade. They believe that such education should at least include discussion about when and how sexual activity can be an enriching experience; abstinence as well as where to get contraceptive services; effective use of condoms, particularly to prevent STIs; understanding heterosexuality, homosexuality, bisexuality, and transgenderism; information about abortion and changes associated with aging. Yet, fewer and fewer programs are doing so, although teachers as well as more than 75 percent of parents surveyed think that these same topics, in addition to abstinence, should be included (Henry J. Kaiser Family Foundation, 2000).

Under these circumstances, one might assume that the restrictions in funding and in the resulting curricula in the schools, emerge from research that supports abstinence-only or the limiting of information about sexuality as most effective, but evidence to the contrary exists. After years of research, indicators are that it is comprehensive sexuality education programs that provide information about both abstinence and contraception that are contributing to the delayed onset of sexual activity among teenagers, the reduction in the number of sexual partners, and the increased use of contraceptives when and if they do become sexually active (Satcher, 2001). Hence, whichever study one chooses to consider, the research community and professional health and sex educators agree that teaching abstinence-only or restricting sexuality education to "keeping kids out of trouble" is too little, too late.

WHERE AND HOW IS SEXUALITY EDUCATION TAUGHT?

School curricula are developed around the various disciplines that have been deemed important, including math, science, technology, language arts, social studies, health, and physical education. Moreover, in recent times, curricula in each of these disciplines have been rewritten to meet what have been defined as "national standards" that students who complete their education (K–12) are expected to attain. State education departments, teacher education accrediting agencies, and professional education associations have established these standards. Many states have either adopted them or created their own. In addition, an accountability movement has arisen in education through the development and implementation of assessment instruments that assure that students have met the standards in each discipline by the time they are ready to graduate.

Human sexuality education is most frequently subsumed under the discipline of health education, although in some states it is offered as a component of consumer sciences or one of the other basic science courses. The national health education professional associations and several states have identified many standards within this subject, and they are entirely congruent with sexuality education. Hence, assessment instruments developed or in process will include items about human sexuality.

Sexuality Education as a Component of Health Education: National Health Education Standards, Scope, and Sequences

According to the U.S. Department of Education, comprehensive school health education (CSHE) is "a primary prevention strategy for teaching our nation's children and their parents the skills needed for a healthy lifestyle"

(Greene, Kreuter, Deds, & Artrodge, 1985, p. 335). Health education involves the development of personal decision-making and problem-solving strategies that young people can use to access and incorporate knowledge, clarify personal values, develop and hold attitudes, and choose behaviors that maximize their health and the health of their family and community.

In 1995, the Joint Committee on National Health Education Standards produced a document entitled *Achieving Health Literacy: An Investment in the Future* that calls for health literacy as an outcome of effective health education. It defines the health-literate person as one who is a critical thinker and problem solver; a responsible, productive citizen; a self-directed learner; and an effective communicator. Furthermore, it outlines the seven standards that describe essential knowledge and skills necessary to be considered health-literate, each of which can easily be adapted to sexuality education. The standards identified here represent an outcomes-based model of education, one that determines what students will know and be able to do when they have completed their K–12 education:

- Students will comprehend concepts related to health promotion and disease prevention.
- Students will demonstrate the ability to access valid health information and health-promoting products and services.
- Students will demonstrate the ability to practice health-enhancing behaviors and reduce health risks.
- Students will analyze the influence of culture, media, technology, and other factors on health.
- Students will demonstrate the ability to use interpersonal communication skills to enhance health.
- Students will demonstrate the ability to use goal-setting and decision-making skills to enhance health.
- Students will demonstrate the ability to advocate for personal, family, and community health.

As mentioned earlier, health curricula are commonly organized around several subcontent areas, including Personal Growth and Development; Family Life and Human Sexuality; Environmental Health; Preventing Violence and Abuse; Community Health; Preventing Chronic and Communicable Disease; Prevention of Alcohol and Other Drug Abuse; Nutrition; Mental Health; Preventing Injury; First Aid and Safety; Consumer Health; Exercise and Physical Fitness. The CDC (1998) suggests a somewhat different organizing structure including the six adolescent risk behaviors as follows:

- Tobacco use
- Dietary patterns that contribute to disease
- Sedentary lifestyles
- Sexual behaviors that result in HIV infection, other sexually transmitted infections, and unintended pregnancy
- Alcohol and other drug use
- Behaviors that result in intentional and unintentional injury

Still other curricula designs include the application of personal life skills to the various subcontent areas. We believe that a combination of content knowledge and life skills approaches to curricula reap the most educational benefit in developing an individual who understands human sexuality and is able to enact behaviors and adopt attitudes and values that will optimize his or her sexual health and life.

Through a health education lens, one can see how sexuality education in school health curricula can contribute to meeting the national health education standards. Since teacher preparation requires that prospective health educators master the many subdisciplines within health, preprofessional and professional preparation programs often require courses to cover the content and teaching methods associated with sexuality education. Although programs around the United States specialize in the preparation of professional sexuality educators only, they are usually unable to meet all of the requirements for certification to teach health, and therefore graduates are less able to secure teaching positions in public education.

Like health education, the several subcontent areas that constitute comprehensive sexuality education (also known as the "scope") and the organization of the curriculum sequences constitute what is commonly referred to as the "scope and sequence" of curricula. In addition to scope and sequence, the organization of the curriculum considers developmental levels, cultural backgrounds, level of inquiry, and teaching methods (activities) used to deliver the content. A comprehensive sexuality education program respects the diversity of values and beliefs represented in the community and will complement and augment the sexuality education young people receive from their families. According to SIECUS (1996), a comprehensive sexuality education (CSE) program covers:

1. human development, relationships,
2. personal skills,
3. sexual behavior,
4. sexual health,
5. society and culture. (pp. 95–96)

Within the subcontent areas, one can address the multidisciplinary perspectives among them:

- A biological perspective concerned with anatomical and physiological characteristics
- A psychosocial perspective concerned with developmental aspects and the interaction of cognitive, affective, and social domains
- A behavioral perspective concerned with cognition and emotional responses
- A clinical perspective concerned with sexual dysfunctions and disorders
- A sociological perspective concerned with the social environment including social organizations and socioeconomic status
- An anthropological perspective concerned with evolutionary and cultural influences on sexual meanings and behaviors including underlying skills, attitudes, beliefs, and values (Bolin & Whelehan, 2001).

Readers can peruse the table of contents of this text to observe still another scope and sequence of the various content and subcontent areas. Content and subcontent areas are but one way to organize curricula. As for other areas of health education, one could also design curricula through a personal life skills application to sexuality content. This text is designed with a "skills to content" bias.

A PERSONAL LIFE SKILLS APPROACH TO SEXUALITY EDUCATION

Knowledge in and of itself is not power. Combining a knowledge base of content/information with personal life skills applied to real-life situations gives power to knowledge. Knowing does not necessarily mean doing. If I know, for example, that I can get HIV from participating in unprotected sexual intercourse (anal, oral, or vaginal), will I be able to apply refusal skills or communicate my insistence for safer sexual practices when I am being pressured to participate?

Mastery of several personal life skills has been identified as important to achieving and maintaining health status. We believe that being a sexually healthy person requires that one is able to implement personal life skills in sexuality-related situations that involve the individual, the family, and the community. Building competence in these skills results in young people having more control over their lives and decreasing their likelihood of acting in high-risk situations.

There is still no universal agreement about the particular set of personal life skills to be developed in sexuality or health education curricula or what constitutes "all" of the skills one would want to include in a teaching environment. Many times the skills are identified in different ways. Some can stand alone, whereas others are subsets of the initial skill. It is expected that the reader will be familiar with and have previously discussed various personal life skills as they apply to health and sexuality education disciplines. A discussion of a selected set of personal life skills appears in each chapter as it applies to the subcontent area, and these are included in each chapter's learning experiences (lessons), to provide prospective teachers with activities and information that will increase their future students' knowledge about sexual issues while increasing their ability to act on that knowledge, using the skills. For the purposes of a quick overview, the particular personal life skills selected for this text are briefly discussed in the following sections.

Communication/Refusal Skills

A common cliché is that "sex is something we do, not something we talk about." Nothing could be further from the truth. At the root of many sexual problems is an inability to communicate feelings, fears, desires, and other emotions with one another.

Communicating is a recursive activity whereby one person relays information to another person and the other person is able to receive the intended information. The means by which that information is transferred is one component of communication, and listening/receiving skills are another. Hence, the techniques used to transfer and receive are another component of communication. Communication is also how we share our feelings, attitudes, values, knowledge, and so forth. It is one of the most essential skills— if not the most essential—in supporting self-confidence and building and maintaining relationships. One can only imagine the enormous effect communication has on human sexuality, particularly the ability to communicate what pleases us, what doesn't, what we want to do, with whom, when, and how (see also Chapter 3).

Seemingly simple, effective communication is a complex phenomenon that takes place on many levels and through many sources. One may give and receive messages through the written or spoken word or through silent gestures. Messages can be transmitted in both the public or private arena. In this technologically diverse world, we are increasingly communicating through electronic media.

We receive and give messages in verbal and nonverbal ways. *Verbal* communication includes the intonations of speech (tones of voice, speed of delivery, and so forth) and the language used (common discourse, slang, cultural expressions, and so on). *Nonverbal* communication includes body and facial expressions, stance at delivery (distance or closeness), and the use of recognizable symbols or signs. Each of these factors influences the ways in which a message is transferred. In addition to the speaker factors, the listening skills of the receiver also determine the level of communication. One way to assure that the communication loop has been successfully closed (or opened) is that the listener is able to reflect back and receive confirmation that the speaker's intended message has been received (for example, "This is what I heard you say").

The environment in which communication occurs plays a significant role in the success of the communication itself. For example, when a personal message is being transferred in a public place, the surroundings may determine how it is expressed and how it is received, as well as the level of noise and distractions. How much emotion the message evokes can also influence the success of the communication. One's vulnerability or the level of the relationship between the parties communicating can also be deciding factors in successful communication. For example, the sharing of feelings or self-disclosure has inherently different risks than does the sharing of information.

Other obstacles to communication often have to be overcome as well. Some of these obstacles, including sociocultural factors such as age, ethnicity, gender, economic status, and level of cognition may affect the transfer of messages. For example, it is acceptable, if not expected, that boys will joke about sex, but serious talk, especially when it includes emotion, is often considered a sign of weakness or ignorance. Girls who talk about sex may be considered as portraying a certain "knowing" that is often considered inappropriate for "nice girls" in some cultures. Seeking sex information from an older person is sometimes inhibited by what might be considered the "appropriateness" or the "correctness" of the words that constitute the inquiry. Factors such as differences in perceptions, experiences, strong differences of opinion, flexibility, personal bias, and general personality characteristics may also present their distinct obstacles. A stubborn person, who has made up his or her mind about an issue, will often not use good listening skills but rather be involved in preparing his or her rebuff.

Among the communication skills worth developing as they apply to sexual decisions are acceptance/refusal skills. Young people are often pressured to participate in sexual activities that they might not be comfortable with but feel unable to refuse. This is especially characteristic of teens who want to belong, to be accepted, and who have low self-confidence. It is also a characteristic of immaturity and conflict in one's value system and morals. The ability to say no when one wants to suggests a certain freedom and ego strength, as does the ability to say yes without pressure or coercion. Thus, practice activities for developing acceptance and refusal skills will be included in various learning experiences throughout this book.

Activities should encourage students to be effective speakers and listeners; recognize and overcome obstacles to communication; accept or refuse participation in behaviors that put them at risk; use language to overcome conflict and get information in respectful, caring, relationship-enhancing ways; and collaborate with others to resolve complex sexuality related issues (*Health Education Skills Matrix,* 2002). Mastering these skills will likely increase students' self-esteem, enhance their relationships, and provide a greater chance that they will be heard and understood.

Decision-Making/Problem-Solving Skills

We make decisions every day, some more important than others. Sometimes the decisions we make seem to just happen. Oftentimes we do not realize that we have actually gone through a thought process that emerges in one position or another. Young people's decision-making skills are often limited by adults who believe that, left to their own decision, younger people will make too many wrong ones—hence, better they are told what to do and when to do it.

When it comes to important life matters, people must develop skills in decision making and practice and hone them so that they can make well-informed, well-thought-out decisions as they become more complicated over time. Whether we decide to eat an apple or a pear will probably have few long-term consequences; whether we decide to become sexually active or not can have many consequences.

There is a direct relationship between making one's own decisions and accepting responsibility for them. There is also a relationship between our decision-making ability and our ability to resolve problems effectively. Our ability to make decisions is influenced by several factors. One, discussed earlier, is the amount of experience we have in making decisions for ourselves. Another is the experience we have with the factors or situation about which we will make a decision. Still another influence is the input and pressures we experience from those who are involved or will be affected by our decisions.

We rarely make important decisions without feeling pressure from our peers, partners, family members, employers, religious leaders, teachers, doctors, and other important individuals in our lives. It is especially complicated when these influential others have differing opinions about us and differing influences that affect us.

Incorporating some of the various decision-making processes that exist in the literature, providing practice opportunities during role playing and other classroom activities, will develop this skill. One such process of decision making requires that students

- Learn how to clearly identify the problem or situation that requires a decision.
- Identify the persons and situations that will influence or be influenced by their decisions.
- Gather the information they will need to make their decisions from reliable sources.
- Identify and acknowledge the potential consequences and level of risk of their decisions.
- Recognize how future decisions will be influenced by this decision or its outcome.
- Evaluate their personal strengths and weaknesses with regard to their ability to carry out their decisions.
- Be prepared to take responsibility for the outcome of their decision.

Classroom activities can provide opportunities for young students to apply decision-making skills to less complicated decisions and then increase the complexity of the practice situations, developmentally. Younger students may be making social decisions about who they want to be their "best" friend. Later in their development they will make decisions about whom they want to be intimate with. In sexuality education, more benign circumstances can be offered for practice in early socialization experiences such as decisions about dating or touching or kissing. Then, as students age, classroom exercises can incorporate the more complicated sexual behavior choices such as which sexual activities they will participate in and with whom. Activities for practicing decision making will be included in the learning experiences incorporated in the various chapters of this text.

Conflict Management Skills

What do we do when things happen to us over which we feel unsettled, angered, or frustrated? Conflict can be intrapersonal or interpersonal. *Intrapersonally,* we can be conflicted about decisions we have to make that have implications for our lives and future but do not necessarily involve another person. *Interpersonally,* we may be at what seems to be an immovable difference between ourselves and another person or persons. How do we resolve differences when they occur in important relationships or require us to make a decision about that which we are unclear? Resolving conflicts can mean surrendering, leaving or walking away, committing violence or bullying, suing an individual, or seeking an outside source for mediation.

The notion of conflict resolution is to develop skills that help people overcome a conflict without violence. Among the skills to be developed are the following:

- *Negotiating:* discussing the conflict and finding a mutually agreeable solution.
- *Mediating:* involving an outside person to the conflict who helps those involved find a mutually agreeable resolution. The outsider does not make any decisions but rather creates an environment for communication. He or she usually encourages both parties to gather information; reframe the problem to be more acceptable; and create, discuss, and formalize an agreement.
- *Arbitrating:* selecting an outside person who will listen to the various sides of the conflict and make a specific decision that will be adhered to by the parties involved. An arbitrator can be a peer or a group of peers who are selected by the people involved or by an outside agency (such as a teacher, a school administrator, or a parent) to resolve a conflict. An arbitrator can help parties make a decision on their own, but, if one cannot be reached, then the uninvolved person makes the decision.
- *Legal conflict resolvers:* tapping into a variety of legal systems—lawyers, the courts, the government—to resolve a conflict.

Young people generally resolve conflict in similar ways to those that have been modeled for them. If their family or friends resolve conflict by fighting or crying, for example, they will initially implement these same skills. If they are continually successful, then they are less likely to seek other strategies. If they are continuously unsuccessful in resolving their conflicts in self-satisfying ways, their self-esteem and self-confidence may be challenged. Hence, an educational environment that provides opportunities to observe and practice new strategies is useful.

In cases where conflict is recognized as unmanageable or irresolvable, outside sources can be sought. Hence, conflict management education includes identifying sources in the family, immediate social environment, and the larger community that are available, accessible, and authentic.

Stress Management Skills

We cannot live without stress, either physiologically or psychologically. Stress is what motivates us to take action and to regain the body's homeostasis when we are biologically or psychologically shifted off course. There is a relationship between stress and the way we live our lives, our health, and our sexuality. Hans Selye (1956), one of the pioneers of stress theory, explains that stress is the nonspecific response of the body to any stressor put on it. Moreover, he theorizes that the physiological response of the body or general adaptation to accommodate for the stress occurs in stages, whether the stressor is positive (eustress) or negative (distress). Others have perceived stress as a more emotional response to some environmental change that the person may perceive as a danger or threat. The emotional response or the perception of the stressor becomes the mediating factor (Lazarus & Finkelor, 1984; Mason, 1975). From this research comes a variety of notions about what kinds of experiences create stress, what effect stress has on our heath and well-being, and who is more likely to experience more or prolonged reactions to stress.

Unmanaged stress results in illness (physical and emotional) and possibly death. It affects the immune system, resulting in a compromised health status and mental health condition. For school-age people, it may result in a range of feelings such as worthlessness, apathy, loneliness, anger, hostility, and low self esteem. These feelings support the likelihood of behavior problems like truancy, substance abuse, low academic achievement, attention disorders, and the potential for high-risk sexual activities (Anspaugh & Ezell, 2000).

Our personality, environment, and physiology impact on the ways stress affects our sexual health and behavior. The human sexual response cycle occurs as a stress response, and our desire for and our body's very ability to participate in sexual behaviors are related to our level of stress. Making decisions about what behaviors we will do and with whom often occurs under stressful circumstances, and these result in taking chances that we might not ordinarily take if our stress level was not high. Hence, recognizing that we need stress to live, the importance of managing stress becomes particularly important.

What does it mean to "manage stress"? Managing stress does not mean eliminating all stress from one's life, even if that were possible. Experiencing nothing that is unexpected or different than the usual would not only be boring but stressful in and of itself. Hence, managing stress means maintaining stress at an optimal level for living an interesting life without causing disease (Greenberg, 2003). How well we cope with the stressors that occur in our lives determines how well we manage stress. Sometimes temporary relief of stress enables an individual to take some time to deal more effectively with a stressor. Temporary stress relief includes such strategies as distraction, avoidance, and escape (Fetro, 2002). In situations where more long-term solutions are necessary, other stress management skills are necessary, including the following:

- Knowing the difference between positive and negative stress and being able to prioritize personal stressors.
- Being able to analyze the impact of the stressors we experience from sources such as family, friends, employment, and so forth, on our health and well-being.
- Being able to recognize and evaluate stressful situations and ways of dealing with them.

- Clarifying self-expectations and the expectation of others.
- Knowing one's capabilities and limitations.
- Being able to use healthy stress management strategies such as relaxation techniques, a support system, time management, and therapy (New York State Education Department/Coordinated School Health [NYSED/CSH], 2002).

Relationship Management Skills

Relationship management suggests that one can use a variety of the life skills at the interpersonal and intrapersonal level to develop, maintain, and enhance personal, professional, and community relationships. Here are some of the important skills associated with managing relationships:

- Developing and evaluating one's own relationship capabilities, including nurturing, empathy, respect, and responsibility.
- Being able to assess the importance of these characteristics as they operate in ourselves and in the persons with whom we create relationships.
- Being able to communicate self- and other's expectations of the relationship.
- Being willing and able to make and enact commitments.
- Being able to create mutually acceptable boundaries that maintain the relationship and the individuality of the people involved.
- Being able to resolve conflicts in constructive, relationship-enhancing ways.
- Being able to experience and demonstrate the range of human emotions as they are appropriate to the particular relationship (levels of love, intimacy, anger, caring, and so forth).

Chapter 6 is devoted to the various types of relationships one might expect to encounter and how sexual behaviors occur in these relationships. The chapter discusses how one develops and maintains relationships at various levels of intimacy. Managing each relationship as it develops, and throughout its existence, requires an understanding of the skills described here and the ability to apply them wherever appropriate.

Goal-Setting Skills

The process of setting goals and planning to achieve the goals is another personal life skill that has important implications to one's sexual self, family, and community. Goal setting is related to decision making in that one needs to decide which goals are worth achieving, at what cost, and at what benefit.

Goals may be short-term or long-term. Very young children can learn to create achievable short-term goals. They would become overwhelmed with long-term or more global goals. Success often brings success; hence, young children who are encouraged to set reasonable and achievable short-term goals and do step-by-step planning for their achievement will be better equipped to set and achieve longer-term goals as they mature. During adolescence, more life-planning and longer-term goals become important. Hence, recognizable rewards for the achievement of the steps and the ultimate goals tend to reinforce the implementation of the skill. The more achievable the goals, the more in control people feel over their lives and behaviors.

Among the components of successful goal setting is an ability to evaluate one's personal assets as they relate to the goal and to incorporate into one's goals self-expectations and the expectations of important others such as family and friends (Fetro, 2000). Important skills that make goal setting manageable include the ability to do the following:

- Identify the planning steps that could lead to successful achievement and accept their importance in the process.
- Be flexible enough to adjust the plan as needed.
- Be able to make commitments and carry them out.
- Analyze the barriers to achieving a goal and develop strategies to overcome them.
- Predict the potential outcomes (Fetro, 2000) and their effect on future goals.
- Recognize one's support systems and analyze their importance in achieving the goal (NYSED/CSH, 2002).

Adolescents' goal setting will impact their decisions about such things as when they will become sexually active and what impact an unplanned pregnancy or STI might have on their ability to go to college, travel, and so forth.

Resource Management Skills

Many health and information services are associated with human sexuality. Some are medical, others pharmacological, and still others psychological. One of the greatest difficulties is assessing the reliability and validity of the information supplied or the quality and appropriateness of the services. It is especially important for young people, who are bombarded with sexual messages, to determine which resources they can depend on and who they can trust. Even more important is that, too often, when they seek medical or mental health assistance for a related problem, they do so in an emergency, sometimes in secrecy and without knowing how to select a reliable service. Here are some resource management skills worth developing:

- Evaluating information, products, and services related to human sexuality for validity and reliability.
- Analyzing how cultural beliefs influence sexual behaviors and the use of products and services related to human sexuality.
- Accessing services related to sexual health for self and others.

- Evaluating the messages received from technology and the public media.
- Becoming an advocate for the availability of quality services related to sexual health.

Overall Skills Development

A variety of influences operate in the successful development of personal life skills. Fetro (2000) suggests that it is an ongoing process involving the following steps:

1. *Introducing the skill:* Develop an understanding of the importance of the skill, its similarities and differences from other learned skills, and how it relates to other skills previously mastered.
2. *Modeling the skill:* Have the learner observe the skill in others as it occurs in different situations. The students may be called upon to share examples of the skill in use, or the teacher may model the use of the skill.
3. *Practicing and rehearsing the skill:* Have the students role-play the skill in pairs, small groups, and then larger situations until they feel confident in their ability to implement the skill. The learners can be encouraged to report on outside events where they practiced implementing the skill.
4. *Providing feedback and reinforcement:* Provide frequent peer and teacher feedback that identifies the successes and discusses the various alternatives rather than the failures in implementation. Have the students identify their own successes and alternatives to experiences in implementing the skill.
5. *Discussing obstacles to implementing a skill:* Where learners are unable to implement a skill or where they are uncomfortable with the skill, help them to identify the obstacles, and generate suggestions for overcoming them.

Although these personal life skills can be applied to any area of education, they have particular relevance to developing a healthy sexuality. Providing school-age students with developmentally appropriate experiences that enhance their ability to use personal life skills as they learn about the various subcontent areas of human sexuality will increase the likelihood that they will use the skills effectively throughout their sexual lives.

OTHER TEACHING CONSIDERATIONS

Developmental Appropriateness

In no other content area of health is recognizing the developmental appropriateness of subject matter and classroom learning activities more important than in sexuality education. Although enormous variability in cultural influences, intelligence, personality, and so forth, can be observed among students at each grade level, general patterns exist and should be considered. Teachers, armed with a knowledge of these general patterns and the uniqueness of each student's values, attitudes, religious beliefs, and other qualities, can plan and implement developmentally appropriate sexuality education programs.

Information and experiences are *developmentally appropriate* when they are within the intellectual and experiential realm of understanding of the learner. For example, knowing that babies are made from the joining of the woman's egg and the male's sperm is far more appropriate in early grades than learning about the part sexual intercourse plays in delivering the sperm to the egg, which is more developmentally appropriate later. Knowing about germs and how they are transmitted from one person to another is far more appropriate in second or third grade than learning about the relationship between oral, anal, and vaginal intercourse and the transfer of HIV. Although it is beyond the scope of this text to discuss developmental psychology, developmental learning patterns, or developmental theory, it is expected that prospective teachers will understand these concepts from their professional education studies and be able to apply them to sexuality education. Developmentally appropriate information and learning experiences will be applied throughout this text.

Teaching Methods

It is expected that readers have become familiar with the diversity of generic methods found to be effective in teaching K–12 students in their general education methods courses. Moreover, readers will have read about and be familiar with the varied learner styles associated with the concepts of multiple intelligence, recognizing that some learners are more visual, others more auditory, some more introspective, others more interpersonal. The teaching of sexuality education incorporates all of the methods used by classroom teachers in every discipline. Learning occurs when teachers take an inquiring journey with their students. It calls for interacting and learning in a recursive, information-sharing, and experiential manner between students and teacher where various opportunities for individual successes are provided.

Although no single teaching strategy has been identified as most effective with all types of populations, combinations of cognitive and affective models tend to be successful in increasing decision-making and problem-solving capabilities. Much like counseling, teachers are least effective when they are strictly lecturing, giving wrong or right "advice," or inhibiting exploration, reflection, and critical thinking.

Some strategies that involve students in active learning through storytelling, role playing, and other such "hands-on" activities enhance opportunities for self-discovery. They provide students with opportunities to share, explore, and be accepting of attitudes and values that are different from their own. Personal involvement in active learning requires students to self-assess and self-explore, and to recognize and embrace aspects of their belief system that are sometimes not easily acknowledged. These self-discovering activities can enhance self-esteem and self-confidence. It may be effective to follow active learning experiences with writing in personal journals or logs. Keeping a journal or a log requires that students personally debrief the activity and reflect on their experiences.

Cooperative learning activities, in which students work in groups to achieve a task, each taking a different component and then merging each of them to achieve an overall goal, is particularly effective. In sexuality, it increases awareness of the cooperation needed among family, friends, partners, and the community to maintain optimal sexual health. It enhances the individual's ability to communicate, negotiate, and ultimately develop a successful and respectful working relationship. Hence, the cooperative design of the activities themselves is an important aspect of the learning experience in addition to the content and life skills being developed.

Components of Learning Experiences / Lesson Plans

Earlier, the various content and subcontent areas that constitute the human sexuality scope and sequence of a health education curriculum were presented. Unit information is delivered through a sequentially planned set of lessons or learning experiences (which may be several lessons) that relate to one another in an organized manner and build upon each other. Each subcontent area includes information that the student will be expected to know; the objectives or learner outcomes to be achieved; the strategies and activities that will be implemented to develop the desired skills or deliver the information; the methods, materials, time, and environment that will support the learning; as well as the assessment tools that will be used to determine whether the desired learning standards are being achieved.

Although it is outside the realm of this book to develop the reader's initial understanding of generic curricula outlines, unit plans, and the writing of lesson plans, a brief description of a useful format and a discussion of the components of an effective learning experience (to replace the traditional lesson plan format) will be described here. Several other formats for developing lessons are also acceptable and widely used. Learning experiences different from traditional lesson plans are particularly useful because they do not restrict the teaching plan to single sessions. For this reason, the prospective teacher will find this format to be particularly helpful when developing a human sexuality curriculum where content builds from one session to the next. The following format will be used in the learning experiences sections of each chapter in this text.

A Learning Experience Format

TITLE

LEARNING CONTEXT
- The purpose, objective, or focus of the experience
- The learning standard(s) being addressed (national learning standards)

- The performance indicators that would be assessed
- Description of where this experience fits into the curriculum
- What students need to know or be able to do to succeed in this experience

PROCEDURE

A narrative description of

- What the student(s) will do individually, with one another, and with the teacher.
- What the teacher will do.
- How the activities support attainment of the learning standard(s).
- Which current scholarship and "best classroom" practices have been included, and how.
- How technology is or can be used to enhance learning or assess performance.

INSTRUCTIONAL/ENVIRONMENTAL MODIFICATIONS

- How will the range of intellectual, physical, emotional, and cultural learning styles and abilities be accommodated for in this lesson?
- What modification needs to be made to accommodate for students with various challenges (for example, language proficiency, physical disabilities, and the like)?

TIME REQUIREMENTS

Identify

- The total time required (number of sessions).
- The time required for each component.
- Time required for assessment.

RESOURCES

- For the teacher: handouts, speakers, media, computers, reading materials, equipment, and so forth.
- For the student: notebooks, reading material, articles, paste, pencils, and so forth.

ASSESSMENT PLAN

Describe

- How students will be involved in their own assessment (creating rubrics, contracts, peer assessments, and so forth).
- Techniques used to collect evidence of student progress toward meeting the learning standards, performance indicators (for instance, observation, group discussion, journal writing, and logs).
- Tools used to document student progress (such as scoring guides, rubrics, and rating scales).

STUDENT WORK

- Collect student work that represents the various levels of student performance.
- Include comments reflecting the basis of the assessment on these works.

REFLECTION

Your personal comments regarding

- Why this lesson was chosen.
- How effectively it meets the intended learning standard(s) and performance indicator(s).

- What the teacher learned from developing (and implementing) the learning experience.
- What peer review was implemented, and how it was reflected in the learning experience.

(Note: Students can visit the website of the New York State Academy for Teaching and Learning at www.nysed.gov to view learning experiences and to gather additional information on assessment, portfolio development, rubrics, other authentic assessment strategies, paper-and-pencil testing, and more.)

More about Assessment/Evaluation

We expect that the readers of this text will have a basic understanding of educational assessment and evaluation strategies emerging from various courses in their preservice education. These same strategies, used by classroom teachers and health educators, can be incorporated into sexuality education. Assessment and evaluation provides the teacher with an understanding of what the learner has learned and how well the "learning experience" accomplished its stated goals and objectives.

Frequently, measures of a student's knowledge of specific content do not address the student's ability to use the knowledge constructively to affect his or her sexual health. To use current educational terminology, what sexuality educators must seek to measure is how students are progressing toward their goals (benchmarks), their ability to engage in activities that model real-life situations or challenges (authentic assessments), their performance (behaviors) or knowledge in use (performance assessments), and the quality of those behaviors based on criteria preestablished for the task (performance standards).

Performance assessments get at the very essence of sexuality education, whether content or skills: translating information to action. They tell students what they are expected to be able to do and how they will do it as participants in their own learning. The teacher engages the student in his or her own progress and provides continuous feedback.

Like health educators, some sexuality educators are moving toward the use of the portfolio as a project that assesses a student's performance. A *portfolio* is a collection of the student's work that represents his or her progress through the learning experience, unit, or entire curriculum. It should include an array of work that indicates the student's knowledge, critical thinking skills, development toward being able to access and evaluate accuracy of research and other health information, ability to engage in reflection, and so on. Assessing portfolios is a type of performance assessment whose criteria for judging should be preestablished in consultation with the student. The contents of the portfolio can be assessed in process (at various times in the curriculum) and at the culmination of the entire course of study. The student and his or her parents then have an understanding of how he or she is progressing and what he or she can do to achieve more. The emphasis is less on the curriculum and more on the student's progress.

Using an array of paper-and-pencil short-answer or essay tests or performance assessments, including portfolios, rubrics, and different scoring devices that clearly define the criteria and differentiate levels of performance, is important to assess student progress and to determine the success of the curriculum in meeting the specified goals and standards. Assessment may also be instructional. Although assessment tools can be developed by the teacher or by the student, they are most effective when they are generated by a student–teacher partnership. Rubrics are assessment tools that clearly define what students will be expected to do maximally and minimally because they are presented in levels of achievement. Using a Likert-type scale, the highest level represents all of the expected work in the highest possible performance for the specific task, and the lowest level represents the least work possible. Rubrics help students clarify what they must do to achieve the highest grade. Among other benefits, students can monitor their own progress, and they are equally understood by parents and others who are observant or have a stake in the student's progress.

In addition to setting the stage for more reliable grading, a broad range of assessment techniques provides the teacher with ongoing opportunities to reflect on the curriculum, in both content and teaching strategies, and make the necessary changes to create more effective learning environments and experiences.

SUMMARY

The data are clear: Sexuality education is not only an important component of the learning of school-age children but also one that is necessary and desired by students and their families. There are many models for delivering effective sexuality education in a free and democratic society. One that is supported by the sexuality and health education professions is comprehensive sexuality education. Sexuality education curricula must not be driven solely by the curtailment of sexually related problems and diseases (although the outcome should have a decreasing impact on these problems) but also by a need to help students initiate and maintain behaviors, develop attitudes and values, and implement personal life skills that enhance their healthy sexuality. Understanding that positive primary behaviors are easier to develop than changing risky behaviors, the curriculum must take a primarily preventive and sexually positive orientation. A powerful curriculum will provide students with content knowledge in the various subcontent areas of human sexuality and the personal life skills to implement this knowledge in their lives.

Sexuality education incorporates the positive and healthy influences on human beings that sexual intimacy can engender, including when sexual intimacy is appropriate to the person's situation, age, culture, religion, and relationships; when it occurs in respectful and noncoercive situations; and when it will not result in physical or psychological harm. In such environments, students will feel empowered to make decisions that support their well-being, develop a healthy sexuality, limit or abstain from risky behaviors, and combat peer pressure.

Sexuality education needs to be current, reflective, and scholarly. It must be inclusive of the cultural, intellectual, and developmental issues operating in schools. Teachers' knowledge base must include the most recent information on teaching, learning tools, and assessment strategies, and they must have at their fingertips resources, curricula, media, and other technology that are both flexible and useful to the variety of learner types they will encounter in their classes. Above all, teachers of human sexuality must be able to allay the fears of school administrators and parents regarding the dissemination of controversial information in order to engender in their constituents a feeling of safety with complicated and personal subjects.

The following chapters will prepare readers with the knowledge base, personal life skills, and developmentally appropriate learning experiences for their prospective students in the K–12 grades. Also available are resources and references to professional associations and literature that can be used in the future. It would behoove teachers of sexuality education to continue their professional development by attending the many national, regional, and local conferences available in the discipline.

REFERENCES

Alan Guttmacher Institute. (2003). *State policies brief*. New York: Author.

Anspaugh, D. J., & Ezell, G. (2000). *Teaching today's health*. Boston: Allyn & Bacon.

Bolin, A., & Whelehan, P. (2001). Perspectives in human sexuality. In K. J. Davidson & N. B. Moore (Eds.), *Speaking of sexuality: Interdisciplinary readings* (pp. 16–24). Los Angeles: Roxbury.

Centers for Disease Control and Prevention. (1998, September 18). Trends in sexual risk behaviors among high school students—United States, 1991–1997. *Morbidity and Mortality Weekly Report, 47*(36), 749–752.

Centers for Disease Control and Prevention. (2002a). Youth Risk Behavior Surveillance System—U.S. *Morbidity and Mortality Weekly Report, 51*(4).

Centers for Disease Control and Prevention. (2002b, June 28). Youth Risk Behavior Surveillance System—United States, 2001: Curriculum update (Winter, 2002). *Morbidity and Mortality Weekly Report, 51* (SS-4), 3–68.

Centers for Disease Control and Prevention. (2004). Youth Risk Behavior Surveillance System U.S. 2003. *Morbidity and Mortality Weekly Report, 53* (SS2), 2–91.

Fetro, J. V. (2000). *Personal and social skills: Understanding and integrating competencies across health content*. Santa Cruz, CA: ETR Associates.

Freire, P. (1972). *Pedagogy of the oppressed*. New York: Herder & Herder.

Greene, L. W., Kreuter, M., Deds, S. G., & Artrodge, L. B. (1985). Thoughts from the School Health Education Evaluation Advisory Panel. *Journal of School Health, 55*(8), 335.

Greenberg, J. S. (2003). Stress and health counseling. In J. Donnely (Ed.), *Health counseling*. Belmont, CA: Wadsworth/Thomson Learning.

Health Education Skills Matrix. (2002, July). Alexandria, VA: Association for Supervision and Curriculum Development.

Henry J. Kaiser Family Foundation. (2000a). *Fact sheet: Teen sexual activity*. Menlo Park, CA: Author.

Henry J. Kaiser Family Foundation. (2000b). *Sex education in America: A view from inside the nation's classrooms*. Menlo Park, CA: Author.

Henshaw, S. K. (1998). Unintended pregnancy in the United States. *Family Planning Perspectives, 30*(1), 24–29, 46.

Hite, S. (1976). *The Hite Report: A nationwide study of female sexuality*. New York: Macmillan.

Joint Committee on National Health Education Standards. (1995). *National Health*

Education Standards: Achieving health literacy: An investment in the future. Atlanta: American School Health Association, Association for the Advancement of Health Education, & American Cancer Society.

Kaplan, H. S. (1979). *Disorders of sexual desire.* New York: Simon & Schuster.

Kelly, G. F. (2004). *Sexuality today: The human perspective.* Guilford, CT: Dushkin.

Kinsey, A., Pomeroy, W., & Martin, C. (1948). *Sexual behavior in the human male.* Philadelphia: Saunders.

Kinsey, A., Pomeroy, W., Martin, C., & Gebhard, P. (1953). *Sexual behavior in the human female.* Philadelphia: Saunders.

Kohlberg, L. (1964). Development of moral character and moral ideology. In L. Hoffman & M. Hoffman (Eds.), *Research* (Vol. 1). New York: Russell Sage Foundation.

Ladas, A. K., Whipple, B., & Perry, J. D. (1983). *The G spot and other recent discoveries about human sexuality.* New York: Dell.

Laumann, E. O., Gagnon, J. H., Michael, R. T., & Michaels, S. (1994). *The social organization of sexuality: Sexual practices in the U.S.* Chicago: University of Chicago Press.

Lazarus, R. S., & Finkelor, S. (1984). *Stress appraisal and coping.* New York: Springer.

Mason, H. W. (1975). A historical view of the stress field. *Journal of Human Stress, 1,* 22–36.

Masters, W., & Johnson, V. (1966). *Human sexual response.* Boston: Little, Brown.

Masters, W., & Johnson, V. (1970). *Human sexual inadequacy.* Boston: Little, Brown.

McKay, A. (1999). *Sexual ideology and schooling: Towards a democratic sexuality education.* New York: State University of New York Press. Also in J. P. Elia (2000), Democratic sexuality education: A departure from the sexual ideologies and traditional schooling. *Journal of Sex Education & Therapy, 25*(2&3), 122–129.

National Public Radio, the Henry J. Kaiser Family Foundation, and the Harvard University Kennedy School of Government Representatives. (2003). *Sex education in America.* Menlo Park, CA: Henry J. Kaiser Family Foundation.

New York State Education Department/Coordinated School Health. (2002). *Design draft documents.* Center For Health Education Curriculum and Assessment Leadership Team. Albany: New York State Education Department.

Reiss, I. L., & Reiss, H. M. (1997). *Solving America's sexual crises.* Amherst, NY: Prometheus.

Satcher, D. (2001, June). *Call to action to promote sexual health and responsible sexual behavior.* Washington, DC: Office of the Surgeon General.

Selye, H. (1956). *The stress of life.* New York: Bantam.

Sexuality Information and Education Council of the United States. (1996). *National Guidelines Task Force: The SIECUS guidelines for comprehensive sexuality education: K–12.* New York: Author.

Silverstone, R. (2000). On governance, psychology, education and sexuality. *Journal of Sex Education & Therapy, 25* (2&3), 114–121.

Terry, E., & Manlove, J. (2000). *Trends in sexual activity and contraceptive use among teens.* Washington, DC: National Campaign to Prevent Teen Pregnancy.

Westheimer, R. K., & Lopater, S. (2004). *Human sexuality: A psychosocial perspective* (2nd ed.). Baltimore, MD: Lippincott, Williams & Wilkins.

MALE AND FEMALE SEXUALITY DEVELOPMENT THROUGH THE LIFE CYCLE: BIRTH TO AGING

EFREM ROSEN

OBJECTIVES

After active involvement in the learning experiences from this chapter, students will be able to

1. Name the reproductive body parts and their biological functions throughout the life cycle.
2. Name the sexual parts of the body and how they develop and function.
3. Know how psychological development affects sexuality.
4. Explain the process of fertilization, fetal development, and childbirth.
5. Relate the complexities of puberty to themselves and others.
6. Describe some of the developmental changes that occur during adulthood and aging.

REFLECTIVE QUESTIONS

Elementary School

1. Why do some girls have different-sized breasts than others?
2. Why do some boys have different-sized penises than others?
3. Does the size of a person's genitals have anything to do with how masculine or feminine he or she is?
4. When do girls start to menstruate?
5. How much menstrual flow comes out when a girl or woman menstruates? Is too much "bleeding" dangerous?
6. What is a "wet dream"?
7. Can a boy or man control himself from getting an erection when he doesn't want to?
8. What does it mean "to have sex"?
9. Do all people have sex?

Middle School/High School

1. What are the changes that occur during puberty?
2. How do I know if the changes that are happening to me are normal?
3. When does puberty end?
4. When can a girl become pregnant for the first time?
5. What happens to the body during pregnancy?
6. How does the baby develop?
7. What happens during childbirth?
8. What is menopause?
9. Do men have a menopause?
10. What happens to female and male sexuality as people get older?

—————————— **SCENARIO 1: MALE** ——————————

Joseph has just finished ninth grade. He knows he is growing up because he has begun to grow hair around his genitals and even some fuzz on his face. His father has a black beard and mustache. Joseph hopes he can have a full beard one day. He is a really good athlete and loves to play sports. His parents just don't understand why he doesn't want to go away to a 2-week sleep-away sports camp this year. Recently some strange things are happening to Joseph that he doesn't want anyone to know about, including his parents. Most mornings he wakes up with an erection that goes away after he urinates. Just the other night he woke up and found that he had wet his bed. He was mortified. He quietly went into the bathroom, got the hair blower, and dried everything before anyone woke up. This is not the first time this happened to him. After the first time, he was invited to his friend's house for a sleepover and he stayed up all night afraid to go to sleep.

What are the physical changes that are happening to Joseph?
Did Joseph urinate in his bed? If not, what did happen?
What are some of the other changes Joseph can expect?
If you were Joseph, whom could you talk to about the changes that are
  happening that you do not understand?

—————————— **SCENARIO 2: FEMALE** ——————————

Germaine is 11 and has begun puberty. Her breasts are beginning to develop, and she has noticed some pubic hair. She knows about menstruation but has not gotten her period yet. Her mother told her that it is likely to happen very soon. None of Germaine's friends have breasts, and none of them have had their period yet. Germaine is embarrassed. She doesn't want anyone to know that she has begun her development. She worries about taking a shower after swim class and doesn't sleep over at her friends' houses anymore, always making some excuse or another. The other thing that Germaine can't stop worrying about is getting her period while she is sitting in class. What will she do? What if she stains her clothing and others see? She doesn't want to carry menstrual pads in her school bag for fear that someone will see, so she wears a thin pad everyday to school and checks often.

What are the physical changes that are happening to Germaine?
What are some of the other changes she can expect?
If you were Germaine, to whom might you talk about these changes?

INTRODUCTION

What constitutes human sexual development? When does that development begin? How do individuals develop into sexual beings? These are among the many questions that young people may ask when learning about human sexuality.

Some would argue that human sexuality begins at conception since, for example, there is some evidence that indicates that, even before birth, a female's vagina will lubricate and a male's penis will become erect (Rathus, Nevid, & Fichner-Rathus, 2002), resulting in the creation of a human sexual being at birth. Sexuality continues to develop throughout life and is affected by the many complex interactions between our biology/physiology, psychology, and environment. Also affecting our psychosexual development are sociological, cultural, and spiritual influences. Therefore, it is the basic premise of this chapter that humans are sexual beings from the day they are born until the day they die (Family Planning Queensland, 2002).

To better understand human sexual development, one must know how the body develops and works. It is important that young people learn about their genitals and reproductive anatomy and are able to name the parts and speak about them without shame and discomfort. Understanding how their bodies will perform sexually and recognizing the sexual changes that occur over their lifetime can increase communication and comfort between themselves and others. Hence, this chapter begins by identifying the genital and reproductive systems that influence sexual development, followed by a presentation of the theories of development, and a description of the characteristics of behavior and sexual growth over the life cycle, including those that influence psychosexual health.

FEMALE AND MALE GENITAL AND REPRODUCTIVE SYSTEMS

A most important part of how and when young people learn information about their internal and external sexual anatomy and physiology is age-dependent. For example, early in children's lives, prekindergarten children (2–4 years of age) can be encouraged to know the correct names of the basic body parts, such as *penis* or *vagina*. As they mature, they learn more about the external genitals and some rudimentary functions. The function of the genitals in sexual behaviors, such as intercourse, would not be understood, nor would it be appropriate to teach about them, until much later in development. Too complex or too much information may simply go over a child's head and be dismissed or rejected until the child is ready to understand it. Thus, it is necessary to assess children's developmental ability to grasp and use information and the contexts in which the information appears in order to teach this material effectively.

Associated with teaching appropriate information about sexual anatomy and physiology is incorporating the life skills presented in Chapter 1. For example, if brothers and sisters close in age are being bathed together, they may be aware of and call attention to the differences in their genitals, but they still need communication, decision-making, and refusal skills to avoid inappropriate touching or fondling and to feel a sense of control over their body. Preadolescents need to know the names and functions of both external and internal male and female genitalia in preparation for the changes of puberty (discussed later in this chapter). As young people approach adolescence, they also need to learn about the functions of the genitals as components of the reproductive and sexual systems. Older adolescents and adults who are choosing to be sexually active must understand their body parts and functions in order to experience pleasure and prevent pregnancy and STIs.

Like other body parts, it is important to emphasize that the genitalia of males and females vary in size and shape. Diversity is normal! Young people can be encouraged to recognize that while their faces have similar body parts (a nose, lips, eyes, etc), they do not all look exactly alike. Similarly, there is wide variation among men and women in what their genitals look like. Knowing that such differences are normal, adolescents' common concerns about differences can be diminished. What follows is a description of the male and female genitalia along with their corresponding reproductive and sexual functions.

Female Sexual Anatomy and Physiology

EXTERNAL GENITAL ORGANS

External genital organs on the female include the vulva, which consists of the mons veneris, labia majora, labia minora, Bartholin's glands, clitoris, vestibule, breasts, and urethra.

The *mons veneris,* which means the "Mound of Venus," is a pad of fatty tissue that lies over the area where the two pubic bones come together on the front of the body (pubic symphysis). It protects the pubic area during intercourse and becomes covered with hair during puberty. It contains several nerve endings that can be stimulated during sexual stimulation.

The *labia majora* ("outer lips") are two elongated folds of fatty tissue that extend from the mons veneris to the perineum, an area of skin between the vagina and the anus. At the anterior end, the labia majora form a cover over the clitoris.

The *labia minora* (inner lips) are two thin folds of skin that lie within the labia majora and cover the separate vaginal and urethral openings. The anterior or front end of the labia minora forms a cover or hood over the clitoris (similar to the foreskin of the male's penis) and is called the *prepuce.* These folds of skin have numerous nerve endings that are sensitive to tactile stimulation and become engorged with blood during sexual stimulation, causing them to take on somewhat of a bluish color, swell, and open, making the vagina more accessible.

Bartholin's glands are two small glands found at the base of the labia minora that secrete small amounts of fluid during stimulation. The function of this fluid is unknown.

The *clitoris* is made up of the shaft, which is hidden under the hood, and the glans, which is probably the most sensitive structure on the female body, responding to touch, pressure, and temperature. The clitoris develops from the same embryonic structure as the penis, also fills with blood during sexual arousal, and is partly responsible for the orgasmic response (see Chapter 3 on sexual behavior). The clitoral hood (similar to the foreskin in the male) secretes a fluid (smegma) that becomes calcified and sticky, sometimes causing adhesions between the hood and the clitoris. Bathing with care and cleaning the area eliminates smegmal adhesions.

The *vestibule* is the area within the labia minora that contains both the urethral and vaginal openings. The urethral opening allows the passage of urine from the bladder to the outside of the body. The vaginal opening is the entrance to the female's internal genital organs and is surrounded by a ring of muscles that can expand sufficiently for the passage of a baby or the insertion of tampons or an erect penis. The vaginal opening is also partially covered by the *hymen,* a traditional symbol of virginity. However, its function is not known. By adolescence, the hymen is a thinly and delicately stretched tissue that has openings through which menstruation can flow. Because of the delicacy of this tissue, it is often ruptured as a result of vigorous activity, the use of tampons, masturbation, gynecological examination, or sexual intercourse. On rare occasions, it may need to be surgically removed. Thus, it is not a true symbol of virginity.

Females have two *breasts,* as do males, at birth. Female breasts develop and grow during puberty. The size and shape of the breasts differ from one woman to another and change over a woman's lifetime. For many women, breasts are sensitive and respond to sexual stimulations. As in all mammals, the female breasts are also designed to produce milk for nourishing babies. The main structures within the breasts are the mammary glands where milk is manufactured. There are also ducts where the milk collects and is transported outside the body via the nipples. The nipples are surrounded by the areola, which change shape and color after delivery of a baby and secrete an oily substance to facilitate breastfeeding.

INTERNAL GENITAL ORGANS

These consist of the vagina, cervix, uterus, Fallopian tubes, and ovaries.

The *vagina* is a muscular tube, collapsed in its relaxed state, that extends about 3.5 inches from the vaginal opening just past the *cervix.* The vagina expands to accommodate a tampon, finger, or an erect penis during intercourse. It is also the canal through which the baby can pass out of the body during childbirth and through which menstrual flow exits the body. Like other muscles in the body, its muscle tone can be maintained through a series of special exercises, known as Kegel exercises, if done on a regular basis. This outer third is particularly sensitive to sexual stimulation.

The *cervix* is the muscular opening to the uterus near the upper end of the vagina. The cervix contains the opening (called the *os*) between the uterus and the vagina though which semen, menstrual fluid, and a baby passes during childbirth. The cervix secretes mucus that changes in consistency during different stages of the menstrual cycle. The dilation of the cervix is an indicator of a fetus's stage of delivery.

The *uterus* is about the size and shape of an upside-down pear. The anterior end is *the fundus*. The fundus consists of three layers of tissue. The innermost layer is the *endometrium*. This layer contains the blood vessels necessary for the nourishment of the developing fetus. It builds up and sloughs off with the menstrual cycle, unless a pregnancy occurs, at which time the cycle usually stops for the duration of the pregnancy.

At the upper end of the fundus, the uterus opens into two very thin tubes, the *Fallopian tubes/oviducts*. Just beyond, but not attached to the other end of each tube, is an ovary. Each month, one or more ova (commonly known as *eggs*) pass into one of the tubes through the *fimbriae*, hairlike projections that sweep the egg into the tube. The egg is moved by *cilia* (hairlike projections) to the upper third of the tube where, in the presence of sperm, fertilization normally takes place. The ovum, if fertilized, will continue its journey and implant in the *endometrium* of the uterus. If the fertilized ovum does not complete its journey, a potentially dangerous *ectopic pregnancy* (fetal development outside the uterus) can occur that requires surgical removal. If unfertilized, the ova will exit the body as part of the menstrual flow.

A female is born with each of her *ovaries* containing about 400,000 immature eggs or *follicles* (commonly known as ova). After puberty, an egg ripens in one ovary every other month, breaks out of the follicle, and passes through the ovarian wall (*ovulation*) into the fallopian tube. Before ovulation, the egg develops inside this capsule, the *Graafian follicle*, which secretes the hormone *estrogen*. Once ovulation occurs, the follicle becomes the *corpus luteum* and begins to secrete the hormone *progesterone*. Both estrogen and progesterone play a role in menstruation, birth, growth, and aging and are responsible for the buildup of the endometrium that is required to receive the fertilized egg and maintain the ensuing pregnancy.

Male Sexual Anatomy and Physiology

EXTERNAL GENITAL ORGANS

A male's external genitals include the penis and scrotum.

The *penis* consists of the *root* that attaches it to the body, the *shaft* that makes up its major length, and the *glans*, or head, which contains the urethral opening and where the foreskin attaches. The penis changes in size from the relaxed (flaccid) state to the erect state when sexually stimulated, when its tissues (the *corpus spongiosum* and *corpora cavernosa*) fill with blood.

The *scrotum* is a sac of skin located beneath the penis that contains the *testicles* and sperm ducts. The outer layer of the scrotum is covered with hair and sweat glands, and the inner layer consists of muscle and connective tissue that can contract or relax depending on the external temperature. Shortly before birth, the testes descend into the scrotum since normal sperm production requires a temperature that is lower than body temperature. If the testicles do not descend into the scrotum, surgery is required, or the male will be sterile. After puberty, when sperm production begins (and may continue till old age), the muscles of the scrotum maintain the temperature by elongating away from the body or contracting close to the body, so that normal sperm can be produced. At the time of ejaculation, it contracts, moving closer to the body.

INTERNAL GENITAL ORGANS

These consist of the testes, epididymis, vas deferens or sperm duct, prostate and Cowper's glands, seminal vesicles, and urethra.

The *testes* (or *testicles*) produce sperm within, and male hormones between, the *seminiferous tubules,* which are highly coiled structures within the testes. Once the sperm mature, they pass into the *epididymis* where they are stored for a short period of time.

The sperm leave the testes during the process of *ejaculation* by entering a tube known as the *vas deferens,* which carries the sperm to the urethra. On the way, fluid from the *seminal vesicles* and *prostate gland* add nutrients to the sperm, forming *semen.*

The *urethra* is the tube that goes from the bladder through the penis. It carries the semen out of the body in the final stage of ejaculation. The urethra also carries urine out of the body, but not at the same time since the muscles of the prostate gland contract during ejaculation, thus preventing semen and urine from mixing.

Finally, *Cowper's glands* add alkaline fluid and nutrients that activate the sperm and help protect them from the acidic environment of the urethra and the vagina. These glands can also store live sperm that can be secreted before ejaculation (the preejaculate) and can cause a pregnancy.

THEORIES OF SEXUAL DEVELOPMENT

The development of sexuality includes a sequential set of stages that involve biological, intellectual, emotional, social, and environmental components. Each stage—childhood, adolescence, and adulthood—manifests the onset of interacting components. Within each stage, there are the physical components, such as brain differentiation and creeping, crawling, and walking, and the psychological components, such as giving language and meaning to feelings and attitudes as evidenced in the childhood stage. These constitute psychosexual development.

In the development of erotic responses, it has been hypothesized that there is a normal distribution of variation in the population (Haroian, 2000). Therefore, some people will focus on sexual concerns where sexual expression dominates the various stages of development. Other people will give a low priority to sexual concerns in response to life events. Both of these extremes are affected by culture, the double standard, the attitudes of peers and adults, and other factors. In any case, knowing what to expect in human growth and development helps people understand changes in themselves and others and thus allows them to plan for the future.

The following theories and theorists have been used to explain the complicated development of human sexuality. Many others have made substantial contributions, but because it is not within the parameters of this text to provide a full discussion of each theory, it behooves the reader to seek additional information from the vast library of available psychological materials.

The Freudian View of Psychosexual Development

A widely popular view, especially among psychoanalytic psychotherapists, developed by Freud and Strachey (1975), focused on sexual pleasure drives, libido, erogenous zones, and fixation as they affect personality development (Stevenson, 1992). Freud's work suggests that our sexuality and our personality development are concluded by about age 6 with little that can change them throughout the remainder of our lives. His work explains that our pleasures are an outcome of meeting our biological drives, and our frustrations are a result of not meeting them. Throughout infancy and early childhood, children strive to meet those needs through stimulation of their erogenous zones (the mouth, genitals, and anus) without an understanding of, or concern for, what society deems "acceptable" behavior.

Freud described five developmental stages:

The oral stage. This stage concerns pleasures derived from oral stimulation. It begins at birth and lasts about 1.5 years when the child is preoccupied with nursing or suckling. If the needs and demands for these sensations are refused by the mother or caretaker, the child develops pessimism, envy, suspicion, and sarcasm. If, on the other hand, the child is overindulged and is excessively satisfied, he or she becomes optimistic, gullible, and full of admiration for others. The stage ends with weaning.

The anal stage. During this stage, pleasure is derived from stimulation of the anus through the control and release of material from the rectum. This includes the conflict of toilet training representing the need to control bodily functions. The child meets the conflict between the parent's demands and the child's desires, resulting in either an *anal-expulsive* character that is unorganized, reckless, careless, and defiant or an *anal-retentive* character that is neat, orderly, careful, and passive-aggressive. Proper toilet training resolves this stage and affects the child's attitudes toward possessions and authority. This stage lasts about 2.5 years.

The phallic stage. During this stage, pleasures are derived from genital contact. This stage contains the potential for the most crucial sexual conflict that focuses on the genitals. The conflict, labeled the Oedipus complex (in males) and the Electra complex (in females), involves the child's unconscious desire to sexually possess the parent of the opposite sex and the fears relating to this drive and identification with the same-sex parent. This dilemma is resolved when gender roles are learned. Fixation in this stage results in a personality that is reckless, self-assured, and narcissistic. Failure to resolve this period results in a fear of incapability of love. Resolution allows boys and girls to pass into the latency period.

The latency period. Freud believed that sexual development concludes after 6 years of age, and the period from 6 until puberty is one where little if any sexual development occurs. He described a period in which the sex drive lies dormant, when sexual desires and erogenous impulses are totally repressed. Behaviors are focused on nonsexual energies and same-sex relationships. As soon as the physical changes of puberty arrive, this period ends.

The genital stage. As the child's energies once again focus on his or her genitals, interest turns to sexual and erotic relationships and the fulfillment of sexual desires. Freud believed that to complete this period successfully, the child must experience sexual intercourse in a heterosexual relationship.

Although extensively criticized by more recent research, Freud's concepts are still valuable in the understanding of psychosexual development.

Erikson's Developmental Theory

Erikson (1963) took a more psychosocial view of development and explained that infants, children, adolescents, and adults face a series of ongoing developmental tasks. He suggested that development results from drives and behaviors that are within one's experience and influenced by the social context within which they occur. Unlike Freud, Erikson believed that development can be influenced and changed in each stage and the anticipation of expectations for each stage can also influence these changes.

In infancy (birth–1 year), the conflict is between trust and mistrust; during early childhood (1–3 years), it is between autonomy and shame and doubt. In preschool (3–6 years), the conflict is between initiative and guilt, while during school age (6–12) years, it is between industry and inferiority. In adolescence, the conflict is between identity and identity confusion; in young adulthood, between intimacy and isolation; in middle adulthood, between creativity and stagnation; and, finally, in older adulthood, between integrity and despair. To continue to grow, these opposing psychological forces must be resolved. Inadequate resolution results in thwarted development, leaving the person with a lack of certain skills and attributes essential to later life. For example, if, as an infant, a sense of trust in self and others doesn't develop, the person will grow up with a strong sense of mistrust making it difficult to establish and maintain intimate relationships.

Sexually Supportive Growth

Haroian (2000) considers sexual development to occur in four stages. The first is from birth to 6 years of age, in which the physical changes are primary, and sexual interests and behaviors are expressed spontaneously unless repressed or inhibited. The second stage is from about age 6 to the onset of puberty at about age 12. Physical growth slows, with a shift toward mental growth characterized by the need for privacy and autonomy and the desire for sexual pleasure. The third stage, from puberty to early adolescence, seems to be controlled by the sex hormones with growth spurts, the development of secondary sex characteristics, and a new awareness of self and others. The fourth stage is mid- to late adolescence, from about 16 to adulthood. Growth again slows, the body image is consolidated through hormonal balance, the sex response cycle is achieved primarily through masturbation or coupling, and sexual gratification is integrated into relationships.

Sexual Growth as an Ongoing Process

Others consider sexual development as an ongoing process that begins very early in life, even before birth. The potential for a complex set of interactions allows for the development of a complex sexuality. This is the gradual construction of a system of sexual meanings. Gagnon and Simon (1973) view the process as the construction of associations or assemblies that are actively formulated by the person rather than being acquired by biology. For example, there is the formation of a specific gender identity, the emergence of a sense of modesty, or the learning of a specific set of mechanisms that become the basis for sexual arousal and other feelings and behaviors.

The Social Constructionist View of Psychosexual Development

More recently, from the work of social constructionists, emerges a view of "childhood sexualities" (Plummer, 1991). According to this perspective, at birth, sexuality is simply a biological potential that awaits a social context to become significant. It is not fixed in the child awaiting repression or liberation, but rather it is something that is socially constructed. The culture furnishes the scripts that help define the nature of a developing sexuality (Gagnon & Simon, 1973). This process continues throughout the life cycle and varies according to class, race, and gender. The child learns the meaning of sexuality through sexual encounters with parents, siblings, and peers. For example, a 3-month-old baby may experience an orgasm, but a meaning has to be given to it. Thus, the experience may be very different for a 3-month-old, a 5-year-old, a 15-year-old, or an adult. The biological experience is the same, but the meanings shift and change depending on the child's prior experiences and culture. Sexual meanings are constructed from these experiences, and sexual scripts are built. Thus, a language is added

(Plummer, 1991). This process also includes the development of a "gender identity," the sense of being a boy or a girl (see Chapter 4).

Social constructionists, therefore, view sexual development as a highly variable, ever-changing process that depends on forever-altering contexts.

> And herein lies a dilemma. It is precisely because of this "developmental" imagery being so pervasive that many children and adults collectively construct the sexual worlds of childhood around such a theme. Cross-generational sexuality may serve to reinforce such assumptions; "the child is a child, the adult is an adult." But it also harbors the potential to suggest that the child is an adult and the adult is a child; that such categories are neither fixed nor universal. Such meanings are likely to be relatively rare, given the dominance of our developmental view of age. But the constructionist view of age at least signposts a greater flexibility than is usually thought. (Plummer, 1991, p. 9)

CHARACTERISTICS AND BEHAVIORS IN SEXUAL GROWTH

Before Birth

At conception, sexual development begins with the interactions of a unique set of genes, half contributed by the woman and the other half by the man. These genes interact in an environment that "includes other genes from the same genome, and their products; the physical conditions, nutrients, hormones, toxins, and disease agents present during fetal life and the life experiences to which the genes' owner is exposed after birth" (Levay & Valente, 2002, p. 122). During fertilization, a sperm from the man fuses with the egg from the woman and produces the fertilized egg or zygote. Gender differences begin when the parental chromosomes normally recombine, producing either the male (XY) or female (XX) body plan. This allows the embryonic gonads to differentiate (under normal circumstances) into the appropriate genital structures (for example, penis and testes in males and vagina and ovaries in females).

Further male differentiation occurs with the production of the hormone *testosterone* as a result of the action of at least three genes on the Y chromosome. In the absence of testosterone, female embryonic gender differentiation occurs (see Chapter 4 for more on gender). Extensive research on the development of gender leads to the conclusion that, in the presence of testosterone, male differentiation occurs regardless of sex chromosomes. The absence of this hormone produces the female (for a more extensive presentation of the normal and abnormal differentiation of gender, see Levay & Valente, 2002). This process also triggers rapid cell divisions (*mitoses*) of the zygote from one cell into many cells, the *morula*. By the 32-cell stage, this fertilized egg is called a *blastocyst*. During this period of cell divisions, which begin to occur immediately after fertilization and continue for several days, the egg is moving down from the upper end of the Fallopian tube to where it implants in the *endometrial lining* of the uterus and continues to develop for about the next 40 weeks.

Brain development also shows gender differences. Research on mammals by Gorski and his associates clearly shows gender differences in the growth of specific nuclei, neurological centers in the central nervous system. These also seem to be a result of circulating fetal testosterone (Davis, Shryne, & Gorski, 1996). Also, "hormone levels during development not only guide the development of anatomical differences between male and female brains, but also influence an animal's or person's sexual behavior in adulthood" (Levay & Valenti, 2002, p. 146). The extent to which animal research is also applicable to human behavior, and the extent to which this physical development affects or causes differences in the sexual behavior of humans, requires much more extensive research.

The Neonate: Birth to 1 Year Old

At the time of birth, or as a result of genetic or visual testing during pregnancy, a gender is assigned by either the parents or a physician. At this stage of development, infants focus almost solely on their physical parts. They quickly learn that touch feels good, and their nervous system focuses on physical tasks such as coordination, visual acuity, and the differentiation of self from the rest of the world. A most important component during this stage of development is the formation of a bond between the caretaker and the child. By 4 weeks of age, there is interest in bodily functions. Infants seem to enjoy contact with their caretaker's body, display contentment after a meal, enjoy a bath, and respond positively upon being wrapped snugly or held. They also respond contentedly to the caretaker's voice, closeness, movement, and sensations from their own body. They vocalize demands and discomforts through crying and also use body language, including pelvic thrusting, which may be comforting. At about 4 months, infants will cry for social stimulation and will gaze intently at a caretaker's face. They will grab fingers and hands and touch body parts. During the second 6 months, they will grasp and hold objects. The process of self-discovery develops. Near the end of the 1st year, they will evoke emotions of affection, jealousy, and sympathy (Haroian, 2000).

Some infants, at 4 to 5 months, seem capable of having sexual responses that resemble orgasms (Kinsey, Pomeroy, & Martin, 1948). Typically, self pleasuring of the genitals (masturbation) starts at 6 to 12 months. It begins by rubbing the genitals against soft objects such as a pillow or a favorite blanket. Later, genital manipulation is readily observed. Although, at this age, the behavior may not be offensive to caretakers, some will intervene and remove the infant's hand or object. These early messages can cause the child to develop negative feelings toward his or her own body.

One to 3 Years of Age

During this time, children also develop positive or negative messages about their bodies by the way they are cuddled, touched, and spoken to. By watching the behavior of their caretakers and other adults, they learn attitudes about sexuality and relationships (Family Planning Queensland, 2002). They enjoy being the center of attention, which also helps them develop their sense of self. They enjoy nudity, including bathing, and often take off their clothes and run around nude. Genital play is common. They also learn about bowel and bladder control. By the second year, genital play emerges as a recognized source of pleasure accompanied by facial expressions, flushing, rapid respiration, and perspiration with an inward gaze and self-absorbed look (Martinson, 1994). Thus, masturbation seems to be a common experience in the early developmental stages.

During the 2nd year, sometimes referred to as "the terrible two's," growth and development occur rapidly. Manual dexterity and manipulation are achieved so that children can work with small objects effectively. They will romp, fill and empty toys, flee and pursue, tear objects apart, and try to put them together. They love water and doll play, and both boys and girls pretend to be the mothers of their dolls. Anxious caretakers will sometimes interrupt this play in boys, thus affecting their gender identity. Two-year-olds' major focus has to do with bowel and bladder control, thus directing much attention to their genitals.

Year 3 is characterized by a high degree of self-control. Children now develop fine-motor skills like turning pages of a book and appear to spend time "reading." They watch facial expressions of adults, express love, and affirm their own gender. They will question where babies come from and try to relive their own infancy, touching their mother's breasts and asking for a bottle, showing jealousy if there is a new sibling, and talking about imaginary playmates, repeating stories frequently. They will make simple choices with an intense need for attention. Tensions are expressed through nail biting, thumb sucking, masturbating, or chewing on hair or clothing.

Four to 6 Years

Four-year-olds are great talkers, with great imagination and lots of questions. They will make up alibis and dramatize experiences such as wanting "to run away from home." Their interest in death may cause bad dreams. Their sexual interest revolves around babies, especially if there is an infant sibling, thinking that "the baby comes out of their mother's belly." They are often observant of an infant sibling's genitals, especially if different from their own. They may play "show me yours and I will show you mine," expressing more interest in the genitals. They begin to inquire about how babies are made. They like to "play house" in groups, pretending Mommy and Daddy roles, dressing and undressing dolls, especially in preschool or nursery classes. They continue their interest in touching their genitals. Many will masturbate, but by now most have learned that touching their genitals should not be done at all or certainly not in public.

Five-year-olds are focused on "Mommy" with expressions of love and gratitude (if Mommy has been the primary caretaker). Sex, reproduction, and death are their favorite topics, and they can talk about the past and the future (Haroian, 2000). They talk of love and marriage, generally identifying with the same-sex parent (if there is one available). In understanding their gender identity, they compare the differences between boys' and girls' bodies and may express interest in "marrying" someone they know. They are beginning to develop a sense of trust but may appear vulnerable at times, expressing fears of violence with bad dreams. These are the rudimentary developments of life scripts.

Six-year-olds are focused on themselves and considered to be egocentric. They defy and become critical of others, including parents. They are beginning to ask the question "Who am I?" They are better able to process sex information about anatomy, especially the names of body parts, sexual behavior, marriage, and death, and convert physical concerns to mental ones. This is the beginning of the period, described by Freud's followers, as the Freudian latency period, a time thought to include little sexual development. However, many sex researchers (sexologists) find little evidence to support the notion of a latency period's existence but rather believe that sexual interests and behaviors present during this time continue throughout life.

Seven to 9 Years—Preadolescence

Seven-year-olds are self-absorbed "in their own little world," learning the meaning of things and people and developing feelings about them. This self-reflection may be interpreted as moodiness, shyness, or depression. These youngsters may either feel inadequate or assertive and sulk if treated like babies. They have a tendency to get distracted but need reminders to complete chores. Frequently, they blame others or create alibis. Sevens can bathe and dress themselves but still may need help with cleanliness. They are aware of their genitals and can link body functions to sexual feelings; touching feels good.

By 8 years old, same-sex play becomes more common, and peer pressure may be noted. Athletics are often gender segregated. Same-sex play, in the form of comparing or fondling each other's genitals, may occur but does not influence or substantiate the subsequent expression of sexual orientation. Children at this stage are learning adult scripts and behaviors associated with prepubescent changes that will allow them to make the transition to adulthood (Blonna & Levitan, 2000), but they have a long way to go. There may be much confusion over sexual facts and embarrassment in asking adults for information. The start of peer groups as the source of information is observed, but this information is most often *mis*information. These youngsters have curiosity about life in other cultures, procreation, marriage, parenting, and babies and take on an almost intellectual interest in sexual information.

Nine-year-olds are no longer considered children developmentally but are not yet adolescents. Their self-image is still developing, and they are capable of some objective self-appraisal. At times, they can appear self-absorbed, thinking about peer relationships, school, and family. They build strong lasting friendships and identify with same-sex peer groups by using passwords, dress codes, rituals, and taboos, thus establishing a strong sense of brotherhood/sisterhood. Typically, boys roughhouse and wrestle; girls whisper and gossip (Haroian, 2000). Girls are closer to puberty than boys, and both are becoming aware of pending changes and gender role behaviors. If they don't achieve their own expectations in what they consider a timely manner, they may feel guilt or shame. They can be critical and judgmental of others, setting the stage for prejudices.

Ten to 17—The Adolescent Years

Recent observations indicate that although hormonal changes are occurring as early as 6 years of age, physical changes begin to be more visually evident by the 10th and 11th years. While enormous variability occurs in this age group, the visual physical changes begin to be accompanied by psychosexual expressions described as "sexual attractions." These sexual attractions sometimes cause early sexual fantasies and sexual interests that are observable in children's "play." Games begin to encompass flirtatiousness and "teasing" as these youngsters begin to mature. The flirtatiousness and teasing are typically an outgrowth of behavior modeled from older siblings in their family or influenced by the media.

Young adolescents, in their search for sexual maturity, begin to develop an ability to communicate intimately, share feelings, and identify societal and personally acceptable sexual behaviors. They also begin to understand their own and their partner's values, including messages about trust and fidelity. This is a time when mixed messages, rampant in society, become confusing to them. To accomplish these developmental tasks, young adolescents need

- A great deal of information,
- Effective communication with their parents,
- The ability to make progress toward independence,
- A personal value system,
- A positive self-image, and
- The ability to differentiate between what is healthy from what is unhealthy in their lives (Weinstein & Rosen, 2002).

While adolescents grapple with a new, expanding sense of their sexuality, how they ultimately feel about their sexual self will greatly affect their general self-image, confidence, and their ability to construct effective and positive life scripts. The extent to which they become comfortable with their bodies and sexual expression, and clear about their sexual values, is directly related to how effectively they will function in all other areas of their lives (Hass, 1979).

To further understand what is happening during adolescence, the Sarrels (see Sarrel, 1989) describe what they call a "sexual unfolding" whereby the intellectual, moral, and spiritual growth of adolescents is accompanied by the emergence of their sexuality. Through the following series of

10 interactive processes, the Sarrels explain that young people develop a sexual identity and an increased capacity for emotional and sexual maturity:

1. An evolving sense of the body (toward a body image) that is gender-specific and fairly free of distortion (particularly about the genitals);
2. The ability to overcome or modulate guilt, shame, fear, and childhood inhibitions associated with sexual thoughts and behavior;
3. A gradual loosening of the primary emotional ties to parents and siblings;
4. Learning to recognize what is erotically pleasing and displeasing and being able to communicate this to a partner;
5. Resolving conflict and confusion about sexual orientation;
6. A sexual life free of sexual dysfunction or compulsion;
7. A growing awareness of being a sexual person and of the place and value of sex in one's life, including options such as celibacy;
8. Becoming responsible about oneself, one's partner, and society (for example, using contraception and not using sex as a means of exploitation of another);
9. A gradually increasing ability to experience eroticism as one aspect of intimacy with another person—not that all eroticism occurs in an intimate relationship, but that this fusion of sex and love is possible; and
10. Experiencing first sexual intercourse and, in some cases, oral or anal sex.

When adolescents are searching for their independent identities, they are also attempting to find meaning for their sexual feelings and changing relationships. The themes that predominate during adolescence include resolving the relationship between body image and self-image; knowing their body and its sensual and sexual responses; creating a sexual identity that acknowledges and can overcome socially limiting gender roles and expectations; recognizing and accepting their sexual orientation; learning about themselves in intimate relationships; and developing a sexual value system (Masters, Johnson, & Kolodny, 1988).

Puberty: The Biology of Adolescence

The rapid onset of hormone flow from the hypothalamus and pituitary gland triggers a complex set of biological and psychological responses that characterize an extremely rapid period of growth and development. What determines when this sudden flow of hormones will begin is probably established during fetal development, but the biological changes that it produces have been clearly described (Katchadourian & Lunde, 1989). The timing is uniquely individual and characteristically unrelated to a specific gender.

PUBERTY IN BOYS

Briefly, puberty in boys is observed by the development of secondary sex characteristics such as the beginning growth of facial hair (usually seen initially around the upper lip), followed by signs of the voice deepening. At the same time, growth of the penis, testes, and scrotum occurs, and pubic hair appears. This is followed by a general body growth spurt that begins at about 11, continues for 2 to 3 years, and then slows until adulthood. On the average, the genitals reach adult size by about 15 years of age. This pattern, however, is just an average and often of great concern for boys going through the process.

Erections are not a phenomenon of adolescence; they are observed *in utero*. Hence, it is not the fear of being unable to achieve an erection but rather the size of the erect penis that is often of concern for young men as they develop. Considerable variation exists in penis size. The size of the flaccid penis is not correlated with the size of the erect penis. Yet, the assumed relationship between penis size and "manliness" seems to cause much stress.

A first ejaculation is commonly experienced early in puberty, usually during sleep, but sometimes during masturbation. These nocturnal emissions, commonly known as "wet dreams," are a particular source of anxiety and confusion to the uninformed adolescent. Unprepared for these events, young men may awake alarmed, thinking that they have lost urinary control and wet their bed. They are often embarrassed and will suddenly become fearful about sleep in general and especially sleeping at a friend's or relative's. Nocturnal emissions are frequently accompanied by erotic dreams and fantasies. These dreams and fantasies occur during the REM stage of sleep and can repeat four to five times during the night.

Boys may also experience spontaneous orgasms from nonsexual physical activities as well as from viewing sexual materials or nude people. The capability for spontaneous orgasm is a phenomenon of early adolescence that is usually lost in almost all males by late adolescence. These occurrences, coupled to the changes that occur in their genitals, intensifies their ever-increasing interest in sexual behavior. This is called *sex drive* or *libido* and is also under the influence of the male hormone, testosterone. In girls (discussed later), this same hormone begins to be secreted at puberty and also affects sex drive. But there remains much confusion about the relationship between testosterone and sex drive. It is not a higher concentration of testosterone that correlates to more sex drive. One needs a critical amount of testosterone to initiate sex drive, along with such factors as sexual desire, decreased performance stress, and healthy attitudes about sex.

Typically, boys achieve their full adult height later than girls. Yet, there is no correlation between the beginning of the growth spurt and when final adult height is achieved. The deepening of the voice occurs at about the same time. Associated with these changes are skin problems (usually acne) in both boys and girls. As with the timing of the onset of pubertal changes, there is a great disparity as to which parts of the body will grow when, which boys will begin growth before others and when the full changes will be completed.

PUBERTY IN GIRLS

For girls, hormonal changes (menarche and the secretion of the pituitary hormones, follicle stimulating hormone [FSH] and luteinizing hormone [LH], as well as estrogen and progesterone) trigger breast development and the appearance of pubic hair, the first signs of sexual maturity. Many young girls have their first menstrual period at 10 years of age and others at 15 or 16. The average age of menarche in the United States is around 12. This onset of puberty is usually 2 years earlier than it is in boys and tends to perpetuate the physical and emotional separation between boys and girls of the same age.

Breast development may begin with the appearance of a small lump or mound in only one breast and continues to include increases in the size of the nipple and areola. This perfectly normal unevenness in initial breast growth sometimes causes alarm to unknowing girls and their parents. How large one's breasts will be and at what age they will be fully developed is associated with one's genetics. At the same time, other physical changes are occurring in the vagina but are not easily observable. Pubic hair, a more visible sign, is also developing at this time.

Menarche begins around the same time as the growth spurt. It is not an indication of reproductive maturity. Initial menstrual cycles are usually sporadic and irregular and generally do not include ovulation. A regularized menstrual cycle takes about 1 year to achieve. Overall growth in height will be completed after about 1 year. Because ovulations do sometimes occur, although irregularly at the beginning, young girls must be cautioned about the possibility of an unwanted pregnancy. The average age of menarche is decreasing as the general health status of girls is increasing. Although predominantly controlled by genetic factors and hormonal changes, the relationships between the onset of menarche and body fat, nutrition, and general health status are becoming better understood.

Both male and female teenagers need to know about the process of menstruation. Many myths persist concerning the amount of bleeding that occurs; the dangers of bathing, swimming, and other intense physical activities; the effects on behavior; and the like. Expressions such as "the curse," "on the rag," or "PMSing" are descriptors that reflect negative feelings about the process of menstruation. Thus, young women need to know what to expect, what is normal for them, and how to care for their sexual health. They can be helped to see menstruation as a normal, healthy part of female functioning. Young men also need to know that menstruation is a normal body process and does not usually render a woman sick or unable to cope, nor is she "bleeding to death."

At the same time that the sex hormones (estrogen and progesterone) are being secreted and development is occurring in girls, there is an awareness of vaginal secretions often accompanied by spontaneous sexual thoughts and sexual activities. The ability to experience spontaneous orgasms by fantasizing and viewing sexually explicit materials exists in some female adolescents, as it does in males, and may continue throughout adulthood. As with boys, girls are very concerned about the meaning of their physical changes and experiences. They are sometimes worried about whether they will be first or last among their friends to develop and about such things as "who knows" when they are menstruating. These concerns are a common part of early puberty and generally resolve as the process continues and the adolescent becomes more knowledgeable.

Other Adolescent Developmental Issues

The wide range of variation in development among individuals takes on special concern when a teen's growth pattern is significantly different from his or her peers. Peer group acceptance or rejection is important to the development of a positive self-image and is closely associated with the feedback teens believe they are receiving from their friends. Regardless of whether an individual's maturation is early or late, a teenager will frequently ask, "Am I normal?" Late developers may not understand why they have not yet begun to change. Early developers may feel uncomfortable because they are noticed as fully mature. Thus, either group may believe that something is wrong. Good education and information are usually all that is needed to reassure adolescents about how normal their physical development really is, especially when other psychosocial factors are accounted for.

The profound biological changes of puberty engender extremes in feelings of vulnerability and sensitivity. Young adolescents are intensely preoccupied with the questions "Who is this new person I have become?" and "How do I measure up, physically?" They are overly involved with grooming, dieting, dressing, and exercise behaviors (their hair, their makeup, their clothing), which reflects their concern about their changing bodies. They have a heightened need for privacy, particularly about their physical being. This is often at a time when their parents are feeling disconnected and somewhat out of control. The result may be a heightened need by parents for more vigilant observations and direct information in contrast to the desire, by the adolescent, for independence displayed as personal secrecy. The closed doors while dressing or bathing, the request for parents to leave the room during medical examinations, and the reluctance to change clothes during physical education classes become sources of stress related to puberty.

PSYCHOLOGICAL FACTORS

Puberty is not only a period of biological growth but also a stage of rapid personality development and psychological maturation. Havighurst (1972) identified a series of seven life tasks that adolescents are expected to successfully master in order to make the transition into adulthood. Each of these tasks, in some way, affects their sexuality.

Accepting One's Body.   The ideal presented in the media is youthful beauty and perfection, without flaws, scars, or flab. In a multicultural society such as ours, the cultural definitions of physical perfection become even more complicated as the media acknowledges little, if any, cultural diversity.

Using media norms, teens experience a general dissatisfaction with their physical appearance, feeling either too big or too small (whether in height or in the size of their breasts, hips, penis, or nose). Young men in U.S. society often view their bodies as performance tools and instruments used for proving their masculinity. Young women, on the other hand, may see their bodies as instruments of attraction needing outside validation of their desirability. Because body image is directly associated with sexual identity, adolescents can be encouraged to accept what they have rather than what others think they should have—in other words, to develop an internal locus of control and personal identity rather than one dependent on the scripts of others.

Changing Sex Roles.   From birth, people begin to develop their sense of masculinity and femininity as a result of strong environmental influences (see Chapter 4). Many have accepted socially defined meanings for the ways in which boys and girls are encouraged to be different in their gender roles, their family responsibilities, their career choices, and their sexual behavior. Changes in traditional gender roles have certainly been observed, and sex-role stereotypes, values, and standards are no longer so clearly defined. Also, these often represent enormous divergence from the cultural and familial messages adolescents are receiving at home and in their communities. Hence, many occupations, tasks, and behaviors no longer carry a strictly masculine or feminine label. For some young people, these changes have allowed them more freedom and expanded their opportunities for self-exploration. For others, the changes leave them perplexed, guilt ridden, and, perhaps, distraught about the future.

Research suggests that women reach adulthood with more skills for developing trusting and intimate relationships than men because they are encouraged to disclose experiences and share personal feelings with same-sex friends in their earlier years. Young men are frequently discouraged from these same behaviors because of the embarrassment and fear of being labeled gay or unmanly. Consequently, they are less prepared for emotional intimacy in adulthood. Yet, sexual learning requires an ability to participate in varying levels of intimacy, sharing, and self-disclosure.

These socially constructed realities and routines in behavior, assigned by gender, often determine an individual's sexual definitions, roles, and reciprocal behavior choices. In a society filled with change and growing diversity, individual possibilities still remain somewhat limited. The challenge for adolescents is to establish a personal sense of comfort with whatever social roles they will identify with and then to find individualized expressions, careers, and interpersonal and sexual relationships that are congruent with their individually constructed life scripts.

Establishing Peer Relationships.   As stated earlier, in later childhood, social groups are frequently exclusively same-gender where play and activities are the learning field for relationships. Later in adolescence, other gender relationships are more available, and the rules and roles become somewhat confusing. The influence of family, peer, and other cultural factors promotes the development of social scripts and interactions. Relationships within the family and the community provide initial models for future relationships. In religious contexts, young people learn about the rules of their church regarding intimacy, fun, sex, and so forth. At the same time, the peer group provides a new, and perhaps conflicting, set of rules.

In early adolescence, the primary social learning environment for sexual expressions shifts to become the school and sports or other after school activities that are fairly well supervised. In middle adolescence, there is less supervision and thus more opportunity for intimate peer relationships. Among older teenagers, the learning field becomes a social proving ground where experimentation with learned realities in peer relationships occurs.

The meanings and boundaries that peer relationships provide vary dramatically from group to group and from context to context. Sexually intimate expressions also range from fun, where sexual urges can be acted on, to serious emotional attachments. In any case, these and other social situations provide an opportunity for young people to experiment while developing their sociosexual scripts. Whereas most of this explains the processes experienced by heterosexual youth, far less opportunity is available for homosexual youth since they come to terms with their sexual orientation frequently in hostile and unacceptable environments (for more, see Chapter 5).

Resolving Dependence on Parents.   It is not uncommon for adolescents to spend less time with parents and family than they did as children. They can become intensely involved with friends and depend on them for interests, goals, ideas, and values. This influence is commonly known as peer pressure. From observing and modeling one another's behaviors, including their sexual identity, adolescents can become quite vulnerable. Adult rules of behavior are replaced with peer-influenced or individual motivations and boundaries. At the same time that teenagers feel independent, they continue to demonstrate family dependency. The confusion between independence and dependence and between the adult self and the child self contributes to the conflict. The family controls and rules are usually ineffective and can precipitate sexual acting-out as a means of expressing indepedence. The absence of parental understanding and the presence of strong control mechanisms act to decrease communication and inhibit the learning environment often resulting in family disengagement or destructive triangulations.

While teens are concerned with their peer group's acceptance, the parents' system must stay in touch with the adolescent; resist power plays; clearly define their understanding of the family's ideas about choices, risks, and needs; and reinforce self-esteem. In many cases, it is parents who need help in communicating positively and constructively. Responsibility and morality are difficult concepts to communicate clearly. When a working dialogue between parent and teenager is not accomplished, alienation and hostility can result.

Choosing a Career.   The appropriate choice of a career has become a more difficult and personal decision to make. Increased technology and efforts to reduce sexual discrimination have increased the range of choices available, especially for women. Yet many people still feel the effects of gender role stereotypes. For example, too many young heterosexual men define their future primary role as "breadwinner," limiting their choices of careers to only those that have the best financial possibilities. Their "masculinity" is then defined by their ability to achieve financial success. Many young heterosexual women select careers so that they fit with future childbearing responsibilities, or they may have to delay marriage and childbearing in order to achieve success in high-powered jobs. Strong, aggressive and competitive behaviors on the job may create confusion for women in terms of their feminine identity.

Planning a Family.   Planning for family living as an adult has become extremely difficult since the meaning of family continues to undergo change in American society. Alternative living styles (for example, staying single, being homosexual, living in an extended family, cohabiting, and living in a nonparenting family) are more socially acceptable but more complicated to negotiate successfully than is the more traditional family system. With increased exposure to the diversity of family structures, adolescents are creating new definitions of a "healthy family." The various boundaries, including sexual boundaries, distribution of power, and ways families deal with conflict, also are being expanded.

Achieving Socially Responsible Behavior.   Moral development, like intellectual or personality development, is believed to proceed in sequential steps (Kohlberg, 1964; Piaget, 1971). Resolving moral conflicts and developing a value system and personal ideology that allows for a fruitful life are among the tasks associated with adolescent development. Within this framework, choices about sexual behavior follow a process of reasoning that is first heavily influenced by the family, then by peer groups and society, and, finally, for those who achieve some autonomy of moral reasoning, by personal standards and values organized in a self-established meaning system. Conflicts occur when adolescents' values and morals seem to be divergent from those of their immediate family or close friends.

SOCIAL FACTORS THAT INFLUENCE ADOLESCENT SEXUALITY

The biological and psychological factors that influence adolescent sexuality appear in several social contexts. As external influences, they affect adolescent sexual values, attitudes, and behaviors. For example, few people would deny that the mass media influence adolescents, but the degree and type of influence it has on an adolescent's perception of his or her sexuality constitutes an ongoing investigation. The amount of exposure to the media (especially television, the movies, and literature) is often determined by early patterns in the home. It is not uncommon for adolescents to watch television for several hours each day, frequently unsupervised. Even those adults who supervise them are often unable to control viewing outside the home. Because of the visual nature of television and movies, messages are strong and clear, leaving little to the viewer's imagination. What implicit effects they have are also unclear. Yet, soap operas and their overt statements about sex in relationships, the more covert influences of advertising on sex roles, and the availability of male-dominated violence on sitcoms and in movies are not to be underestimated.

Unrealistic goals influence sexual expectations at vulnerable times in psychosexual development. Listening to popular songs is an activity embedded in adolescent culture. The words and their messages often explain notions of love and sex. With the addition of video, CDs, and DVDs to the music scene, the messages directed at several human senses are ever more powerful. There is great controversy about the power of the media's influence on behavior. Research is still indecisive. However, the media are still a source of both factual and mythical misinformation.

Although we concern ourselves with understanding the potential harm of the media on sexual behavior, we can also recognize its benefits. The technological revolution has made it easy to access all sorts of useful information, especially on the Internet. It also provides an abundance of material for conversation within the family, the peer group, and in therapeutic sessions. In each of these contexts, adolescents can use observed situations and commonly shared popular programs to discuss their values and attitudes, create their meanings, and establish their boundaries.

SOURCES OF SEXUAL ANXIETY AMONG ADOLESCENTS

After a great deal of research, Laumann, Gagnon, Michael, and Michaels (1994) agree that adolescents seem to be concerned about the following biological, psychological, and social factors:

- Worry about sexual development and the physical and emotional changes that accompany it
- How sexual behavior will fit into close relationships with other people
- Variations in sexual orientations and behaviors that vary from what they have been taught are acceptable
- Decision making with regard to sexual intercourse, and associated information such as birth control methods
- Problems associated with unwanted pregnancy and abortion
- The meaning of masculinity and femininity and how sex roles become a part of an individual's life
- Their health state and the body not functioning sexually as desired or expected
- Sexual fantasies, masturbation, and other self-exploratory activities

Four specific sexual concerns stand out as common contributors to personal and family conflict and misinformation: masturbation, homosexuality, premarital sexual intercourse, and unwanted pregnancy.

Adulthood

The process of sexual development continues through adulthood. One part of the process involves the learning of effective communication with intimate partners. People spend a portion of their adult lives in uncommitted, nonpermanent relationships, many of which include intimate sexual activity. Some adults choose to remain single, others commit to marriage or other long-term arrangements, and still others follow a pattern of "serial monogamy," involving sexual fidelity for a period of time between two or more partners. For some couples, living together or cohabitation is a preferable alternative to marriage. Yet, for others, marriage is the only legal choice. Still others may return to single living as a result of separation, divorce, or death of a spouse. However, marriage is still the statistically preferable living style for heterosexual couples in the United States (U.S Bureau of the Census, 2002).

The frequency and behaviors of married/cohabitated and same-sex couple's sexual activity show great variability. The average heterosexual couple engages in sexual intercourse two to three times per week early in the relationship in addition to a variety of other sexual activities including oral-genital sex, anal intercourse, and hand–genital stimulation. The data seem to indicate that frequency declines to about once per week as the years in the relationship grow. Many adults continue to masturbate, even in long-term relationships (Laumann et al., 1994).

Several variables account for the frequency of sexual intercourse, in addition to length of time the couple (whether homosexual or heterosexual) is together, including general health status, cultural and religious influences, childbearing and parenting responsibilities, work habits, and so forth. But the number of times a couple has sexual intercourse is not necessarily a measure of their satisfaction with their sexual relationship. For example, sometimes couples have sex more often because they think it is what they are supposed to be doing if they are happy or because they think it is their responsibility to satisfy their partner. Also, for many married or cohabitating couples, sexual satisfaction may be derived from many other sexual activities other than sexual intercourse, particularly later in life. Sexual satisfaction in a relationship is an important component of sexual health. Many factors, such as the level of open and honest communication, self-image, and partner sensitivity, may contribute to sexual health. Issues such as extramarital sexual activity, dissatisfaction in the sexual relationship, and conflicts contribute to a decline in sexual health (Delamater & Friedrich, 2002). An unsatisfactory sex life seems to be among the primary reasons for divorce/separation.

The frequency of sexual relationships outside the committed relationship varies considerably by gender, age, culture, and data-reporting systems. Many will only engage in outside sexual activity once while they are married, but the incidence varies widely by ethnicity and culture. Some reasons for infidelity, in addition to individual intimacy problems, include dissatisfaction with the sexual component of the relationship, revenge after a partner's infidelity or other transgression, and simply experimentation or a release from boredom.

Another part of the process of sexual development in adults is making informed decisions about planning for a family and the prevention of sexually transmitted diseases including HIV/AIDS. For heterosexual couples, in many cases having an unexpected pregnancy negates any family plan that might have been put into place. Such questions as "How many years after marriage (heterosexual or homosexual) should a pregnancy be planned?" "What should our financial status be before we have children?" "What do we know about parenting?" (see Chapter 7), "How much does it cost to raise a child?" "What kind of assistance is available to the family and in the community?" "How will becoming parents affect our careers?" and others need to be addressed as part of the planning process. An unwanted pregnancy places sexual health at risk, as does engaging in sexual activities that may cause STIs and/or HIV/AIDS (see Chapter 11). Engaging in risky sexual activity with casual or multiple partners and having vaginal, oral, or anal intercourse without using a condom or dental dam enhances the potential for infection.

Many challenges face adults as they negotiate their early to middle adult years. How successfully they will overcome or deal with the challenges will influence their personal sense of self, their interpersonal relationships, and their psychosexual development. Each life event, including their general health status, the health status of their partner, their family, and their career successes, will have implications about how they interact with their partners and how they deal with the myriad of sexual issues that arise throughout life.

Aging

As stated at the beginning of this chapter, the process of sexual development is lifelong and includes aging. Not dissimilar to middle adulthood, being interested and participating in sexual activity in later life is a product of such factors as level of earlier interest, partner availability, interest in sexual activity by the partner, the general health status of both participants, and other cultural factors. Influencing these factors are the stages of aging. At this time in our history, aging is viewed in three stages: early aging, middle aging, and late aging; sexual interest and frequency of activity change and decline over these stages.

As in other developmental stages, sexual relationships in later life have their own problems and issues. One of these is simply based on prejudice. Sex is still too often seen in our society as the purview of youth. Older people, who display sexual interests or talk about them, are labeled either as "cute" or as "dirty old men/women." With this societal attitude, many older people live out the self-fulfilling prophecy that sex is inappropriate for older people. But desire may still remain. As the population ages (and it is doing so at an extraordinarily rapid rate), older people are remaining healthier for longer periods of time. They are accepting themselves as people who desire the full range of human experiences, including sexual activity, and they are recognizing and adjusting to the limitations that aging might place on sexual abilities.

Once again, as in childhood and adolescence, biology plays a major role in the aging process as it relates to sexuality. In women, the decline in estrogen production, which can begin anytime between 40 and 60 years of age, leads to menopause (most commonly between the 50th and 53rd year). The process lasts about 2 years and varies in intensity depending on genetic factors and the woman's health status. A good diet and physical activity may minimize the degree of stress and the symptoms associated with menopause. Several symptoms accompany the onset of menopause, such as night sweats, hot flashes, anxiety, irritability, depression, and sleep problems. But the severity of these is very individual. Some women are overwhelmed and their life activities are affected, while others experience very little change. Over time, there is a thinning and loss of elasticity of the vaginal wall and a decrease in vaginal lubrication. These symptoms can sometimes make penetration during intercourse uncomfortable, resulting in a decline in sexual desire. Some women learn that using an effective lubricant and receiving more stimulation before intercourse are very helpful. Loss of elasticity of the body's skin and sagging of the breasts may also occur over time. These sometimes have a negative affect on women's perception of themselves. To control or minimize physical changes may include estrogen replacement therapy and testosterone treatments (Delamater & Friedrich, 2002). Several other medications are available to help women overcome psychological problems.

Women's attitudes about the meaning of menopause will also affect their interpersonal relationships, including their sexual relationships. If they see postmenopause as a period that marks their decline, they may become disinterested. But if they see this time as a release from possible pregnancy and a freeing of themselves from the monthly cycle, they will maintain their desire and interest in sex. Women's frequency and interest in sexual behaviors after menopause is also associated with their premenopausal interest and frequency. Very sexually inclined women will continue to be more sexually interested, and those who had a low desire will be less interested. Moreover, several medications, including testosterone derivatives, are being studied that will influence women's sexual desire and ability to achieve orgasm. Unlike Viagra, currently used primarily for men but being tested in women, they are just becoming available.

What happens to men as they age? Is there a male menopause? The research has not been able to identify a single moment in time when "things stop" in the same way that the menstrual cycle stops in women. For men, aging and changes in their sexuality are gradual, and decline is evidenced over time. It is accompanied by a gradual decline in testosterone production that may begin as early as 40 years of age. The decreased testosterone level results in decreased sperm production (although it may continue into the 80s or 90s), reduced erections, erections that occur more slowly, a longer refractory period following orgasm, and a decline in sexual desire. Not all of these symptoms are directly related to the decrease in male hormones. Some are related to decreased health status that has an effect on blood flow to the penis (heart disease, diabetes, hypertension, and so on), partner availability, and fear of failure to perform (often due to the unrealistic expectations placed on men). Also, as women's does, men's physical appearance changes (usually a decline in height and a tendency toward an increase in weight). These changes are sometimes internalized. Being less attractive and "sexy," men may find that the pressure to perform as they did when they were younger, without the same physical responses, becomes difficult, and, unlike for women, their inability to achieve and maintain an erection is obvious. Erectile failure experiences and an inflexibility to change the sexual repertoire to include other sexual behaviors without intercourse sometimes negatively influence men's sexual desires.

Much is happening in the treatment of erectile and desire problems in men. Although it is still unclear as to how much testosterone replacement is appropriate and effective, it is one of the interventions being used and studied. Along with Viagra, Cialis, and Levitra, several other medications are presently coming to the pharmaceutical marketplace. These medications have made a considerable difference in men's abilities to achieve and maintain erections, but they are not effective for all men, and at this time, they require sexual desire to be effective.

For many older people, negotiating the variety of social changes associated with aging has enormous influence on their interest in sexual behavior. Aging can be a period marked by death of a spouse or lover, retirement, an empty nest, financial changes, health problems, and often the added responsibilities of helping raise grandchildren. Many older couples find that it is a time to reestablish their relationship, find a new partner or spouse after the loss of their lifetime partner or spouse, find a second career, or develop a variety of new athletic and play activities. For some, this time of change represents having the time, money, and privacy to do new things. For others, it represents the end. Aging in our society is taking on new meaning, and, as the population of older and healthier adults continues to grow, new understandings about this stage of the life cycle will emerge.

SUMMARY

The process of human sexual growth and development involves a complex set of interactions among genes, hormones, and brain and physical development with a host of environmental, experiential, cultural, and familial processes. It all begins with the fertilized egg followed by a rapid series of cell divisions and the implantation of the egg into the uterus where the development continues for about 40 weeks. After birth, human sexual growth and development continue throughout life.

A great deal of research has been conducted on the development of sexuality, resulting in several theories, a few of which have been highlighted in this chapter. Two views emerge: sexuality is either a series of integrated stages or a continuous process. Regardless of which view is preferred, much more research is needed. Described in this chapter are the major characteristics of growth and behaviors according to age, from the early embryonic processes to the aging of adults. Because of the biological, psychological, and social complexities of puberty and adolescence, this period of sexual growth is emphasized.

Teaching the process of sexual development can be considered a sensitive matter because of the ways that U.S. culture views the privacy of most sex-related information. The challenge for the teacher is to keep parents informed, present information accurately, and address students' questions directly and comfortably. There is a very close relationship between human sexual development and general growth. Both are essential to long-term health. The study of genital and reproductive anatomy and physiology cannot be considered different from the study of any other aspect of human anatomy and physiology. Students learn about body systems in health science or biology classes, and so the human sexuality teacher must determine what has been learned and what has not before embarking on this unit. Because we have already established that sexuality begins before birth and continues throughout adulthood, essential information and personal life skills that are developmentally appropriate can be integrated throughout the K–12 curriculum (K–3, 4–6, 7–9, and 10–12).

By the time children reach kindergarten, they have already been influenced by attitudes and behaviors about their bodies, their sensuality, and their notions of the same and different gender. Children are inquisitive about their own anatomy, especially their genitals, and, as their world expands beyond the family, the anatomy of others. This is the time when children ask questions about their body parts and functions and often use childhood labels (*pee pee* or *wee wee*) or street language (*tool* or *dick*) to express themselves. Children at this level can be introduced to more appropriate terminology in nonthreatening, nonjudgmental ways. They can also begin to learn about modesty, privacy, and appropriateness of the setting for self-exploration.

When they move from kindergarten through second grade, students are interested in the very bare basics of reproduction, pregnancy, birth, love, and marriage. Myths that the stork delivers babies or that babies come right out of Mommy's belly button can be addressed. Children at this age sometimes talk about marrying their mother, father, or grandparent. This is an ideal time for students to begin to learn about family life and family roles and responsibilities.

WEBSITES

Abstinence Programs for Children and Parents: www.etr.org

Alan Guttmacher Institute: www.agi-usa.com

All about Sex Discussion: www.allaboutsex.org

Advocates for Youth: www.advocatesforyouth.org

Children's Health and Parenting: www.kidshealth.org/index2.html

Coalition for a Positive Sexuality: www.positive.org

Electronic Journal of Human Sexuality: www.ejhs.org.

Family Planning Queensland: www.fpq.asn.au

Go Ask Alice: www.goaskalice.columbia.edu

Kaiser Family Foundation: www
.talkingwithkids.org

Male Health Center:
www.malehealthcenter.com

Mental Health Net: Dating, Love, Marriage,
and Sex: www.cmhc.com

National Campaign to Prevent Teen Pregnancy: www.teenpregnancy.org

National Parenting Center: www.tnpc.com

Sexuality Information and Education Council
of the United States (SIECUS): www
.siecus.org

REFERENCES

Blonna, R., & Levitan, J. (2000). *Healthy sexuality.* Englewood, CO.: Morton.

Davis, E. C., Shryne, J. E., & Gorski, E. C. (1996). Structural sexual dimorphisms in the anteroventral periventricular nucleus of the rat hypothalamus are sensitive to gonadal steroids perinatally, but develop peripubertally. *Neuroendocrinology, 63,* 142–148.

Delamater, J., & Friedrich, W. N. (2002). Human sexual development. *Journal of Sex Research, 39*(1), 10–14.

Erikson, E. (1963). *Childhood and society.* New York: Norton.

Family Planning Queensland. (2002). Sexual development in early childhood. *FPQ Fact Sheet.* Available online: www.fpq.asn.au.

Freud, S., & Strachey, J. (1975). *Three essays on the theory of sexuality.* New York: Basic Books.

Gagnon, J. H., & Simon, W. (1973). *Sexual conduct: The social resources of human sexuality.* Chicago: Aldine-Atherton.

Haroian, L. (2000). Child sexual development. *Electronic Journal of Human Sexuality, 3,* 1–28. Available online: www.ejhs.org.

Hass, A. (1979). *Teenage sex.* New York: Macmillan.

Havighurst, R. J. (1972). *Developmental tasks and education* (3rd ed.). New York: McKay.

Katchadourian, H., & Lunde, D. (1989). *Fundamentals of human sexuality* (5th ed.). New York: Holt, Rinehart & Winston.

Kelly, G. (1994). *Sexuality today* (4th ed.). Guilford, CT.: Dushkin.

Kinsey, A., Pomeroy, W., & Martin, C. (1948). *Sexual behavior in the human male.* Philadelphia: Saunders.

Kohlberg, L. (1964). Development of moral character and moral ideology. In L. Hoffman & M. Hoffman (Eds.), *Research* (Vol. 1). New York: Russell Sage Foundation.

Laumann, E. O., Gagnon, J. H., Michael, R. T., & Michaels, S. (1994). *The social organization of sexuality: Sexual practices in the United States.* Chicago: University of Chicago Press.

Levay, S., & Valente, S. M. (2003). *Human sexuality.* Sunderland, MA: Sinauer.

Martinson, F. (1994). *The sexual life of children.* Westport, CT: Bergin & Garvey.

Masters, W., Johnson, V., & Kolodny, R. (1988). *Heterosexual behavior in the age of AIDS.* New York: Grove.

Piaget, J. (1971). *Science of education and the psychology of the child.* New York: Viking.

Plummer, K. (1991). *Understanding childhood sexualities.* Available online: www.ipce .info/library/file/plummer.htm.

Rathus, S. A., Nevid, J. S., & Fichner-Rathus, L. (2002). *Human sexuality in a world of diversity.* Boston: Allyn & Bacon.

Sarrel, L. (1989). Sexual unfolding revisited. *SIECUS Report, 17*(5), 4–5.

Stevenson, D. B. (1992). *Freud's psychosexual stages of development.* Available online: 65.107.211.206/science/Freud/ Psychosexual Development.html.

U.S. Bureau of the Census. (2002). *Statistical abstract of the United States.* Washington, DC: U.S. Government Printing Office.

Weinstein, E., & Rosen, E. (2002). Treating adolescents. In *Critical issues in sexuality: Implications for psychotherapy* (Chap. 3). Boston: American Press.

LEARNING EXPERIENCES

The following learning experiences will prepare students in the earliest grades to

- Correctly name the genital body parts in males and females and describe their location.
- Rudimentarily explain where babies develop.
- Describe new responsibilities and life changes when a baby arrives.

Later elementary school children will be able to

- Name and describe the various genital and reproductive body parts and their functions.
- Describe the changes for both males and females, including secondary sexual characteristics, accompanying puberty.
- Identify the emotional changes that can accompany puberty.
- Describe the physical and emotional factors surrounding menstruation.
- Explain nocturnal emissions.
- Explain rudimentary concepts of pregnancy and fetal development.

By middle school, students will be able to

- Communicate effectively the parts and functions of the reproductive parts of the human body.
- Relate the nature of changes in their own body to family patterns.
- Analyze how their physical appearance such as body size and stature are related to family patterns.
- Understand how the physical differences between males and females contribute to their roles in reproduction.
- Explain normal pubertal development.
- Describe pregnancy, fetal development, and childbirth.

By the end of high school, the students will be able to

- Appreciate the unique patterns of sexual development that occur throughout the life cycle.
- List the responsibilities associated with sexuality throughout the life cycle.
- Describe the difference between the mature and immature stages of sexual development.
- Evaluate the personal, emotional and physical benefits of delaying sexual activity.
- Connect personal health practices with the changes in sexuality that occur throughout the life cycle.
- Know the community resources available to maintain sexual health.
- Describe pregnancy, fetal development, and childbirth.

LEARNING EXPERIENCE 1

TITLE: Where Do Babies Come From?

GRADE LEVELS: K–3

TIME REQUIREMENTS: Two to four sessions

LEARNING CONTEXT

Following this activity, students will be able to

- Describe how different animals reproduce and care for their offspring.
- Be aware that human babies develop inside their mothers.
- Explain where human babies come from.

NATIONAL LEARNING STANDARDS

3:   Students will demonstrate the ability to practice health-enhancing behaviors and reduce health risks.

5:   Students will demonstrate the ability to use interpersonal communication skills to enhance health.

7:   Students will demonstrate the ability to advocate for personal, family, and community health.

PROCEDURE

The class has a lesson on reproduction. The teacher demonstrates how any one or all of the following animals reproduce. For example, a chick comes from an egg that is laid by the mother hen. Fish come from a fertilized egg that is in their mother's body. The teacher identifies similarities in human families.

Questions for Discussion

How are babies similar to their parents?

How are they like other species?

How are they different from other species?

RESOURCES

Chicken eggs; fish bowl with fish that reproduce (such as guppies); pregnant gerbils, rabbits, rats, or mice

HOMEWORK

Children, with parents' help, collect pictures of a variety of animals and human families that resemble each other.

ASSESSMENT PLAN

The teacher can use a rubric or scale that includes the following criteria for measuring learner outcomes.

For a grade of A, students will be able to
- Identify at least four ways babies are similar to their parent(s).
- Identify at least three ways they are similar to rabbits, gerbils, or other animals.
- Identify at least two ways they are different from the other species above.
- Simply explain that an egg and sperm that meet begin the development of a baby, and identify where the baby grows.
- Correctly spell all of the new words the teacher chooses from the activity.

For a grade of B, students will be able to
- Identify at least three ways babies are similar to their parent(s).
- Identify at least two ways they are similar to rabbits, gerbils, or other animals.
- Identify at least one way they are different from the other species above.
- Simply explain that an egg and sperm that meet begin the development of a baby, and identify where the baby grows.
- Correctly spell most of the new words the teacher chooses from the activity.

For a grade of C, students will be able to
- Identify at least two ways babies are similar to their parent(s).
- Identify at least one way they are similar to rabbits, gerbils, or other animals.
- Identify at least one way they are different from the other species above.
- Simply explain that an egg and sperm that meet begin the development of a baby, and identify where the baby grows.
- Correctly spell some of the new words the teacher chooses from the activity.

For a grade of D, students will not be able to
- Identify at least one way babies are similar to their parent(s).
- Identify at least one way they are similar to rabbits, gerbils, or other animals.
- Identify ways they are different from the other species above.
- Simply explain that an egg and sperm that meet begin the development of a baby, and identify where the baby grows correctly.
- Spell only one or two of the new words the teacher chooses from the activity.

REFERENCE

Contributed in part by Cheryl Lyn Funk, Honolulu, Hawaii.

LEARNING EXPERIENCE 2

TITLE: My Body

GRADE LEVELS: 4–6

TIME REQUIREMENTS: Two sessions (total 90 minutes)

LEARNING CONTEXT
Following this activity, students will be able to sort and identify the external sexual anatomy of the male and female body.

NATIONAL LEARNING STANDARDS
3:   Students will demonstrate the ability to practice health-enhancing behaviors and reduce health risks.

5:   Students will demonstrate the ability to use interpersonal communication skills to enhance health.

PROCEDURE
Students brainstorm a list of the external genitalia for males and females. Students put each body part on an index card. The teacher holds up a picture of each body part, and the students hold up the corresponding card naming the part of the body.

RESOURCES
Index cards and pictures of body parts

ASSESSMENT PLAN
The students will keep a piece of paper on their desks folded down the middle with their name on the top. The heading on the left column reads correct answer; on the right, incorrect answer. Each time the student holds up the correct body part, the student gives him- or herself a mark in the left column. Wrong answers are marked in the right column. At the end of the activity, the students will add up their answers and turn in the papers.

LEARNING EXPERIENCE 3

TITLE: Growth and Development: Puberty

GRADE LEVELS: 4–6

TIME REQUIREMENTS: Two sessions (90 minutes total)

LEARNING CONTEXT
Following this activity, students will be able to
- Describe how the body grows.
- List the changes associated with puberty.
- Identify the gender differences as boys and girls grow.

NATIONAL LEARNING STANDARDS
1: Students will comprehend concepts related to health promotion and disease prevention.
3: Students will demonstrate the ability to practice health-enhancing behaviors and reduce health risks.
5: Students will demonstrate the ability to use interpersonal communication skills to enhance health.

PROCEDURE
Students bring in a baby picture and current picture of themselves and a picture of a parent, grandparent, sibling, or close cousin of the same sex without showing them to others in the class. The teacher numbers the pictures and places them on the bulletin board. The students try to match the families from the pictures. On a piece of paper they write the numbers on the pictures and the names of the students that they think are a match.

The teacher places the correct name next to each picture on the bulletin board so the students can see how many they identified correctly. The class discusses how the students have changed since the pictures were taken and how they might still change to look like their parent(s) or other family members. The class lists the changes involved for girls and boys in growing up.

RESOURCES
Bulletin board, pictures of students when they were babies or young children, and slips of paper with each student's name

HOMEWORK
Students collect baby pictures several days before this activity.

ASSESSMENT PLAN

The teacher can use a rubric or scale that includes the following criteria for measuring learner outcomes.

For a grade of A, students will be able to

- Identify at least five ways parents and children in a family may be alike.
- Identify at least five ways parents and children in a family may be different.
- Explain at least four changes that occur during puberty for girls and for boys.
- Identify at least four similarities between males and females.
- Identify at least three differences between males and females.

For a grade of B, students will be able to

- Identify at least four ways parents and children in a family may be alike.
- Identify at least four ways parents and children in a family may be different.
- Explain at least three changes that occur during puberty for girls and for boys.
- Identify at least three similarities between males and females.
- Identify at least two differences between males and females.

For a grade of C, students will be able to

- Identify at least three ways parents and children in a family may be alike.
- Identify at least three ways parents and children in a family may be different.
- Explain at least two changes that occur during puberty for girls and for boys.
- Identify at least two similarities between males and females.
- Identify at least one difference between males and females.

For a grade of D, student will not be able to

- Identify at least one way parents and children in a family may be alike.
- Identify at least one way parents and children in a family may be different.
- Explain at least one change that occurs during puberty for girls and for boys.
- Identify at least one similarity between males and females.
- Identify at least one difference between males and females.

LEARNING EXPERIENCE 4

TITLE: The Female Reproductive System

GRADE LEVELS: 7–9

TIME REQUIREMENTS: Two sessions (90 minutes)

LEARNING CONTEXT
Following this activity, students will be able to
- Identify the female's pelvic organs.
- Understand the changes that occur during puberty and what specific organs are involved during these changes.
- Follow the path that an ova takes after ovulation.
- Explain the process of menstruation.

NATIONAL LEARNING STANDARDS
1: Students will comprehend concepts related to health promotion and disease prevention.
2: Students will demonstrate the ability to access valid health information and health-promoting products and services.
5: Students will demonstrate the ability to use interpersonal communication skills to enhance health.

PROCEDURE
The students will be asked to label the parts of the female reproductive system on the handout provided and put their name at the top. Then, in small groups, they will be asked to describe the function of each part on the handout provided. From the handouts, they will label the parts of the body an ova will pass through after it is released from the ovary and describe the changes that occur during menstruation.

Using transparencies, the teacher will review with the class the various overheads with the labels and descriptions included.

RESOURCES
Transparencies, information charts, and handouts of the female reproductive system; a model of the ovary, Fallopian tube, uterus, and vagina (Attach fill-in-the-blank diagrams of female reproductive systems.)

ASSESSMENT PLAN
The teacher will collect the individually filled-out handouts and review the students' knowledge. A paper-and-pencil test can be administered.

FEMALE
Describe the function of each of the following:

Endometrium _____

Ovaries _____

Ova _____

Fallopian tubes _____

Grafenberg spot _____

Gynecologist _____

Hysterectomy _____

Menopause _____

Menarche _____

PMS _____

Labia manora _____

Labia majora _____

Toxic shock syndrome (TSS) _____

Uterus _____

Vagina _____

Bladder _____

Urethra _____

Anus _____

Rectum _____

Female Internal and External Genitalia

Label the parts of the female internal genitalia

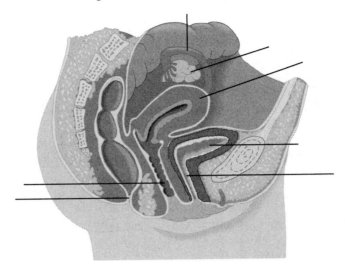

Label the parts of the female external genitalia

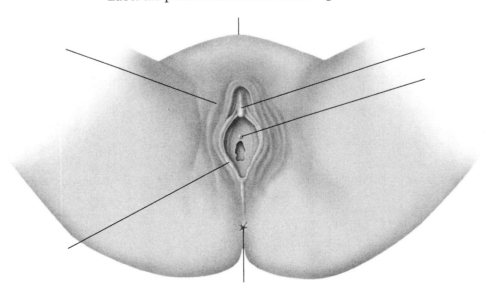

LEARNING EXPERIENCE 5

TITLE: The Male Reproductive System

GRADE LEVELS: 7–9

TIME REQUIREMENTS: Two periods (90 minutes)

LEARNING CONTEXT
Following this activity, students will be able to
- Identify the male's genital structures.
- Understand the changes that occur during puberty and what specific organs are involved during these changes.
- Follow the path that sperm take from the testes to leaving the body during ejaculation.
- Explain the process of ejaculation.

NATIONAL LEARNING STANDARDS
1:   Students will comprehend concepts related to health promotion and disease prevention.
2:   Students will demonstrate the ability to access valid health information and health-promoting products and services.
5:   Students will demonstrate the ability to use interpersonal communication skills to enhance health.

PROCEDURE
The students will be asked to label the parts of the male reproductive system on the handout provided and put their name at the top. Then in small groups they will be asked to describe the function of each part on the handout provided. From the handouts, they will label the parts of the body that sperm passes through.

Using transparencies, the teacher will review with the class the various overheads with the labels and descriptions included and discuss the changes that occur during puberty.

RESOURCES
Transparencies, information charts, and handouts of the male reproductive system; a model of the internal and external organs, including a section model of the testes (Attach fill-in-the-blank diagrams of male reproductive systems, the secondary sex characteristics, and the route that sperm travels.)

ASSESSMENT PLAN
The teacher will collect the individually filled-out handouts and review the students' knowledge. A paper-and-pencil test can be administered.

MALE
Describe the function of each of the following:

Semen _____

Seminal vesicles _____

Sperm _____

Testes _____

Urethra _____

Vas deferens _____

Rectum _____

Anus _____

Castration _____

Circumcision _____

Cowper's gland _____

Ejaculation _____

Epididymis _____

Foreskin (prepuce) _____

Hernia _____

Penis _____

Prostate gland _____

Scrotum _____

Bladder _____

Nocturnal emission _____

Sterility _____

Urologist _____

Impotence _____

Secondary sex characteristics _____

Male Internal and External Genitalia

Label the parts of the male internal genitalia

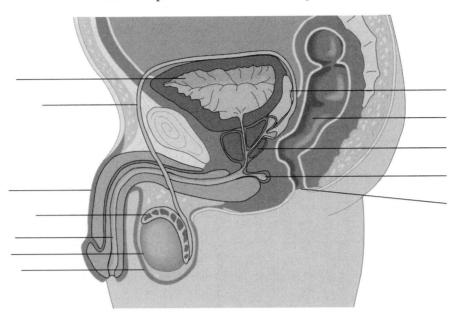

Label the parts of the male external genitalia

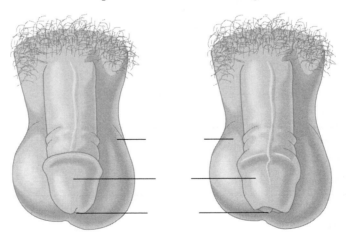

LEARNING EXPERIENCE 6

TITLE: The Growing Diary: Changes during Puberty

GRADE LEVELS: 7–9

TIME REQUIREMENTS: Learning about a different gender: One period (45 minutes). [Accurate record keeping is required throughout the semester or year. Set up during the first session with a letter home to parents.]

LEARNING CONTEXT
By the end of the semester, students will
- Be able to track body changes during puberty.
- Understand the process of rigorous research and keeping accurate records.

NATIONAL LEARNING STANDARDS
1: Students will comprehend concepts related to health promotion and disease prevention.
2: Students will demonstrate the ability to access valid health information and health-promoting products and services.
4: Students will analyze the influence of culture, media, technology, and other factors on health.
7: Students will demonstrate the ability to advocate for personal, family, and community health.

PROCEDURE
Students will keep a growth diary for observation and self-reflection that remains confidential. At the beginning of the year, each student will take a photo of him- or herself that can be used for a beginning analysis and an audiotape for recording his or her observations. The teacher will show the students how to set up their notebook for regularly collecting data on height, weight, chest, waist, and hip measurements; skin condition; voice timbre; and other characteristics. Students should also keep a journal on their emotional reactions to their physical changes. In this journal, they should collect clippings, poems, and song lyrics that reflect on what is happening to them as they grow.

Throughout the semester, the following questions may be discussed in class:

Is puberty a roller coaster ride? What are the ups and downs?

How are the experiences of boys and girls similar? Different?

To what extent are the changes noticed in themselves similar or different from the changes observed in others?

How will the physical and intellectual changes that they are experiencing serve them for the rest of their lives?

How have these experiences affected your relationships with parents and other adults (authority figures, celebrities, religious figures, and so forth)?

What other qualities do adults acquire during puberty?

RESOURCES
Notebook, pictures, clippings, and recordings

ASSESSMENT PLAN

Near the end of the semester, the teacher will have the students write a personal essay about the process of keeping a diary and scrapbook for the semester or year and their reactions to doing this project. A three-point rubric can be used to evaluate the personal essay:

> *Three points:* A strong thesis statement with coherent and organized paragraphs; substantial supporting details and content
>
> *Two points:* Adequate thesis statement, somewhat coherent with some supportive details
>
> *One point:* Inadequate thesis statement, lacking coherence and unity with insufficient supportive data

REFLECTION

As an extension of this activity, the teacher might have students identify the hormones, their source, and the effect they have on the changes that occur during puberty. Students may be asked to locate hormone centers such as the hypothalamus, pituitary gland, adrenal gland, thyroid gland, testes, and ovaries and note how each of these hormones affect puberty.

LEARNING EXPERIENCE 7

TITLE: Body Image

GRADE LEVELS: 7–9

TIME REQUIREMENTS: One period (about 45 minutes)

LEARNING CONTEXT
- Encourage students to reflect on how they feel about their bodies.
- What aspects of their body image would they like to change?
- What strategies could they use to deal with their body image gap?

NATIONAL LEARNING STANDARDS
1: Students will comprehend concepts related to health promotion and disease prevention.
2: Students will demonstrate the ability to access valid health information and health-promoting products and services.
4: Students will analyze the influence of culture, media, technology, and other factors on health.
5: Students will demonstrate the ability to use interpersonal communication skills to enhance health.
7: Students will demonstrate the ability to advocate for personal, family, and community health.

PROCEDURE

In their journal, students describe their own body image in writing, confidentially. They will reflect on how they think their body matches up to the their ideal notion of someone their age. Then have the students reflect on what influenced their notion of the "ideal" body. Also, they will reflect on how they think others view them specifically (their closest friends, their family, members of the opposite gender, and others).

Individually have the students select several pictures from magazines that reflect their idea of the ideal American look for men and for women. In small groups of four, have the students take along their selections and come up with a group representation that they can all agree on. Be sure their pictures represent different cultures. In small groups of four, have the students discuss some of the following questions:

What were some of the characteristics that their group considered ideal?

How does culture and age influence the ideal body?

How similar and different were the images offered by men from those offered by women?

Where do notions of an "ideal body" come from?

Why is there so much focus on body image, especially for women, in our society?

Is the ideal image of men and women different in different cultures?

How has the ideal image changed over time?

How important is it to look a certain way?

RESOURCES

A variety of magazines that reflect age, culture, and so forth

ASSESSMENT PLAN
Have the students hand in a written reflection on some of the concerns they have about their own appearance and some of the concerns for young people who try to achieve an "ideal" body image.

REFERENCE
Adapted from the Media Awareness Network of Canada, www.media-awareness.ca

LEARNING EXPERIENCE 8

TITLE: What Belongs to Whom?

GRADE LEVELS: 7–9

TIME REQUIREMENTS: May include three sessions, the time required for each component.

LEARNING CONTEXT
Following these lessons, students will be able to
- Identify the parts of the reproductive and sexual systems.
- Describe the function of each body part.
- Identify which gender the part of the body belongs to.
- Feel comfortable discussing the human reproductive and sexual system.

NATIONAL LEARNING STANDARDS
1: Students will comprehend concepts related to health promotion and disease prevention
2: Students will demonstrate the ability to access valid health information and health-promoting products and services.
3: Students will demonstrate the ability to practice health-enhancing behaviors and reduce health risks.
5: Students will demonstrate the ability to use interpersonal communication skills to enhance health.

PROCEDURE

Session 1

The students will practice their vocabulary skills. They will fill in the blanks on Handout A. The teacher will then review the answers by calling on volunteers to offer their answers. Each student will add up the number correct and hand in the sheets.

Handout A

Put a letter *F* for female, *M* for male, and *B* for both next to each body part or function that correctly represents the correct gender that it appears in.

_____ labia minora	_____ semen	_____ Fallopian tubes
_____ penis	_____ epidymus	_____ cervix
_____ ureter	_____ urethra	_____ menstruation
_____ ovaries	_____ vagina	_____ hymen
_____ labia majora	_____ sperm	_____ uterus
_____ vulva	_____ testicles	_____ bladder
_____ estrogen	_____ prostate	_____ foreskin
_____ testosterone	_____ clitoris	_____ Cowper's gland
_____ progesterone	_____ seminal vesicles	_____ preejaculatory fluid
_____ ova	_____ ejaculation	_____ vas deferens

Session 2

In small groups, have the students write one sentence explaining where the body part exists and what its function is. Review with the class.

Session 3

Using Handout B, have the students select the one term in each numbered point that does not fit with the other two. In small groups, have the students indicate what each item does and why the item they have selected does not fit.

Handout B

Select the one term for each number that does not fit with the other two.

1. clitoris   vagina   uterus

2. ova   ovaries   vulva

3. ejaculation   erection   cervix

4. hymen   cervix   foreskin

5. menstruation   preejaculatory fluid   estrogen

6. estrogen   progesterone   Fallopian tubes

7. sperm   vas deferens   bladder

8. testicles   scrotum   cervix

9. Cowper's gland   menstruation   uterus

10. uterus   ovaries   prostate

(Other words can be added as determined.)

RESOURCES
Handouts A and B

ASSESSMENT PLAN
The activities themselves should be done after the unit on growth and development is completed and will provide the teacher with an informal assessment of the extent of learning.

REFLECTION
These activities can incorporate a variety pieces of information and can be applied to other units.

SEXUAL BEHAVIORS

JENINE DEMARZO AND SHANNON WHALEN

OBJECTIVES

After reading this chapter, students will be able to

1. Identify behavioral content that is appropriate for and understandable at the different grade levels.
2. Begin a dialogue related to the brain's function in sexual arousal.
3. Identify how the five senses contribute to sexual arousal.
4. Identify appropriate terminology and definitions related to sexual arousal, sexual communication, sexual behavior, sexual response cycle, sexual variation, and sexual dysfunction.
5. Promote communication skills in sexual relationships.
6. Discuss influences on sexual communication.
7. Discuss masturbation as a form of sexual activity.
8. Identify types of shared sexual behaviors.
9. Identify types of noncoital and coital sexual behaviors.
10. Discuss prostitution in a contemporary and historical context.
11. Compare and contrast the four phases of the sexual response cycle.
12. Identify changes that occur in the body during each of the phases of the sexual response cycle.
13. Identify different types of sexual variation.
14. Discuss sexual dysfunctions in men and women.

REFLECTIVE QUESTIONS

Middle School Students

1. Why are candy, roses, candlelight dinners, and moonlit walks all considered romantic? Who do you think thought this up? Are there other things that are automatically considered romantic?
2. Are there any things that are definitely a turn-off in a relationship? What are they? Are they the same for all boys and girls?
3. If someone liked you, how would you like to find out?
4. What do you say to someone if you like them?
5. What behaviors are appropriate for middle school students to do in a relationship?
6. Do parents of middle school students believe the same behaviors are appropriate as the middle school students themselves? Why or why not?

High School Students

1. Are there certain sights, sounds, smells, tastes, and touches that can be counted on to stimulate everyone? If not, why not? If yes, what are they?
2. What behaviors are appropriate for high school students in a relationship?
3. Do parents of high school students believe the same behaviors are appropriate as the high school students themselves? Why or why not?
4. Have any students had a conversation with their families about values and sexuality? If so, do you hold the same values as your family? Why or why not?
5. Why is it important to set sexual boundaries for yourself before you get in a situation that may turn sexual?
6. If a person wants to remain abstinent, does that mean that he or she cannot participate in any sexual activity?

High School, *continued*

7. Does sexual fantasy help a person remain abstinent or tempt a person to do more because he or she is thinking about it all the time?

8. What is the sexual response cycle, and why should all people know about the phases of the cycle?

9. What are some sexual variations? Are there behaviors that people in this society participate in that would be considered abnormal in other cultures?

10. What are the different types of sexual dysfunction? Does sexual dysfunction only happen to older people, or can it happen to younger people, too?

SCENARIO

Todd, Kevin, Brad, and RJ were sitting around a picnic table. All four boys were working at the town pool for the summer. Todd and Kevin were lifeguards, Brad worked the desk, and RJ was on the landscaping crew. As had become the custom, the boys were "shooting the breeze" during their lunch break. As usual, the topic centered around girls. The boys were complaining to each other about how they could never tell whether a girl liked them. They all agreed that it would be so much easier if the girls would just come right out and tell them who they liked. Instead, the boys had to struggle to interpret small gestures and phrases, as if they were a foreign language. Even if they knew a girl liked them, they could never count on it lasting. One minute he and she were an item, and the next minute, he was dumped. Who could figure it out? All four boys agreed that they knew what they liked—the smell, the touch, and the "look" of a certain girl could make them crazy—but what did the girls like?

Kevin was the only one of the boys with an older sister, so he was considered the expert of the bunch. Kevin spent a lot of time eavesdropping on his sister and her friends, trying to figure them out. From what he could tell, each girl liked different stuff. Today he was telling his friends that he heard one conversation where the older girls were complaining about their boyfriends. One girl said she liked to be kissed on the neck, and another girl complained that she hated it when her boyfriend did that. One girl said she liked a foot massage, and another girl said she couldn't stand getting a foot massage. She was too ticklish. The boys were not happy when they heard this information. They all agreed that it would be a lot simpler if there was a "recipe" for making a girl happy, but it didn't seem like that was the case. Would they ever know the right thing to do to make their partner happy?

Have you ever experienced the confusion that the boys are talking about?

Is it just boys who are in the dark, or do girls wonder what boys like?

Do same-sex couples have the same confusion, or is it easier because they know what their own gender likes and doesn't like?

What does body language tell us about whether someone finds us attractive or not? What are some signals to look for that indicate a positive or a negative response?

Why don't people simply tell their partners what turns them on and off? Why is that something that has to be "figured out"?

INTRODUCTION

Scientific research has contributed much to what we know about sexual arousal and somewhat less to what we know about sexual attraction. One way we have come to understand the phenomenon of *sexual arousal* is by research conducted to identify the physical changes that the body undergoes during sexual excitement. Scientists have been able to clearly illustrate these changes due to the fact that most humans experience sexual arousal in fairly similar ways. Not all of these changes are easy to observe, but they all influence erection, vaginal lubrication, and orgasm. Most often we come to understand these changes by the use of models (which will be utilized later in the chapter). These physical changes are triggered by physiological factors, such as hormones, as well as by psychological factors, such as thinking someone is attractive. Most often people can readily identify these physical changes. However, they have more difficulty understanding the psychological influences that affect these changes.

Our psychological perceptions of sexual arousal greatly influence how we respond to these physical changes. It has often been said that the brain is the organ most responsible for triggering our sexual arousal. How our brain interprets these physical changes will ultimately influence whether the body gets the "green light" to allow the sexual response to continue or the "red light," if the brain interprets the sexual response/arousal as inappropriate or unwanted. The phenomenon of *sexual attraction* is truly directed, more often than not, by the thinking brain. Scientists have realized this in light of the fact that what one person finds erotic or stimulating may not at all stimulate another person. Sexual attraction is most often shaped by cultural standards of beauty and desirability, cultural gender expectations, individual comfort levels, and experience (Reinisch, 1990; Westheimer & Lopater, 2004).

PATTERNS OF SEXUAL AROUSAL AND SEXUAL ATTRACTION

The Brain

We know that the brain is crucial to the body's sexual functioning. Two areas of the brain seem to be the most predominant in affecting sexual arousal: the cerebral cortex and the limbic system.

The *cerebral cortex* is the wrinkly matter that covers most of the brain. The cortex is the area in which conscious behaviors take place, such as perception, communication, memory, understanding, and voluntary movement. The cortex is responsible for sexual fantasies, desires, thoughts, and images. When the brain receives arousing images or messages, it sends a message through the spinal cord to the *autonomic nervous system,* causing an increase in heartbeat, rise in respiration, pronounced muscle tension, engorgement of the genitals, and increase in skin sensitivity.

Just beneath the cortex is the *limbic system,* which consists of several parts that are associated with emotions and feelings. The limbic system contains the *thalamus* and *hypothalamus,* which play a vital role in the expression and experience of emotion (DeKoker, 1996).

Sex and the Five Senses

The brain receives stimuli from the five senses: sight, smell, touch, hearing, and taste.

Sight: Visual information plays a huge role in sexual arousal for humans. Contemporary fashion, cultural ideals concerning body weight and appearance, use of cosmetics and hair care products, as well as the tremendous market for erotic visuals, pictures, websites, and movies, reflect the emphasis our culture places on visual stimulation. For many people, it is often "love at first sight" if they are pleased or sexually aroused at first glance. Chances are they will allow themselves to get closer to the prospective sexual partner.

Smell: Recent research has indicated that odor may control some human sexual activities. Our olfactory senses may bring us sexual messages that are beyond our capability to identify (Stern & McClintock, 1998). Chemicals called *pheromones,* released through our skin and transmitted into the air, have been found to stimulate sexual interest in both animals and humans. In U.S. culture, body odors are not considered sexually appealing. Americans often use deodorants to conceal these odors. However, this is not the case in all cultures. In some societies, the smell of sweat is very appealing, as is the natural odor of a moist vagina.

Touch: The skin is the largest organ in the body. It has nerve endings throughout its surface that render it sensitive to even the softest touch. There are particular areas of the body, called *erogenous zones,* that are highly sensitive. These areas include the genitals, lips, breasts, nipples, ears, neck, buttocks, and inner thighs. The sense of touch is the most frequent method of sexual arousal and has the most direct effect on arousal in both men and women.

Hearing: Our sense of hearing can also influence sexual arousal and response. For some people, the sound of their partner's voice, romantic music, or "sexy talk" during lovemaking may set the mood. Sex and love have been major themes of music for centuries throughout the world.

Taste: The sense of taste and its role in sexual arousal have not been studied with the same fervor as the other senses. Perhaps this is due to individual variations and cultural implications. Basically we all like and dislike different things, and not everyone has the same capacity for taste. Smokers and older individuals often complain that their sense of taste has diminished or that it is less sensitive to particular nuances of some foods. Some foods such as chocolate, strawberries, and shellfish have been said to have an arousing effect. However, it may be that there is some psychological association with the food and/or some past sexual experiences.

Aphrodisiacs are substances that allegedly enhance erotic feelings and sexual capacity. In all cultures throughout the world, at one time or another, particular foods or mysterious combinations of substances have been sought and powerful effects have been attributed to them. However, it is controversial whether any particular food can indeed enhance erotic sensations and sexual performance. It is known that some legal and illegal drugs cause biological changes in the body that affect sexual arousal and response. Some of these cause increased blood flow to the erogenous zones and increase skin sensitivity. Drugs, whether legal or illegal, are usually dangerous and may have many negative and possibly irreversible side effects, even death.

Experiencing Sexual Arousal

For both sexes, sexual arousal means experiencing physiological changes in the body. These changes are primarily due to two processes, vasocongestion and myotonia. *Vasocongestion* is the increase of blood flow to the genital regions in both men and women. This increase in blood flow results in the engorgement or erection of the penis in men and the engorgement and erection of the labia and clitoris in women. The enlargement of these tissues promotes arousal and increases sensitivity. *Myotonia* is the increase in muscular tension that accompanies arousal. Myotonia is influenced by neural excitement. The nerve endings are stimulated and send messages to the brain; the body responds with involuntary muscular contractions. The increasing muscular tension will reach a point where it can no longer escalate. It is at this time that *orgasm* occurs for most people. Humans of either sex undergo similar changes in the body during this process, also called the *sexual response cycle,* which will be fully discussed later in this chapter.

Both men and women may also exhibit other signs and symptoms of sexual arousal. Breathing may become more shallow and rapid, accompanied by an increase in heart rate. Some people may begin to perspire down their backs or chests or may exhibit a *sex flush,* which is a temporary reddening of the skin's surface. The sex flush may appear anywhere on the body, but often it is noticed on the ears or cheeks and sometimes across the torso (Masters & Johnson, 1966).

PATTERNS OF SEXUAL COMMUNICATION

Communication is the stronghold of any effective relationship, particularly one that has the added dimension of sexual behavior. Sex within a relationship can often make individuals feel vulnerable and afraid. Good communication can quell these emotions and have a positive influence on the quality of the sexual relationship. Generally, people who communicate well regarding their sexual needs and desires, communicate equally as well across their overall relationship (see also Chapter 1).

Communication is the exchange of words, gestures, and movements that convey meanings, allowing two or more people to exchange ideas or information, all of which occur within cultural, social, and psychological contexts. Understanding and being aware of these contexts will influence one's ability to communicate well with one's partner. Partners who were raised in two distinct locales, regions, or even countries may have some difficulty understanding each other, even though they speak the same language.

Individuals with distinct personalities will have different communication styles; some may be direct, some indirect, aggressive or passive, objective or subjective. Often, the style in which people express themselves will be a reflection of their sense of self-esteem, self-image, gender role, and perhaps life experiences. These *psychological* tenets are just a few of the factors that may influence one's feelings or comfort level regarding communicating about sexual issues. People who have had a positive sexual past will be more willing and likely to openly communicate with their sexual partners.

The *cultural* context in which communication takes place refers to the language, values, and beliefs of the people involved. Historically speaking, in Western culture, discussions regarding human sexuality were most often discouraged. Obtaining knowledge concerning this aspect of human nature was left to those in the medical profession. All other interested individuals were taught that this type of knowledge was off limits. If we simply look at how the English language refers to sexuality, it is evident that Western culture is not truly comfortable with this topic. We see terminology rooted in scientific jargon or slang terms that often are vulgar and sexist in nature. There are very few terms that people would feel comfortable reciting in front of their parents.

Differences in how people communicate about sex certainly exist between ethnic and cultural groups. Some groups will rely on expressing themselves based on direct experience, while others will never engage in a sexual discussion because it is culturally unacceptable to do so. All people need to be aware that these differences do occur and to respect these differing perspectives.

People's social status in their society will also influence how they sexually communicate with partners. Position in a group or relationship has a direct affect on how people talk to each other. Stereotypically, within American culture, both males and females experience a distinct power hierarchy, with males being more powerful, assertive, and verbally explicit, as opposed to women, who tend to be more passive, nonverbal, and emotionally driven, although the stereotypes do not always hold true. Certain cultures are known to have more powerful women. In different parts of the United States, women are raised to be more or less assertive. Family values also have an impact on communication. There are also differences in sexual communication between heterosexual and homosexual couples. Unlike heterosexual couples, homosexual couples do not experience the gender-driven power disparity, possibly providing a more equal, positive pattern of communication (Bradshaw, 1994; Quadagno et al., 1998).

People often communicate without the use of words. *Nonverbal* communication is another way people can express thoughts, feelings, and emotions. Silence, facial expressions, body posture, and distance or proximity between partners can be used to communicate sexually. Unfortunately, nonverbal gestures can be misinterpreted. Silence may seem like a clear message to stay away, yet it may indicate that the partner is planning a next move. Although people have similar facial expressions that accompany certain emotions, generally, body language and facial expressions are highly personalized in such a way that we cannot truly infer how people are feeling or what they are thinking.

Understanding the Parts of Communication

The act of communicating has several parts that can be categorized in four ways: the *message* (includes the words used), the *sound* or *tone* of the voice, *facial expressions,* and *body language.* Choosing appropriate words is an essential aspect of communicating in an effective manner. If a person wants to improve communication skills, the person should take ownership for his or her remarks. For example, use *I,* not *they* or *some people.* This language will personalize the communication and make it less anonymous. Using words that are assertive, not aggressive in nature, can also improve communication between partners. If a person begins a discussion with "fighting words," a fight is exactly what that person is going to get. Often one's tone of voice may convey a message more clearly than the words themselves. Sarcasm and anger are difficult to disguise despite the most careful selection of words. The meaning of a sentence can also be altered dramatically according to which word is emphasized.

Part of being a good communicator is being an active listener. Maintaining eye contact with your partners will encourage them to continue and will let them know you are interested. Be aware, too, that eye contact may be interpreted differently within different cultures. For example, in Western culture, direct eye contact is a characteristic of good communication. However, in some Asian and other cultures, this is seen as aggressive behavior. One's facial expressions may also communicate boredom and indifference. Words said with a smile may indicate one thing; the same words said with a scowl may mean another.

Body position can also influence the message. Leaning forward toward the speaker generally indicates involvement. Listening with one's head cocked to one side accompanied by toe tapping may be misinterpreted as impatience. It is important to be aware of the many factors that affect communication styles. Differences in culture and psychology can influence the patterns of communication between partners, and often it is the misinterpretation of these factors that make communicating between people difficult (Cupach & Metts, 1991; Quadagno et al., 1998).

Self-Pleasuring/Masturbation

Masturbation is the stimulation of one's own genitals or the genitals of a partner, usually to the point of orgasm. This activity is generally done by manual contact or means other than sexual intercourse. Although it is often described as a solitary method of sexual expression and behavior, masturbation is often an integral part of a couple's sexual behavior. Some couples will masturbate themselves or their partners prior to or in concert with sexual intercourse or in lieu of sexual intercourse.

People masturbate for many reasons: to experience pleasure, to relieve tension or anxiety, or to explore their own sexuality. Masturbation may also be done with vibratory aids (vibrators and other sex toys) and/or in conjunction with sexually explicit printed or visual materials.

Much controversy has swirled about masturbation for as long as historians have kept records of this information. Many people feel guilty about masturbation, often based on religious and cultural beliefs about its social acceptance. It was once believed that masturbation drained the body of vital fluids and strength that caused the individual to be more susceptible to debilitating diseases and mental illness. In different cultures, this belief is still held today. It was also believed that excessive self-pleasuring could cause damage to the nervous system and that it would eventually compromise one's eyesight and memory. Historically, masturbation has been linked to epilepsy, tuberculosis, alcohol abuse, and tobacco use. These beliefs were not based on science, and current research has disproved all of them.

Masturbation is one of the most widely practiced forms of sexual behavior but the least discussed. It isn't just an immature form of childhood or adolescent sex that replaces sexual intercourse. People in every age group and from every socioeconomic class masturbate at one time or another. According to one study, 60 percent of American males and 40 percent of American females aged 18 to 59 reported that they have masturbated in the past year (Michael, Gagnon, Laumann, & Kolata, 1994).

Research consistently illustrates the differences in masturbatory behavior between males and females, although reasons for these differences are unclear. Perhaps, the anatomical realities of the male genitalia make masturbation a more socially sanctioned activity. Boys, from the time they toilet train, have their penises in their hand. The male's genitalia are more easily accessible than the female's. Very often the only contact young females have with their genital area is to clean it after using the toilet. For many females, intimate contact with their own genital region comes with the onset of the first menstrual cycle or even much later on in life, after the birth of their first child. That being said, both male and female infants and toddlers can be observed touching their sex organs for pleasure. Recent studies show that masturbatory differences between the genders is slowly narrowing. This change is most likely due to the increased awareness and acceptance of female sexuality by both women and men.

For many women, manual stimulation of the clitoris is the most reliable way to achieve orgasm. This type of sexual behavior can occur simultaneously with, before, or after sexual intercourse. There is wide variation in technique; women may use their own fingers to stroke the clitoris or vulva or to penetrate the vagina. Some women may rub the clitoral region on a pillow or their partner's hips, thighs, or virtually any other accessible body part. Some women may utilize objects or "sex toys" to masturbate to orgasm. Other women may stimulate their nipples, perineum, or anal region.

There is no right or wrong way to masturbate and there is wide diversity in technique and method (Quinlan, 1994).

Seemingly, male masturbatory technique entails less variation, although some might argue differently. Generally, men will stroke the shaft of the penis or stimulate the head of the penis. This can be done simultaneously or individually. Some may also choose to stimulate the scrotum, frenulum, perineum, or anal region. Once an erection is achieved, generally the motion and tension will speed up until orgasm is achieved. As with women, men often report that their strongest orgasms are through this method of sexual behavior (Hite, 1981; Leitenberg, Detzer, & Srebnik, 1993).

Some people may worry that, if their partner masturbates, there is something wrong with the relationship. No studies confirm this point of view. On the contrary, masturbation may have a positive influence on a couple's sexual relationship. Masturbation could conceivably relieve the pressure for sexual intercourse. In some relationships, however, the role of masturbation is not a substitute for sexual activity but a naturally occurring, complementary component of one's sexual lifestyle.

SHARED SEXUAL BEHAVIORS

Abstinence

Abstinence means refraining from all types of sexual intercourse, including vaginal, anal, and oral intercourse. Some people may decide not to have first intercourse until they marry or identify a lifetime partner. Others may take time off or temporarily refrain from sexual intercourse. Some may never have intercourse. Abstinence is a personal choice not to engage in sexual intercourse, which may or may not include masturbation. Many people choose abstinence for religious or spiritual reasons—for example, not having sexual relations before marriage or only when the couple is planning to start a family. Others may use periodic abstinence within and between relationships, possibly using this time to contemplate the direction in which the relationship is headed.

Erogenous Touching

Some areas of the body, when stimulated, provide sexual arousal and heightened sexual pleasure. There are *primary erogenous zones,* which include the mouth, buttocks, genitals, perineum, breasts, inner thighs, back of the neck, and anal region. The *secondary erogenous zones* may include the ears, navel, lower back, and other areas. Most people have the same primary erogenous zones, and most sexual experiences involve some of these areas. The secondary erogenous zones are more likely to reflect individual preferences, past experimentation, and experience.

During *foreplay,* many couples will engage in erotic touching, which can include soft caresses or more vigorous movements, like rubbing or applying pressure to any of the sensitive areas. Erogenous touching, often the center of foreplay, can be enjoyed on its own and does not always lead to sexual intercourse. However, foreplay does facilitate more comfortable vaginal penetration. The time spent erotically touching one's partner will allow women to generate appropriate lubrication in the vagina and allows men ample time to become fully erect. Honest communication about this aspect of sexual behavior can stimulate more pleasurable and rewarding sexual experiences.

The sensation of touch is one that drives our sense of *sensuality*—touching for the sake of showing affection and care for another individual. Some people believe sensuality can be achieved without any touching at all—a look, a movement, a phrase can all be sensual. All too often, people's sensual needs are disregarded within their relationships. Erogenous touching most often leads to sexual arousal, which prompts partners to speed up this sensual aspect of touching, so that they can "get down to business." Sensuality should be considered the cornerstone of every sexually intimate relationship and should be consciously and deliberately cultivated for maximum fulfillment.

Noncoital Sexual Behaviors

Noncoital sexual behaviors include both masturbation and erogenous touching and can also include kissing, oral-genital contact, and anal sex. All of these behaviors refer to activities that do not involve penile/vaginal or anal intercourse.

Kissing is a nearly universal pattern of behavior. Although cultural differences do occur, most populations enjoy some variation of this behavior (Fisher, 1992). Kissing can signify many things, from friendship to affection to eroticism, all of which depend on how the kiss is delivered and received. Kissing involves placing together the most sensitive body parts—the mouth, tongue, and face—but is not limited to these regions. It can include other body parts, including breasts, nipples, arms, legs, hands, feet, and the genital region.

Many people have their own set of rules concerning kissing behavior. Some may not kiss on the mouth until there is evidence of an intention to date again. Others feel that a kiss is a very intimate sexual behavior and should only be permitted if there is a mutual level of sharing. Kissing is often a precursor to more involved sexual behaviors like intercourse, and "a kiss" may be maintained throughout a shared sexual experience—for example, during sexual intercourse.

The popularity of *oral-genital sex* has increased considerably in the past few years. Oral sex performed on a male is called *fellatio*. Oral sex performed on a female is called *cunnilingus*. This type of sexual stimulation can be done individually or at the same time. Couples may choose to engage in oral sex simultaneously (often called "69" due to the visual similarity); others find that it interferes with their ability to give their partner pleasure.

There are many variations in the technique for performing oral sex, including kissing, sucking, biting, and applying pressure with the tongue. The tongue offers a sensation not experienced with the penis, with the fingers, or anything else. It has the ability to apply pressure more sensitively and directly.

Some individuals choose not to engage in this type of sexual behavior because they find the taste or odor of the male or female genitals unappealing. Due to varying personal preferences, many couples address this issue well before it comes up in the bedroom.

Oral-anal stimulation is similarly exciting to many couples. This type of stimulation is called *analingus*. It is also often referred to as "rimming," which describes the motion of putting one's tongue in or around the anus.

Anal sex includes penetration or manual stimulation of the anus. Anal intercourse is a form of sexual expression enjoyed by many people. Some believe that anal intercourse is the predominant form of sexual expression among gay males and somewhat less so for heterosexual couples and homosexual women. However, many homosexual males do not participate in anal sex, and many heterosexual couples do in order to prevent pregnancy or enhance the sexual experience.

From a sexual health perspective, anal intercourse is potentially the most hazardous form of sexual expression. The anal tissue is composed of very delicate tissue that can easily tear, allowing for the passage of sexually transmitted infections directly into the bloodstream. There is no release of natural lubricant during sexual arousal. Thus, a lubricant should be used with a condom for safety and comfort.

COITAL SEXUAL BEHAVIORS

Coitus, or sexual intercourse, involves the penetration of a woman's vagina by a man's penis. This pattern of sexual expression can be performed in numerous ways. Variations of body positioning may include any, and every, possible combination of arms, legs, and torsos only limited by the flexibility and creativity of the individuals involved. An ancient manual, the *Kama Sutra,* documents some 529 intercourse positions, describing who is in what position, whether on top, on the bottom, side by side, kneeling, sitting, or standing (Tarcher, 1993). There is no one position that is best: personal preference and comfort level will dictate what works best for any couple.

A common face-to-face position is called the *missionary position* in which the man is on top and the woman is lying on her back beneath him, face-up. Many people prefer this position for several possible reasons. This is the traditional or "official" position in Western culture. It allows for making oral contact and for caressing and stimulation of the breasts and nipples. It allows the woman to stimulate her clitoris to assist in her orgasm and also increases the chance of vaginal expulsion.

In the *woman-on-top* position, the woman straddles her partner, sitting, kneeling, or squatting on top of him. This position affords the woman greater control over the penetration and thrusting movements and allows more direct stimulation to the clitoral region. This also allows both the hands to be free for either partner to caress or stroke other parts of the body.

The *rear entry* position is when the man approaches the woman from behind and penetrates the vagina as he faces her from the rear. This can be accomplished by both partners kneeling, by her lying face-down, or by both partners standing with the male penetrating from behind. This position affords deeper penetration of the vagina but disallows for visual and oral contact. This position may also be more comfortable for women in the later stages of pregnancy.

In the *side-to-side* position, partners may face each other lying on their sides; it can be difficult to insert the penis into the vagina from this position. There is also difficulty in achieving a vigorous thrusting motion without the penis slipping out of the vagina. However, the face-to-face contact is stimulating to many couples, as is the ability to touch or fondle other erogenous zones while in this position.

SEXUAL FANTASY

Erotic fantasy or sexual daydreaming is probably one of the most universal sexual behaviors; nearly everyone has experienced such fantasies (Caron, 2003). Because of the intimate nature of these dreams, they are rarely openly discussed. Many of these fantasies often involve sexual behaviors and depictions that would not be part of a person's usual sexual thoughts. Some dreams are highly stimulating and occasionally lead to physical arousal and orgasm. Some people may find this uncontrollable imagery disturbing since most people fantasize about things they would not do in real life. Yet, sexual dreams and fantasy are common and often do not indicate an individual's sexual values or real desires.

Sexual fantasies may help define people's erotic goals. They may also provide material for role play and future sexual interludes. Role plays can alleviate anxiety and help people cope with various situations. Erotic dreams also provide an escape from boredom or routine and can also bring new excitement into a relationship.

Fantasy during sexual intercourse or during masturbation can have a dramatic effect on sexual arousal. Some people may experience guilt if they fantasize during intercourse, perhaps transforming their partners into famous celebrities. Others may find that erotic fantasy can increase sexual arousal and response exponentially. The diverse nature of sexual fantasies is reflective of the variation and creativity of the individuals themselves.

PROSTITUTION

Prostitution is the act or practice of engaging in various sexual or erotic acts for money. Sexual acts may include intercourse, oral sex, anal sex, erotic massage, domination, discipline, and bondage. Both heterosexual and homosexual men and women work as prostitutes, and men and women of all sexual orientations seek their services. Prostitution has been called the "world's oldest profession" due to the fact that just about every civilization throughout recorded history makes reference to its existence. Historically, prostitution has generally been viewed as a necessary evil to abate humans' uncontrollable sexual desires.

In most contemporary societies, prostitution is believed to be publicly abhorred while in reality it is ignored by most and tolerated by many. In some other countries and cultures, prostitution is legal. Some governments play a major role in monitoring the women involved to ensure that they remain disease free. Prostitution is illegal everywhere in the United States with just a few exceptions, such as in the state of Nevada.

In the United States, it is difficult to estimate how many men and women are involved in commercial sex work for several reasons: because it is illegal and punishable by incarceration; because many of the women who engage in this behavior do it irregularly; and because some women who accept drugs or money for sexual activity do not always consider themselves prostitutes. For those women who work regularly, they often identify themselves as "working girls" or "sex workers." The latter term probably is a better representation of how they perceive themselves in relation to the sexual activity. Many, if not most, working women are not sexually insatiable. Most prostitutes do not enjoy the sex with their customers. They see themselves as providing a service that is in high demand regardless of how the economy fares.

Recurring factors seem to be involved in bringing young women into this line of work: poverty, early sexual abuse, familial problems that prompt young people to run away, and involvement with drugs or alcohol. In every society around the world, poverty seems to be the major reason people become sex workers. Desperate people with no skills or little education may see prostitution as their only chance for survival. The job itself has very little external controls; individuals set their own work schedules and frequently work independently. In addition, people participating in commercial sex work can make a lot more money through this line of work than working at a fast-food restaurant, for example.

Female prostitutes are generally classified by the location and conditions in which they work. *Streetwalkers* are those women who stand or walk in a public location and solicit their customers as they pass by. Very often these sex workers are coerced to work for *pimps* who offer a sense of companionship, protection, and a steady supply of drugs.

Traditionally, in the United States, prostitutes worked in *brothels, bordellos,* or *whorehouses.* These were locations where several women worked and were managed by a *madam* or business manager. The women would share a portion of their earnings in return for a supply of customers and a steady location. *Massage parlors* and *escort services* served similar functions. Women who worked as *call girls* were paid the most. They generally have regular repeat customers. These women, and their services, were also managed by a madam, who took a percentage of their fee for this arrangement. In contemporary society, it is evident that there is a steady supply and demand for their services and women who will provide it.

Prostitution is not limited to women servicing men. There are numerous male prostitutes who provide similar services. However, the majority of these men are selling sex to other men. *Hustlers* are generally male prostitutes who solicit their services to homosexual men on the street. *Gigolos* are male prostitutes who provide sexual services to women, and sometimes they offer social companionship or act as an escort to women clients in exchange for money and gifts. Gigolos, like call girls, are highly paid and usually have regular repeat customers.

THE HUMAN SEXUAL RESPONSE CYCLE

In our Western cultural view, we see sexual responsiveness as a phenomenon that occurs most predominantly in the genital region. Theoretically, we liken this experience to a very goal-oriented occurrence that starts and ends with distinctive physiological responses. It is evident that human response to sexual arousal is not completely predictable and not fully centered in the genitals, but, rather, it involves the entire being, both body and mind. Because the brain is involved in these responses, it is understandable that no two people experience the sexual response cycle exactly the same way. To understand the bodily responses, this phenomenon is often divided into separate phases.

The Masters and Johnson Four-Phase Model

William Masters and Virginia Johnson, two pioneers in the field of sex research, provided the most thorough information about how the body responds to sexual stimulation. In their 1966 book, *Human Sexual Response,* Masters and Johnson report their findings based on the clinical observation and instrumental monitoring of men and women during masturbation. Their study closely observed some 694 people having sexual intercourse in the laboratory where they were monitored and interviewed by a research team. Only individuals who had indicated that they were able to reach orgasm were accepted into the study. They base their model theory on the premise that orgasm is a natural built-in response that can be achieved with proper stimulation for every person. Many scientists believe that this model is not representative of the true human response to sexual stimulation, grounded in the belief that it has never been proven that all humans have the capacity for orgasm. Regardless of this controversy, the Masters and Johnson model is widely accepted as one way to explain this portion of human sexuality.

The model identifies the significant stages of responses as *excitement, plateau, orgasm,* and *resolution.* The excitement phase, the first phase, is characterized by blood rushing to the pelvic region, also called *vasocongestion,* which results in one of the first signs of arousal, an erect penis on a male or an erect clitoris and lubricated vagina in a female. This mounting level of sexual arousal can be maintained for varying amounts of time.

The maintenance level of this state of arousal is called the *plateau phase*. At this point, many people experience what is called the "sex flush" in which a reddish rash or blotches may appear on the chests of males or breasts of females. If maintained for a period of time, the body reacts with varying degrees of stimulation.

This phase builds the body's muscular tension (*myotonia*) toward a pleasurable release called *orgasm* or *climax*. This phase is the briefest, lasting less than a few seconds, perhaps up to a minute. Yet the feelings associated with this moment focuses the mind inward and allows the whole body to experience the rush and sensation of various highly pleasurable, physical sensations. Female orgasm is characterized by contractions of the pelvic muscles that surround the vagina. Contractions may also be felt in the anal region and uterus. Males experience orgasm in two stages. The first is experienced in and around the glands that are responsible for contributing to seminal fluid. As this ejaculatory fluid is gathered, the internal sphincter muscle contracts to prevent semen from entering the bladder. At this time, the man may be experiencing a feeling of impending ejaculation. The second stage is characterized by the relaxing of the external sphincter muscle of the bladder, thus allowing the passage of semen. The muscles surrounding the base of the penis, the urethra, and urethral bulb will contract rhythmically to push out the ejaculate, thus providing the pleasurable sensations associated with orgasm.

Immediately after orgasm the body relaxes and returns to its prearoused state. This is called the *resolution phase*. At this point in the response, both the genitalia of men and women return to the prearoused state. Vasocongestion and myotonia disappear within a few moments after climax. Heart rate, blood pressure, and respiration return to the prearoused state. After resolution, males enter the *refractory period* in which they are physically unable to experience another arousal, orgasm, or ejaculate. This may last a few minutes in younger men to a much longer period in older males. Females do not experience the refractory period. In fact, some women may experience multiple orgasms during a singular sexual experience so that their bodies can quickly return to the plateau phase and reach orgasm again. This can happen several times before the female body enters the resolution phase (Masters & Johnson, 1966).

OTHER SEXUAL VARIATIONS

Our society has been slowly exposed to a greater variety of sexual behaviors and to a broader range of ways in which people sexually express themselves. Behaviors that were once taboo or deviant are thought of as less unusual and within the scale of so called "normative sexual behavior." For example, oral sex was seen as a social and behavioral deviant type of sexual expression. Today, we know that oral sex is an integral part of many relationships. Homosexuality itself was seen as a mental disorder by the American Psychological Association until the early 1970s, when it was removed from its *Diagnostic Statistical Manual (DSM)*, a catalogue used to diagnose mental disorders.

Generally, the psychosocial climate of a society plays a vital role in distinguishing deviant from normative sexual behaviors. This climate is dynamic and is influenced by many factors: the media, whether or not famous people are openly involved, acceptance by professionals, and the lay public.

Fetishism is one area encompassing sexual variations. We often attribute special powers to many things, lucky rabbit's foot, lucky numbers, a lock of hair, or even a vehicle. These objects really reflect a symbolism or fetish. *Fetishism* to an object that stimulates a sexual attraction occurs when a person associates a particular object with a person or part of a person (Mason, 1997). For example, one may gain sexual satisfaction from kissing a shoe or lingerie. These objects become sexual symbols.

Fetishist behavior can be placed on a continuum with varying degrees of preference. A fetish may move from a slight preference to a strong preference, to a necessity for sexual gratification. Most people have slight fetishes for different body parts such as legs, eyes, breasts, and muscles. It is only when these fetishes become so strong that they become a substitute for the real thing that professionals deem them problematic.

Voyeurism is when an individual enjoys and receives some sexual satisfaction from viewing sexual behavior, without others knowing they are being watched. Generally, the problem with voyeurism is that it is nonconsensual. The traditional examples of voyeurs are the "Peeping Tom" peering through a neighbor's window while masturbating, or the department store clerk videotaping women disrobing in a department store changing room. Voyeurism is becoming more popular with the ever-increasing accessibility to the Internet and various media alternatives. America's interest in watching other people have sex has fueled the exponential growth of the sex industry. Sexual images found in magazines and books, topless bars, and erotic dance clubs have always been a way for people to satisfy their voyeuristic urges.

Exhibitionism is the act of displaying one's genitals to an unsuspecting stranger. Most exhibitionists receive sexual gratification from this behavior, often exposing themselves to children, adolescents, or young women. This behavior is very often thwarted if the victim shows any sign of interest. This form of expression is so common that at least half of adult women may have witnessed the display of indecent exposure at least once in their lives (Arndt, 1991; Hollander, 1997). Exhibitionists are predominantly introverted, sexually inadequate, and insecure men (Hollander, 1997; Marshall, Eccles, & Barabee, 1991). Most have poor sexual relationships with their female partners that instigate anger that is expressed toward unsuspecting women.

Pedophilia is the recurrent fantasy or urge to engage in sexual relations with prepubescent children. Generally, these children are 13 or younger. In U.S. society, pedophiles are abhorred and vehemently chastised and pursued by both professional law enforcement agencies and the general public. Many pedophiles have a history of negative early sexual experiences, possibly having been molested themselves.

Sexual addiction is one's inability to control sexual behavior. For some people, sexual activity becomes compulsive. Some researchers liken this compulsive behavior to that of alcoholism or other chemical dependencies (Kafka & Hennen, 2000). Sexual addiction is characterized by the inability to stop a behavior despite serious negative consequences such as pregnancy, disease, incarceration, losing one's job, or sociocultural disapproval. Determining whether someone is a sex addict is often difficult because both professionals and laypeople would consider many of the behaviors elicited by individuals normal. Many individuals who are apparently addicted to sex are adults engaging in consensual sex in private places. Despite the controversy among professionals, most will agree that a persistent, uncontrollable sexual appetite characterizes a sexually addicted individual. Addicts may pursue partners based solely on the objectified nature of their desires. Once attaining these sexual liaisons, most addicts feel unsatisfied, leading them to engage in more negative behavior.

HUMAN SEXUAL DYSFUNCTIONS

Unfortunately, our media culture has us believing that everybody is sexually willing and able, anytime, every time, when the reality for many people is that sexual readiness and sexual capability are not always matters of turning down the lights. One's sexual well-being is influenced by many factors, including some biological, psychological, and social ones. *Sexual dysfunction* is a persistent sexual disorder that impairs sexual arousal, desire, or overall sexual satisfaction.

Common sexual disorders in men may include erectile dysfunction, premature ejaculation, delayed ejaculation, and the inability to ejaculate. Common disorders in females may include *anorgasmia,* the inability to orgasm; *vaginismus,* the tightening of the vagina preventing penetration; and *dyspareunia,* painful intercourse. Both males and females may experience desire dysfunctions and painful intercourse. However, the latter is more common in women. Men often have difficulties in the excitement stages of the sexual response cycle. An ability to maintain an erection and or prevent premature ejaculation are the most common.

Erectile dysfunction, also known as *impotence,* is experienced by nearly half of all adult males at sometime in their sexual lives (Bortolotti, Parazzi, Colli, & Landoni, 1997). As men age, this percentage increases. Men who have never had an erection are classified as experiencing *primary erectile dysfunction,* and those who have erectile dysfunction after a period of normal erectile functioning are classified as having *secondary erectile dysfunction.* Secondary difficulties are more common than primary and are generally easier to treat because they are often the result of a temporary biological, psychological, or social factor. Very often, work stress, fatigue, alcohol consumption, particular medical conditions, side effects from prescriptive drugs, or depression may temporarily interfere with normal sexual functioning. Although this condition is often short-lived, it can seriously compromise a man's self-concept.

Premature ejaculation occurs when a man is unable to control or delay his ejaculation as long as he and his partner would like. This causes problems within relationships because the partner is often left sexually unsatisfied. A man may feel confused, embarrassed, and helpless in this situation. Some men may begin to avoid sexual contact with their partners due to the anxiety they experience.

Anorgasmia, the most common dysfunction among women, is the inability to reach orgasm. There is *primary* dysfunction, in which a woman has never experienced orgasm, and *secondary* dysfunction, in which a woman who has been experiencing orgasm ceases to do so. *Situational* dysfunction occurs when a woman is orgasmic in some situations and not others. Lack of orgasm may be a result of many factors such as lack of effective clitoral stimulation, lack of efficient penile stimulation during sexual activity or intercourse, and, very often, an insufficient comfort level with their own bodies or that of their partners. Also, women require more direct stimulation to the clitoris and more time doing so than their partners generally provide. Women can learn how to facilitate their orgasms through self-exploration, masturbation, and positive sexual experiences.

Vaginismus is a sexual dysfunction experienced by relatively few women. The walls of the vagina go into a spasm that prevents the insertion of the erect penis or sex toy. This disorder is said to be a conditioned response that is reflective of an individual's anxiety toward sexual intercourse (Vanderweil, Jaspers, Schultz, & Gal, 1990). Negative past experiences or negative feelings toward this behavior can cause this to occur. Sex therapy can help women heal from this disorder.

Dyspareunia is painful sexual intercourse. Generally, this occurs because a woman is not fully aroused before a penis or sex toy is inserted into the vagina. Physical disorders, such as endometriosis or sexually transmitted infections, can also contribute to this dysfunction. Without appropriate lubrication, intercourse can produce too much friction causing pain and tearing of vaginal tissues. Menopausal and postmenopausal women also experience insufficient vaginal lubrication. The decrease in estrogen production will limit the amount of natural lubrication secreted in the vagina and compromise the elasticity of the vaginal walls. If proper stimulation or prolonged stimulation does not work, women can use lubricating gels or jellies and or hormonal therapies to induce proper lubrication.

Our bodies are very sensitive to the changing world around us and to the potential changes or disruptions that occur in the environment or within the body. Any one of these factors, or any combination of these, can have adverse effects on our sexual functioning. Luckily, more often than not, the sexual dysfunctions briefly described here are often caused by biological factors and, infrequently, by pathological ones.

SUMMARY

Patterns of sexual arousal and attraction, sexual communication, the sexual response cycle, sexual variation, and sexual dysfunction are all a part of a comprehensive sexuality program. Unfortunately, they often take the backseat to other topics deemed more relevant and/or appropriate to young people, such as contraception and disease transmission. One could argue, however, that one topic is no more important than the other. Unless young people understand how and why their bodies work and respond in the ways that they do, they will never truly become aware of themselves as sexual beings.

Some parents and educators might not want young people to become aware of themselves as sexual beings, but health educators make the argument that the reason young people get themselves into risky situations is that they are not taught how to recognize signs and symptoms in their own bodies.

Health educators teach young people to recognize the signs of stress and anger in order to help them to avoid situations that make them anxious or violent. On the same principle, shouldn't we teach young people the signs of sexual response, so that young people can recognize that they are in a situation that may lead to intercourse? If they choose to do so, they can extricate themselves from that situation similarly to the way they extricate themselves from a situation that causes stress or anger. For those students who make a conscious choice to be sexually active, information on sexual communication, arousal, and response can contribute to healthy sexuality.

Another important part of this chapter is the information on sexual behavior and sexual dysfunction. Many times, young people's only exposure to sexuality is through the media. If the media are to be believed, all people have sexual intercourse in a relationship, there is little foreplay, and multiple orgasms occur all the time. When young people enter relationships, they may be confused or disappointed that they are obtaining little sexual satisfaction compared to what happens on television or in the movies. They may also feel pressure to engage prematurely in sexual behavior because they believe that intercourse is the only sexual option available to them in a relationship. It is important for young people to recognize that there are many behaviors they can participate in that do not lead to pregnancy or disease transmission. In addition, young people should be aware of different types of sexual dysfunction in case they are experiencing problems in their sexual relationship.

Finally, information about sexual variation is important to discuss with young people for two reasons: it serves to promote the theme of tolerance and diversity, and it may prevent cases of sexual abuse among young people.

Sexual arousal and attraction, sexual communication, the sexual response cycle, sexual variation, and sexual dysfunction are all a part of a comprehensive sexuality education program. Several learning experiences are provided in this chapter that can be used by prospective teachers when teaching about these topics in their sexuality education curriculum. As with any health issue, the prospective teacher should modify the learning experiences so that they are applicable to district regulations and the student population they are teaching. Particular attention should be made to age-appropriate information whenever any information related to sexuality is taught in the classroom.

WEBSITES

Alan Guttmacher Institute: www.agi-usa.org

American Association for Sex Education, Counseling and Therapy (AASECT): www.aasect.org

American Board of Sexologists: www .esextherapy.com

American Academy of Clinical Sexologists: www.esextherapy.com

American College of Obstetricians and Gyne-cologists: www.acog.org

American Society for Reproductive Medicine: www.asrm.org

Gay, Lesbian, Bisexual, and Transgender links: www.indiana.edu/-gibserv/global.html

Go Ask Alice: Columbia Universities Health Education and Wellness Program: www.goaskalice.columbia.edu

Men's Health Network: www.menshealth.com/new/guide/index.html

Menopause Matters: www.world.std .com/-susan207

National Institute on Aging: www.nia.nih.gov

National Institutes of Health Women's Health Initiative: www.niaaa.nih.gov

National Kidney and Urologic Diseases Infor-mation Clearinghouse: www.niddk.nih.gov

National Women's Health Information Center: www.4woman.org

National Women's Health Resource Center: www.healthywomen.org

Sexuality Information and Education Council of the United States (SIECUS): www.siecus.org

Society for the Scientific Study of Sex (SSSS): www.ssc.wisc.edu/ssss

Society for Women's Health Research: www.womens-health.org

The Kinsey Institute for Research in Sex, Gen-der, and Reproduction: www.indiana .edu/-kinsey

U.S. National Library of Medicine: www.nlm.nih.gov

REFERENCES

Arndt, W. B. (1991). *Gender disorders and the paraphilias*. Madison, CT: International Universities Press.

Bortolotti, A., Parazzi, F., Colli, E., & Lan-doni, M. (1997). The epidemiology of erectile dysfunction with its risk factors. *International Journal of Androgyny, 20,* 323–334.

Bradshaw, C. (1994). Asia and Asian Ameri-can women: Historical and political con-siderations in psychotherapy. In L. Comas-Diaz & B. Greene (Eds.), *Women of color.* New York: Guilford.

Caron, S. L. (2003). *Sex matters for college students.* Upper Saddle River, NJ: Prentice Hall.

Cupach, W. R., & Metts, S. (1991). Sexuality and communication in close relationships. In K. McKinney & S. Sprecher (Eds.), *Sexuality in close relationships.* Hillsdale, NJ: Erlbaum.

DeKoker, B. (1996). Sex and the spinal cord. *Scientific American, 275,* 30–32.

Fisher, H. (1992). *Anatomy of love: A natural history of monogamy, adultery, and di-vorce.* New York: Norton.

Hite, S. (1981). *The Hite report on male sexuality.* New York: Ballantine.

Hollander, M. H. (1997). General exhibi-tionism in men and women. In L. B. Schlesinger & E. Revitch (Eds.), *Sexual dynamics of anti-social behavior* (2nd ed., pp. 119–131). Springfield, IL: Thomas.

Kafka, M. P., & Hennen, J. (2000). Psycho-stimulant augmentation during treatment with selective serotonin reuptake inhib-itors with men with paraphilias and paraphilia-related disorders: A case se-ries. *Journal of Clinical Psychiatry, 61,* 664–670.

Leitenberg, H., Detzer, M. J., & Srebnik, D. (1993). Gender differences in masturbation and the relation of masturbation experi-ence in preadolescence and/or early adoles-cence to sexual behavior and sexual adjustment in young adulthood. *Archives of Sexual Behavior, 22,* 87–98.

Marshall, W. L., Eccles, A., & Barabee, H. E. (1991). The treatment of exhibitionism: A focus on sexual deviance versus cognitive and relationship features. *Behavior Research and Therapy, 29*(2), 129–135.

Mason, F. L. (1997). Fetishism: Psychopathology and theory. In D. R. Laws & W. O'Donoghue (Eds.), *Sexual deviance. Theory, assessment and treatment* (pp. 75–91). New York: Guilford.

Masters, W., & Johnson, V. (1966). *Human sexual response.* Boston: Little, Brown.

Michael, R. T., Gagnon, J. H., Laumann, E. O., & Kolata, G. (1994). *Sex in America: A definitive survey.* Boston: Little, Brown.

Quadagno, D., et al. (1998). Ethnic differences in sexual decisions and sexual behavior. *Archives of Sexual Behavior, 27,* 57–75.

Quinlan, S. (1994). *Women on sex.* New York: Barricade.

Reinisch, J. M. (1990). *The Kinsey Institute new report on sex: What you must know to be sexually literate.* New York: St. Martin's.

Stern, K. N., & McClintock, M. K. (1996). Individual variations in biological rhythms: Accurate measurement of preovulatory LH surge and menstrual cycle phase. In *Psychopharmacology and women: Sex, gender, and hormones* (pp. 393–413). Washington, DC: American Psychiatric Press.

Tarcher, J. P. (1993). *The yin-yang butterfly: Ancient Chinese sexual secrets for Western lovers.* New York: Putnam.

Vanderweil, H. B. M., Jaspers, J. P. M., Schultz, W. C. M. W., & Gal, J. (1990). Treatment of vaginismus: A review of concepts and treatment modalities. *Journal of Psychosomatic Obstetrics and Gynecology, 11,* 1–18.

Westheimer, R. K., & Lopater, S. (2004). *Human sexuality: A psychosocial perspective* (2nd ed.). Baltimore, MD: Lippincott, Williams & Wilkins.

LEARNING EXPERIENCES

After the learning experiences provided here, young elementary students will be able to

- Identify the human senses (taste, touch, scent, and so forth).
- Explain how they experience pleasure (nonsexual) through the senses.

Later elementary school students can

- Identify appropriate ways that people show affection for one another.
- Describe appropriate ways that people in "special relationships" show affection.

Middle school students can

- Describe the multiple functions of the genitals (procreation, pleasure).
- Describe the appropriate terminology for making love; masturbation; and oral, anal, and vaginal intercourse.
- Identify the ways that nongenital touching can be sensual and sexually arousing.
- Use life skills to deal with peer pressure to participate in sexual behavior.
- Explain how people express intimacy in sexual and nonsexual ways.
- Communicate what touching behaviors are comfortable and which are not comfortable for them.
- Clarify their personal values about sexual intimacy and where they believe it is appropriate and where it is not.

By the end of high school, students will be able to

- Describe the sexual functions of genitals.
- Recognize the changes associated with the stages of the human sexual response cycle.
- Recognize individual differences in desire, attitudes, and values about various sexual behaviors.
- Identify the various sexual dysfunctions.
- Identify resources for people with sexual problems.
- Develop skills for communicating about their sexual needs and limitations with a potential partner.
- Develop skills for dealing with peer pressure to be sexual.
- Understand the changes in sexual anatomy, sexual desire, and response over the life cycle.
- Evaluate potential risks associated with participation in sexual behaviors.
- Describe how sexual behavior contributes to or deters from relationships.
- Identify various fetishes and the level of risk associated with each.

LEARNING EXPERIENCE 1

TITLE: Recognizing and Resisting Lures

GRADE LEVELS: K–3

TIME REQUIREMENT: One period

LEARNING CONTEXT

Following this activity, students will identify and discuss lures that are used by pedophiles/abductors to develop relationships and/or abduct young children, and they will practice resistance to lures.

NATIONAL LEARNING STANDARDS

1: Students will comprehend concepts related to health promotion and disease prevention.

3: Students will demonstrate the ability to practice health-enhancing behaviors and reduce health risks.

7: Students will demonstrate the ability to advocate for personal, family, and community health.

PROCEDURE

1. Ask the students whether they know what a *lure* is. After some discussion, point out that a *lure* is a technique that pedophiles/abductors use to try to capture children to abuse and hurt them.

2. The subject of fishing lures may come up—if so, point out that a fishing lure is a technique to try and "capture" fish, but the type of lures the students will be talking about are lures to capture children. (The teacher may want to bring in an actual fishing lure as a visual aid.)

3. Point out to the class, if they do not ask about the term first, that a *pedophile* is a person—usually a grownup, but it could be a teenager—who wants to become friends with or capture a child so he or she can sexually abuse the child. An abductor can be a pedophile or simply a crazy person who wants to steal a child.

4. Ask students whether they know some things a pedophile/abductor might say to a child to try and lure the child to go with the pedophile/abductor. Following is a list and explanation of common lures that are used. The teacher should share these lures with the students if they do not come up in the discussion:

   • *Emergency lure:* The pedophile/abductor tells the child that there has been an emergency at home, that the parent is in the hospital/incapacitated, and that they were sent to pick the child up and bring them to the parent.

   • *Assistance lure:* The pedophile/abductor asks the child for assistance, provide him or her with directions, help with a chore, find a lost puppy, or some such statement.

   • *Bribery lure:* The pedophile/abductor tries to bribe the child with money, candy, toys, or other desirable items.

   • *Name recognition lure:* The pedophile/abductor calls the child by name, because he reads the name from the jacket, notebook, or lunch box.

- *Adult pressure lure:* The pedophile/abductor pressures the child and tries to make the child do what he says because he is the adult.
- *Friendly lure:* The pedophile/abductor befriends the child who is lonely.
- *Ego/fame lure:* The pedophile/abductor tells the child that he or she is beautiful/handsome and should be a model/actor. Then the abductor tries to convince the child to visit his studio for a photo shoot.
- *Home alone lure:* The pedophile/abductor tries to find out if the child is home alone.
- *Computer/online lure:* The pedophile/abductor pretends to be another child and then arranges to meet the child.
- *Authority lure:* The pedophile/abductor dresses up like a security guard or utility worker and tries to make the child trust him because of the uniform.
- *Pornography lure:* The pedophile/abductor offers the child the chance to view pornography if the child visits him.
- *"Want a ride?" lure:* The pedophile/abductor offers a ride to a child who is walking.

5. If there is time, continue the lesson. If there is no time, take a break at this point and continue the lesson on another day. Once a discussion and explanation of the different types of lures has occurred, hold a discussion with the class about what to do if someone tries to lure them:
   - Immediately run toward safety.
   - Yell "No!" as loudly as possible.
   - Tell a trusted adult what has happened.
   - If a child is by him- or herself, find a safe person to go to, such as a store clerk, a police officer, a bank teller, or a woman (if no one else is around).

6. Point out to the class that many children are victims of lures right on the school playground.

7. Take the class outside to the playground and run lure prevention "drills" similar to safety drills. Tell the class to line up in one line. The teacher should approach the first person in line and try to "lure" that student with one of the lures identified in class.

8. As the student is lured, he or she should turn and run toward the school building yelling "No!" at the same time. The student should go to the other teacher or administrator who has volunteered to help and tell that person what just happened.

9. Once a student has completed these steps, the student should get on the end of the line to wait his or her turn to practice the drill again.

10. The teacher should attempt to "lure" each student. If time allows, students should have the opportunity to practice lure prevention three to five times.

11. Conclude the class session by instructing students to go home and share what they learned with a parent/guardian.

INSTRUCTIONAL/ENVIRONMENTAL MODIFICATION
The teacher should make sure the playground area is available for use for the lure drill.

RESOURCES
Arrange for a teacher or administrator to be present during the lure drill. The teacher may want to have a letter prepared to send home to parents prior to the lesson forewarning them that the lesson is about to take place and providing suggestions on how parents can discuss this topic with their children.

ASSESSMENT PLAN

Students will be assessed through their participation in the lure drill and their class discussion.

REFLECTION

This lesson can be traumatic for students, especially sensitive ones. Parents should receive a letter home forewarning them that the lesson will be occurring and telling them that students may come home disturbed or upset. The lesson is vitally important, however, to teach students about child abuse and abduction.

LEARNING EXPERIENCE 2

TITLE: Communication between Partners

GRADE LEVELS: 7–9

TIME REQUIREMENT: One period

LEARNING CONTEXT
After this activity, students will be able to describe effective techniques for interpersonal communication and practice communicating about sexual behavior.

NATIONAL LEARNING STANDARDS
3:   Students will demonstrate the ability to practice health-enhancing behaviors and reduce health risks.
5:   Students will demonstrate the ability to use interpersonal communication skills to enhance health.
7:   Students will demonstrate the ability to advocate for personal, family, and community health.

PROCEDURE
1. Initiate class discussion by asking, "Why don't partners talk about enjoying sexual behaviors, preventing STIs, and pregnancy?"
2. Write student answers on blackboard. (Some possible answers may be "Embarrassment," "Fear of rejection," "Don't know the person well," "Seems unromantic to talk about it," "Don't know what to say," "Want to avoid subject," and "Don't want to know the truth.") Instruct students to write the responses in their notebooks.
3. Discuss the student responses.
4. Put the "Talking about Sex" transparency on the overhead projector or write the statements on the chalk-/whiteboard. Discuss the suggestions for communication about sexual behavior.
5. Pass out the "Talking about Sex" handout (included at the end of this activity) for students to keep in their notebooks for future reference.
6. Answer any questions the class may have concerning these guidelines.
7. Break the class up into pairs. Distribute one of the scenarios (listed later) to each dyad. Instruct the students to select a role and use the suggestions for communication about sexual behavior to have a discussion with their partner. When partners have finished communicating, ask them to switch roles, so each student has a chance to practice the strategies (the teacher may tell students to swap scenarios so students have an opportunity to practice different situations).
8. If time allows, ask for volunteers to role-play their conversations in front of the class.
9. Discuss what happened, and compare and contrast how the situation was handled with how other dyads handled the same scenario.
10. Conclude the lesson by emphasizing the "Talking about Sex" guidelines that were discussed earlier.

INSTRUCTIONAL/ENVIRONMENTAL MODIFICATIONS

Be sure to check periodically with all groups to make sure that each student understands the lesson. Allow any students with physical disabilities a clear view of all interactions taking place during the class, and make sure they are able to maneuver themselves around the room with ease.

RESOURCES

"Talking about Sex" handout; scenarios, preduplicated and cut out—one per pair of students; chalk or dry-erase marker; chalkboard or whiteboard

ASSESSMENT PLAN

Students will be assessed by their participation in the class discussion and through participation in the communication role plays.

REFLECTION

This lesson will allow students to practice interpersonal communication skills and will provide students with the knowledge and skills to become better communicators. It will hopefully help students to protect themselves against premature sexual activity, pregnancy, and STIs.

"TALKING ABOUT SEX" OVERHEAD

Define the topic.
Pick the right timing.
Give a clear message.
Repeat your message.
Act on your decision.

TALKING ABOUT SEX SCENARIOS

Scenario A

Tracy and Jeff, both age 15, have known each other since elementary school and have been going out for 3 months. Tracy thinks she wants to wait until marriage before having sex. Jeff is ready now and is pressuring Tracy. Tracy really loves Jeff and wants to please him, but she has made a commitment to remain abstinent. How should Tracy communicate her choice with Jeff?

Scenario B

Dakota, age 17 and Kolby, age 19, have been going out for 1 year. Dakota's parents are out of town, so Dakota invites Kolby over for pizza and a movie. They have come close to having sex many times. This could be the big night. Dakota has decided that she wants to use condoms as a method of protection. How should Dakota communicate her choice with Kolby?

Scenario C

Colin and Jasmin, both age 16, have been going out for 9 months. Both have had sex in previous relationships. Jasmin tells Colin she wants to have sex with him. Colin really likes Jasmin but doesn't want to risk getting an STI. How should Colin communicate his concerns to Jasmin?

Scenario D

Maria, age 15 and Julio, age 14, have been going out for 6 months. They are hanging out at the park and have been talking about having sex sometime soon. Maria and Julio know about the risks of STI, HIV, and pregnancy. Julio's previous girlfriend had a pregnancy scare, and he doesn't want to repeat this with Maria. How should Julio communicate his concerns to Maria?

Scenario E

Chris, age 17, and Pat, age 19, have been going out for almost a year. Chris is more than ready to be sexually active, but Pat doesn't feel they are old enough to engage in sexual intercourse. Chris is willing to wait to have intercourse but wants to engage in other sexual behaviors. How should Chris communicate his desires to Pat?

"Talking About Sex" Handout

Define the topic.

Think through what you want to talk about. Do you want information, do you want to share your feelings, do you want help with a problem, or do you just want a listening ear? For example, do you want information about family beliefs, about contraception, sex before marriage, or abstinence, or do you want to talk about a fight you had with your boy-/girlfriend, or do you just want to share something you learned in your family life class?

Pick the right timing.

Have the conversation at a time when you are not in a romantic or sexual situation. It is difficult to talk about your decision and feelings in the heat of the moment. For example, having the conversation while you are taking a walk or having lunch together might be a good time. Having the conversation while you are making out would not be a good time.

Give a clear message.

Keep your message about your decision clear and to the point. For example, you might say, "I have decided not to have sex because I don't feel ready, and I don't want to risk getting an STI or getting pregnant." Or you could say, "I want to have sex with you, but I won't unless we use protection."

Repeat your message.

If your partner resists or pressures you, it often works to repeat the message. For example, you might say, "I feel like you aren't hearing me. I have decided not to have sex yet because I don't feel ready and I don't want to risk getting an STI or getting pregnant." Being firm can be difficult because we often want to please the people we care about.

Act on your decision.

Following through on your decision will be an ongoing process. When you are in a romantic relationship, the decision about sex and protection will come up many times. If your decision has been "no sex," you will need to continue your commitment in spite of your own sexual feelings and/or pressure from your partner. If you choose to use condoms, you will have to always have a supply on hand and use them every time you have sex.

LEARNING EXPERIENCE 3

TITLE: Stages of the Sexual Response Cycle

GRADE LEVELS: 10–12

TIME REQUIREMENT: One period

LEARNING CONTEXT
After this activity, students will
- Arrange and rank changes that occur during the sexual response cycle into the four stages of the Masters and Johnson model.
- Discuss the changes that occur during the four stages of the Masters and Johnson response cycle model.

NATIONAL LEARNING STANDARD
1: Students will comprehend concepts related to health promotion and disease prevention.

PROCEDURE
1. Introduce the class to the lesson by pointing out that sex is such an enormous part of our lives as humans, it is often easy to forget that sex is really just a biological function intended to advance our species.
2. Explain that in their 1966 book *Human Sexual Response,* researchers William Masters and Virginia Johnson reveal four generally accepted biological stages of sexual response: excitement, plateau, orgasm, and resolution.
3. Tell the class that they will be broken up into small groups. Each group will receive a set of cards that represent changes that occur during the sexual response cycle.
4. Groups will sort the changes into the four categories. The teacher may choose to allow students to use their textbooks, or not, if students were supposed to have completed the reading the previous night.
5. Divide the class into small groups and distribute a complete set of changes cards to each group. Allow groups 10 to 12 minutes to complete the sorting process.
6. When the small groups have completed the sorting process, instruct the class to move back to the large-group formation.
7. Ask groups to share the changes they identified for the excitement phase. As students are sharing changes, correct any wrong answers and write the correct answers on the board. Instruct the class to copy the notes into their notebooks.
8. Follow the same procedure for the other three phases.
9. Conclude by reminding the class that even though many people participate in sexual intercourse for pleasure, not procreation, the body still believes procreation is the ultimate goal. This is why abstinence and/or contraception is necessary for those people who do not wish to conceive!

INSTRUCTIONAL/ENVIRONMENTAL MODIFICATIONS

The teacher may want to make sure slower learners are paired with faster learners in small groups. The teacher may also want to make sure that "trouble" students are not placed together in the same groups.

RESOURCES

A set of cards that represent the changes that occur during the sexual response cycle (listed here), duplicated and cut out—one complete set of cards for each group

ASSESSMENT PLAN

Students will be assessed through their sorting of cards and their participation in class discussion.

REFLECTION

The four stages of the sexual response cycle can be a very dry topic for students to learn. By breaking the students into groups, distributing the cards, and asking each group to sort the cards into the four stages, the teacher is able to transform a purely cognitive lesson into a lesson that is more student centered and interactive. The students still obtain the cognitive information, but it is conveyed in an innovative way, rather than through conventional lecture.

Stages of the Sexual Response Cycle

Stage 1: Excitement

- Increasing level of muscle tension
- Quickened heart rate and blood pressure
- Flushed skin or blotches of redness on the chest and back
- Hardened or erect nipples
- Swelling of the woman's clitoris and labia minora
- Erection of the man's penis
- Increased vaginal lubrication
- Elevation and growth of the uterus
- Swelling of the breasts
- Elevation and tightening of the testicles
- Tightening of the scrotal sac
- Lubrication of the Cowper's gland
- Thickened skin of scrotum

Stage 2: Plateau

- Penis fully erect
- Testes engorged (50 percent increase in size)
- Fluid appears at tip of penis
- Maximum breathing rate, pulse rate, blood pressure
- Swelling, thickening of outer third of vagina and pelvic floor muscles
- Clitoris retracted
- Uterus, breasts—maximal changes
- Change in color of labia minora

Stage 3: Orgasm

- Involuntary muscle contractions
- Rapid intake of oxygen
- Sphincter muscle contraction
- Spasms of the carpopedal muscles (feet)
- Sudden forceful release of sexual tension
- Rhythmic uterus muscle contractions
- Tightening of the woman's muscles that assists in male orgasm
- Muscle contractions in the uterus and pelvic areas, opening the way for the man's sperm
- Sudden release of muscle tension in series of contractions followed by relaxation
- In males, orgasm usually marked by ejaculation
- Contraction of penis and internal structures
- Possible contraction in muscles in back, buttocks, arms, legs, hands, and/or feet
- Spike in pulse rate, breathing rate, blood pressure
- In females, usually no external evidence of orgasm

Stage 4: Resolution

- Swelled and erect body parts return to normal
- Skin flushing disappears
- General sense of security and enhanced intimacy
- Possible fatigue
- Clitoris returns to relaxed position; vaginal walls relax
- Loss of erection; testes return to nonaroused position; refractory period
- A return to normal heart rate, blood pressure, breathing, and muscle contraction

LEARNING EXPERIENCE 4

TITLE: Interview with a Specialist

GRADE LEVELS: 10–12

TIME REQUIREMENTS: 1–2 weeks to complete the assignment; one period to share the results of the interviews

LEARNING CONTEXT
After this activity, students will
- Identify a reproductive health specialist in their community.
- Interview a reproductive health specialist about sexual dysfunction.
- Share the information they learned from the specialist with their classmates.

NATIONAL LEARNING STANDARDS
1: Students will comprehend concepts related to health promotion and disease prevention.
2: Students will demonstrate the ability to access valid health information and health-promoting products and services.

PROCEDURE
1. Explain to the class that they are going to be given an assignment that requires them to identify a reproductive health specialist in their community—male students should identify a urologist, and female students should identify a gynecologist.
2. Pass out the directions sheet for this assignment (provided later in this activity).
3. Explain that students will be required to develop 10 or more questions to ask this specialist about sexual dysfunction. The questions should be factual questions, not personal questions. For example, "Please share the most common type of sexual dysfunction for men/women."
4. Tell the class that all of the questions developed should be open-ended questions. In other words, the person has to describe an answer. No questions should be close-ended, or yes-or-no questions.
5. Explain that students must type out the questions and answers to the interview and write a reflection paper about the experience of interviewing a specialist. The questions and answers should be stapled to the reflection paper for submission to the teacher.
6. Identify the due date for the assignment, and tell students to write it in the space provided on top of their directions sheet.
7. On the day that the assignment is due, spend the period having students share their experiences and the knowledge they gained during the interviews. Arrange the room in a U shape or circle so students can see each other when sharing the results of their interview.
8. Collect the completed assignments from students.

INSTRUCTIONAL/ENVIRONMENTAL MODIFICATION
Arrange the room in a U shape or circle so students can see each other when sharing the results of their interview.

RESOURCES
Copies of the assignment with directions—one per student

ASSESSMENT PLAN
Students will be assessed through the completion of their interview, the submission of their written reflection, and their participation in class discussion.

REFLECTION
This lesson not only teaches students about sexual dysfunction but provides students with the opportunity to develop the resource management skills needed to identify and interview health experts. The teacher should make very clear the safety rules associated with assignments that require students to spend time in the community. The teacher should make sure that students understand the importance of involving their parents in this process every step of the way. The teacher may also want to identify health experts that would be willing and able to talk to students.

"Interview a Specialist" Directions Sheet

Due Date: _____

1. Identify a reproductive health specialist in your community—male students should identify a urologist, and female students should identify a gynecologist. If a student would like to interview a different type of health specialist, he or she must obtain permission to do so from their parents and teacher.

2. Arrange for an interview with this specialist. Make sure your parents/guardians are involved in this process and are aware of the date and time of the interview. In-person interviews are preferable, but if none can be arranged, telephone interviews will be accepted.

3. Develop 10 or more questions to ask this specialist about sexual dysfunction. The questions should be factual questions, not personal questions. For example, "Please share the most common type of sexual dysfunction for men/women."

4. All of the questions developed should be open-ended questions. In other words, the person has to describe an answer. No questions should be close-ended, or yes-or-no questions.

5. Type out the questions and answers to your interview.

6. Write a reflection paper about the experience of interviewing a specialist.

7. Staple the questions and answers to the reflection paper for submission to the teacher on the due date.

LEARNING EXPERIENCE 5

TITLE: Sexual Behaviors Risk Continuum

GRADE LEVELS: 10–12

TIME REQUIREMENT: 30–40 minutes

LEARNING CONTEXT

After this activity, students will identify where sexual behaviors fall within a continuum of risk and discuss the risks inherent in participating in sexual activity.

NATIONAL LEARNING STANDARDS

    1:   Students will comprehend concepts related to health promotion and disease prevention.

    6:   Students will demonstrate the ability to use goal-setting and decision-making skills to enhance health.

    7:   Students will demonstrate the ability to advocate for personal, family, and community health.

PROCEDURE

1. Tape "No Risk," "Low Risk," and "High Risk" signs on three different walls in the room, in that order.

2. Pass out the sexual behavior cards (see the list later) with pieces of tape, and ask students to tape their behavior card on the wall in a continuum of order ranging from no risk to high risk. Clarify the directions by pointing out that when finished, the sexual behavior cards should stretch in one continuous line around the room.

3. Tell students that no one is allowed to sit back down until everyone is satisfied that the cards are arranged in the most appropriate continuum.

4. Students may ask, "Risk for what? Pregnancy, HIV, STIs?" Do not answer this question. Simply let students decide where the cards fall on the continuum without further information.

5. Once all the cards are on the wall, discuss the range of sexual behaviors and why students classified them as they did.

6. Correct any misconceptions about the different types of sexual activity and use the activity as a springboard for discussing safer sex.

7. Following are process questions to lead the class discussion following the activity:
   - What made you decide whether your behavior card was no-, low-, or high-risk?
   - What are some of the risks of sexual activity?
   - If a person participates in no or low risk sexual activity, does that tempt the person to participate in high-risk sexual activity?
   - What can a person do to decrease the risk if he or she chooses to participate in high-risk sexual activity?
   - What can a person do if he or she is being pressured to participate in high-risk sexual activity?

INSTRUCTIONAL/ENVIRONMENTAL MODIFICATION

The teacher may want to move all the desks away from the wall to the center of the room so there is space for students to stand and tape their signs on the wall.

RESOURCES

Three large signs reading "High Risk," "Low Risk," and "No Risk"; continuum terms printed in large type on 8.5 × 11 paper, one term per sheet; tape

ASSESSMENT PLAN

Students will be assessed through their participation and their class discussion.

REFLECTION

Students enjoy the opportunity to get out of their seats to participate in this activity, and they will need to participate in problem solving and group processing in order to create the continuum of cards on the wall. The learning takes place both through peer education and class discussion. The teacher should be aware of the policies of the school district, however, and eliminate sexual behavior cards that would not be acceptable for use.

SEXUAL BEHAVIOR CONTINUUM CARDS

1. Abstinence
2. Snuggling
3. Phone Sex
4. Skin Tickling
5. Dry Kissing
6. Hugging
7. Reading Erotica
8. Massage
9. Flirting
10. Fantasy
11. Body Paints
12. Sensuous Feeding
13. Undressing One Another
14. Solo Masturbation
15. Showering Together
16. Bubble Baths
17. French/Deep Kissing
18. Wrestling
19. Mutual Masturbation
20. Body Rubbing
21. Monogamy
22. Fingering
23. Vaginal Intercourse with a Condom and Spermicide with Nonoxynol-9
24. Fisting (Brachioproctic or Brachiovaginal Sex) with a Latex Glove
25. Anal Intercourse with a Condom and a Spermicide with Nonoxynol-9
26. Oral Sex on a Man (Fellatio) with a Condom
27. Oral Sex on a Woman (Cunnilingus) Using a Dental Dam
28. Oral-Anal Contact (Rimming) with a Dental Dam
29. Intercourse between the Thighs
30. Vaginal Intercourse with a Condom
31. Anal Intercourse with a Condom
32. Sharing Sex Toys
33. Oral Sex on a Woman during Menstruation
34. Oral Sex on a Man (Fellatio) without a Condom
35. Oral-Anal Contact (Rimming) without a Dental Dam
36. Intercourse with a Condom and an Oil-Based Lubricant
37. Vaginal Intercourse without a Condom
38. Anal Intercourse without Protection

LEARNING EXPERIENCE 6

TITLE: Ranking Fetishes

GRADE LEVELS: 10–12

TIME REQUIREMENT: One period

LEARNING CONTEXT
After this activity, students will
- Read about a variety of different types of fetishes.
- Rank fetishes from most benign to most dangerous/bizarre.
- Discuss their feelings about the different fetishes with their classmates.

NATIONAL LEARNING STANDARDS
1: Students will comprehend concepts related to health promotion and disease prevention.
2: Students will demonstrate the ability to access valid health information and health-promoting products and services.

PROCEDURE
1. Explain to the class that today's lesson is about fetishes.
2. Ask the class whether they know what a fetish is. Solicit some student responses, and then share the following definition. "*Fetishism* is a fixation on an inanimate object or body part that is not primarily sexual in nature, and there is a compulsive need for its use in order to obtain sexual gratification."
3. Point out that the object of a fetish is almost invariably used during masturbation and may also be incorporated into sexual activity with a partner to produce sexual excitation.
4. Explain that a fetish is a type of paraphilia, which is known as atypical sexual behavior. There are two types of paraphilia, noncoercive and coercive: *Noncoercive* paraphilias are ones in which all individuals participating are willing participants. *Coercive* paraphilias are ones in which all individuals do not give consent. These are obviously dangerous if a person acts out a violent fantasy on someone who does not wish to participate in the activity.
5. Distribute the "Ranking Fetishes" worksheet to each student in the class (provided at the end of this activity). Break the class up into partners or small groups. Instruct the class that they are to read about each of the fetishes and, as a dyad/group, rank most benign (1) to most bizarre/dangerous (25).
6. Allow students 10 to 15 minutes to complete their rank order. Then, bring the small groups back together to the large group to process the activity. Following are some process questions to help facilitate group discussion:
   - What was the most benign fetish? What were some other fetishes that ranked low numbers on your worksheet? Why?
   - What was the strangest fetish to you? What were some other fetishes that ranked high numbers on your worksheet? Why?
   - Which fetishes did your group consider dangerous?

- Which fetishes could be coercive? Noncoercive?
- Would you ever date someone with one of these fetish(es)? Which one(s)? Why or why not?
- Do you think fetishes should be allowed or outlawed? Which one(s)? Why?
- Where could a person go to find out more information about fetishes?

INSTRUCTIONAL/ENVIRONMENTAL MODIFICATIONS

The teacher may want to make sure slower learners are paired with faster learners in small groups. The teacher may also want to make sure that "trouble" students are not placed together in the same groups.

RESOURCES

Copies of the "Ranking Fetishes" worksheet—one per student

ASSESSMENT PLAN

Students will be assessed through their completion of the "Ranking Fetishes" worksheet and their participation in class discussion.

REFLECTION

Fetishism is a touchy issue to talk about with young people—not because young people do not want to talk about fetishes, but because their families do not want them to talk about it! An educator should check with his or her chairperson to make sure the subject area is permissible in the district. If it is permissible, this is a good lesson for the students to participate in the learning experience. It is important for students to learn about the variety of sexual behaviors prevalent in society. Oftentimes, the media only expose young people to one type of "normal" sexual behavior. This activity demonstrates that there is a greater continuum of sexual behavior than is portrayed in the media and allows students to identify sexual behaviors that could be considered dangerous to others.

REFERENCES

Eros Guide San Francisco: www.eros-guide.com/articles/2002-12-10/paraphilias/
University of California–Santa Barbara's SexInfo:
    www.soc.ucsb.edu/sexinfo/?article=activity&refid=014

"Ranking Fetishes" Worksheet

Directions: With your partner or small group, rank the following fetishes from most benign to most bizarre/dangerous. The fetish you think is most benign should be assigned the number 1. The fetish you think is most bizarre/dangerous should be assigned the number 25.

_____ Acomoclitic: Getting turned on by shaved and completely hairless genitals

_____ Altocalciphilia: Becoming excited by high heels

_____ Antholagnia: Becoming aroused by the scent of a flower

_____ Autoerotic asphyxiophilia: Deriving pleasure from cutting off their oxygen supply via strangulation or suffocation

_____ Chremastistophilia: Becoming sexually excited by the idea of being robbed

_____ Doraphilia: Feeling that the touch of fur or skin is sensual and erotic

_____ Exhibitionism: Surprising others by exposing their genitals

_____ Frotterurism: Touching other people in sexual ways without their consent and sometimes without their knowledge

_____ Hirsutophilia: Becoming aroused by body hair

_____ Iatronudia: Exposing oneself to a physician

_____ Maieusiophilia: Being aroused by pregnant women

_____ Martymachlia: Getting aroused by having others watch during sex

_____ Masochism: Experiencing sexual pleasure and arousal from receiving mild or mock pain or humiliation

_____ Nasophilia: Becoming sexually excited about a partner's nose

_____ Oculolinctus: Aroused by licking a partner's eyeball

_____ Ozolagnia: Becoming turned on by powerful scents

_____ Pedophilia: Sexual pleasure from engaging in sexual behavior with children

_____ Podophilia: Fairly common fetish about feet

_____ Retifism: Becoming sexually excited by shoes

_____ Sadism: Experiencing sexual pleasure and arousal from inflicting mild or mock pain or humiliation on others

_____ Scatolophilia: Deriving sexual pleasure from making obscene phone calls and listening to the shock and discomfort of the people they call

_____ Transvestitism: Cross-dressing

_____ Urophilia: Sexual excitement from urinating on others or being urinated on

_____ Voyeurism: Watching other people in the act of dressing/undressing, bathing, participating in intercourse, and other private behaviors

_____ Zoophilia: Fantasies of or actual sexual contact with an animal; also known as *bestiality*

LEARNING EXPERIENCE 7

TITLE: Where Do You Stand?

GRADE LEVELS: 10–12

TIME REQUIREMENT: 30–40 minutes

LEARNING CONTEXT
After this activity, students will identify their opinion on prostitution-related issues by standing under the sign that best represents their opinion. They will debate differing opinions with their classmates.

NATIONAL LEARNING STANDARD
    1:   Students will comprehend concepts related to health promotion and disease prevention.

PROCEDURE
1. Tape five signs on the walls, evenly spaced around the room:
   - Strongly Agree
   - Kind of Agree
   - Neither Agree nor Disagree
   - Kind of Disagree
   - Strongly Disagree
2. Explain that you will be reading a statement; the students are to listen to the statement and then get up and stand under the sign that best represents their opinion. Depending on how enthusiastic and talkative the class is, three to five questions may take up the entire period. Following is a list of statements relevant to prostitution:
   - People have the right to do whatever they want to do with their body.
   - Prostitution should be legalized in the United States.
   - Prostitution is degrading to women.
   - Prostitution should remain illegal because it spreads disease.
   - Prostitution is just another career.
   - Prostitution can prevent rape.
   - Wanting to visit a prostitute is abnormal.
   - Most prostitutes make a lot of money.
   - If prostitution was regulated like it is in other countries, it would be a lot safer.
   - If the majority of prostitutes were men, prostitution would be legal in this country.
3. Read the first statement.
4. After the students have identified their opinion by standing under a sign, ask process questions based on where the students are standing. There are no specific process questions for each statement—the questions will differ depending on what opinions students identify themselves as holding. Process each statement as it is asked instead of asking all the statements and going back to process them.

5. Allow students to debate each other and challenge their classmates as to why they are standing under a sign different to their own.
6. Try to play the devil's advocate and get students to shift where they are standing.
7. Once all the discussion about one statement has been exhausted, read a second statement and repeat the process.
8. Conclude by telling the class that there are no right or wrong answers to the questions posed. Students should think more about what was discussed during the period and about sharing what they talked about with their families. They should remember to value and respect the fact that people have different opinions than they do.

INSTRUCTIONAL/ENVIRONMENTAL MODIFICATIONS
Consider moving all the desks away from the wall to the center of the room so that there is space for students to stand under the signs. Also try reading the statements out loud while at the same time revealing the statement on an overhead so that visual learners don't forget what the statement is.

RESOURCES
Five signs: Strongly Agree, Kind of Agree, Neither Agree nor Disagree, Kind of Disagree, and Strongly Disagree

ASSESSMENT PLAN
Students will be assessed through their participation and class discussion.

REFLECTION
Prostitution is another delicate issue to discuss because students' families typically do not want their children to talk about it. An educator should check with his or her direct supervisor prior to facilitating this lesson to ensure the subject area is permissible in the school district. If so, this is a good lesson for the students to participate in. Many myths about prostitution are perpetuated in society—for example, that prostitutes make a lot of money. Through the class discussion that follows each statement, the teacher has the opportunity to refute the myths related to prostitution and lead the class in discussions related to societal values, power, and personal rights.

GENDER ISSUES IN SEXUALITY EDUCATION

JANICE KOCH AND ESTELLE WEINSTEIN

OBJECTIVES

After reading this chapter, students will be able to

1. Identify the attributes of a gender-equitable environment and be able to create same in classrooms.
2. Describe the socially constructed gender issues informing communication, decision making, and so forth.
3. Examine the social context of the classroom through the lens of gender (explain the ways male and female students may experience the human sexuality curriculum differently).
4. Describe ways in which the classroom can support female and male students being heard equally.
5. Examine sexuality curricula for gender bias.
6. Describe a learning experience in which female and male students explore their gender identities.

REFLECTIVE QUESTIONS

Elementary School

1. In what ways are the tasks and responsibilities of the members of your family related to their being a male or a female?
2. How are the various sports that you and your friends participate in affected by being female or male?
3. In what ways do the programs you watch regularly on television show male or female stereotypes?
4. What do you want to be when you grow up? How are your choices related to gender stereotyping?

Middle and Senior High School

1. Was the world a better place when women's and men's roles and behaviors were specifically assigned and men and women knew what was expected of them?

2. What are the advantages and disadvantages of specifically assigned roles by gender?
3. What are some of the stereotypical roles and behaviors identified with females?
4. What are some of the stereotypical roles and behaviors identified with males?
5. In what ways might gender role stereotyping occur in schools? In relationships? In the workplace?
6. What are your personal attitudes about gender role stereotyping?
7. What are your personal attitudes about gender equality versus gender equity?

─────────────── **SCENARIO** ───────────────

Sydney is 16 years old, almost 6 feet tall, and an excellent athlete playing on the school's varsity basketball team. Sydney is academically among the top 10 percent of students, achieving straight A's in math and science. Sydney works out regularly and is strong and in great shape. Sydney and Jordan have been going out for several months, but Sydney wants to be a doctor someday and is afraid to become seriously involved with any one person until sometime after college. Jordan, on the other hand, loves Sydney and is interested in a long-term commitment.

Is Sydney male or female?
Is Jordan male or female?
What characteristics did you use to identify their gender?
What is this couple's sexual orientation?
What characteristics did you use to identify their sexual orientation?

INTRODUCTION

A discussion of sex and gender is germane to the study of human sexuality. The biophysiological development of males and females from conception through puberty and the subsequent changes that occur throughout adulthood and aging lay a foundation for explaining human sexual response and human sexual dysfunction. Moreover, the psychological and social influences on males and females help people to understand their interactional patterns in relationships within and across such things as ethnocultural membership or sexual orientation.

This chapter explores the way families, schools, and communities influence sex and gender identity. It considers how schools socialize children in gender-specific ways and how sex and gender are associated with the development and implementation of personal life skills as they relate to interpersonal relationships.

EXPLANATION OF TERMS

The terminology used in discussing sex and gender is sometimes confusing. Many people use *sex* and *gender* interchangeably, yet to the professional the two words have different meanings.

Sex is a term used to describe the biological differences between males and females. *Sex assignment,* or an individual's assignment as a female or male, is usually made before birth as a result of information gleaned from a genetic test on the fetus in utero (most commonly by amniocentesis) or at the time of birth by observing the infant's external genitalia. Thus, the assignment of infants with penises to the male sex and infants with vaginas to the female sex is biologically based.

Sometimes errors of sex assignment occur because of unusual genetic or physiological factors that render the assignment incorrect or at least inappropriate. For example, a baby determined to be a boy from the observation of a penis may actually be a girl with an enlarged clitoris. Moreover, sometimes "ambiguous genitalia" occur in which the external genitalia do not match either the internal genitalia or the XX or XY chromosomes. The terminology for this ambiguity in newborns is *intersexed* (see Chapter 5). When a sex assignment is made at birth, several rearing activities are set into motion. (An extensive discussion of biological determinants of sex appears in Chapter 2.)

Sex is different from *gender. Gender* is a term used to describe the psychological and social differences between females and males. Different from sex assignment is *gender identity,* a more complicated phenomenon that is not entirely the result of biology but rather a combination of biology interacting with social and psychological factors. Gender identity is an individual's self-perception as a male or female emerging from a variety of sociocultural influences. Even more confusing than sex assignment or gender identity are the concepts of *masculinity* and *femininity.* These are culturally defined stereotypical ways that society expects males and females to behave. Then there are *gender roles* to consider. Gender roles are those behaviors, attitudes, and beliefs one acts on based on self-identity as male or female.

Some individuals develop with a less dichotomous gender identity and psychologically embrace an *androgynous identity,* one that blends both male and female characteristics and does not necessarily recognize either as belonging to a particular sex or gender. Also, some individuals have a *transgendered identity:* their sex assignment and gender identity are incongruent with one another. This more complicated terminology defines a variety of nontraditional biological and psychological gender-related phenomena that are discussed in detail in Chapter 5.

Two additional terms must also be defined in a comprehensive discussion of sex and gender. *Transsexual* people are those whose anatomical and physiological sex are in conflict with their self-concept as a male or female. Sometimes the term *gender dysphoria* is used to describe transsexuals, or those biological males who recognize themselves as females or those biological females who recognize themselves as males, both describing being "trapped in the wrong body."

Finally, there are transvestites. *Transvestites* are those individuals who cross-dress or present themselves in the typical appearance of the other sex. Because it is more acceptable for women to dress in men's suits and pants, transvestites are more commonly males in female clothing, makeup, and hairdos. (For more, see Chapter 5.)

From the time of birth, the process of social scripting and other socializing factors related to gender identity begin, and these affect the individual's construction of his or her personal gender identity and gender roles. Earlier we talked about child rearing that begins as soon as a sex assignment is made. Social scripting can be observed (and experienced) in the ways infants are handled by adults, beginning in the nursery. Typically rough handling for boys and cuddling for girls are observed, and even the colors in which babies are dressed or wrapped (blue for boys and pink for girls) are evidence of social scripting.

Throughout childhood, various messages are reinforced through play, sports, and other activities. Cultural and religious expectations of men and women play an important role in children's socially constructed gender definition of themselves, as do the traditional or nontraditional value systems operating in the family and community. In traditional families, children's behaviors are often ascribed to their gender in stereotypical ways, expecting boys to do the "heavy" jobs and girls to help with the housework. In nontraditional families, children are often encouraged to be more gender-neutral, and tasks are assigned that relate more to the child's ability.

GENDER SIMILARITIES AND DIFFERENCES

It almost seems as if society has a need to describe males and females in terms of polarized differences, then uses those differences to explain all sorts of behaviors and abilities. Yet, beyond the physical characteristics generally found in males that differ from those found in females (body structure, external genitalia, the presence of semen or ova, and so on), there is little research to support the notion that other major inherent differences exist that are not socially determined. For example, research is attempting to explain task- and cognition-related differences. Are males more capable of mathematical iterations and females more capable of creative conceptualizations? Are these biologically determined? Is one gender inherently more intelligent and more capable than another? Are characteristics such as "nurturing" or "aggressive" more characteristic of one sex or the other? Although much of the research has been about one sex and how it differs from the other, it is becoming more and more apparent that capabilities cannot be assigned to individuals on the basis of sex assignment alone.

The training of individuals through the messages they receive after their initial sex assignment as male or female and through puberty often determine the degree to which adults identify themselves in stereotypically masculine and feminine ways. The self-association with one or the other could drive a host of "expected" behaviors, relationship interactions, and even career choices. For example, among the stereotypical behavior expectations that are considered masculine are that men are stronger, less emotional, more aggressive, more competitive, and more courageous, whereas those considered stereotypically feminine are that women are softer, gentler, more passive, and fragile. In this context of masculinity and femininity, the more masculine a male defines himself, the less accepting and acknowledging he is likely to be of those characteristics in himself that he perceives as "feminine"; and the more feminine a woman defines herself, the less likely she will embrace her "masculine" characteristics.

It is not these concepts of self that are of primary importance here but rather the polarization of them that results in restrictions, the valuing of one gender over the other, the potential decrease in self-concept, and the concept of others that can occur. Stereotypical characteristics establish opposing roles, and the discussions surrounding them often become ones of deciding which is the "winning" or preferred role and therefore which is the "losing" or less desired one. Furthermore, these defined characteristics create inequality and inequities in society, education, and interpersonal relationships. They tend to limit people from reaching their individual potential.

As noted earlier in this chapter, a body of literature explains both masculine and feminine characteristics as human characteristics that can be embraced in one's self by members of both genders (the concept of androgyny), rather than as a polarized conceptualization. Such a self-definition empowers people to embrace more fully the breadth of human behaviors, attitudes, and beliefs, not limited by sex or gender. Many people believe that a society's strict notions of masculinity and femininity have changed to a more androgynous posture over the past 20 years or so. Others believe that there is still a long way to go. Hence, it is the goal of human sexuality education to present the gender-related information in an unbiased manner so that young people can create personally meaningful gender identities and select gender-neutral roles more reflective of their individual characteristics.

GENDER ISSUES IN SCHOOLS

Because children, beginning at least by their 5th year if not earlier, spend a large portion of their waking life in schools, it is important to provide the human sexuality educator with an understanding of relevant gender issues as they are experienced developmentally in elementary, middle, and secondary classrooms. Not only do these experiences have implications for the curriculum and student learning, but, through modeling, they influence children's gender identity, gender roles, behaviors, and attitudes. These gender experiences are practices or policies in schools that differentiate the learning experience in ways that might limit opportunities for children based on their classification as male or female.

Moreover, gender-related experiences address educationally relevant processes and skills that have an impact on an individual's notions of him- or herself as they relate to the person's gender (Koch, 2002). Among the questions educators should ask are: How can teaching practices in sexuality education integrate the understanding of gender issues as part of the learning environment? How might the influence of socialized constructions of students as male or female affect their acquisition of personal life skills?

What Is Gender Equity in Education?

Gender equity in education refers to educational practices that are fair and just, free from gender-related bias or favoritism with concern for all (Klein, Ortman, & Friedman, 2002). An awareness of the role of gender in learning and behavior can help educators avoid the trap of limiting children's growth by making and acting on stereotypical assumptions about individual students' abilities and development.

Although implying quality education, equal opportunities, and access for all students, gender *equity* differs from gender *equality*. Gender equality sets up a comparison between males and females, asking, "Are they receiving the same education?" (American Association of University Women [AAUW], 1998). Gender equity poses a different question for the classroom dynamic: Do students receive the right education to achieve a shared standard of excellence? Gender equity asserts that males and females do *not* necessarily need the same things to achieve shared outcomes. Gender equity is *not* sameness or equality; it is equity of outcomes, access to achievement, and opportunity. Hence, equitable education specifically addresses the needs of all people rather than questioning whether any particular gender group receives the same thing as the other (AAUW, 1998).

The field of gender equity in education generally acknowledges that equitable classroom environments have the following attributes in common (AAUW, 1992, 1995, 1998; McIntosh, 2000):

- Classrooms are caring communities where individuals feel safe.
- Understanding is promoted among peers.
- Classrooms are free from violence and peer or adult harassment.
- Classrooms have routines and procedures that ensure equal access to instructional materials and extracurricular activities.
- Classrooms have a "gender agenda," referring to the deconstruction of gendered expectations for students and encouraging full participation of each student, including the expression of non-stereotyped behaviors.
- Classrooms address the avoided curriculum by exploring those who have been omitted and by integrating avoided topics such as sexuality, violence, abuse, and gender politics.
- Classrooms address the lived experience of students by providing assignments or projects that develop all students' capacities to see their life experiences as part of knowledge, where students are authorities of their own experiences and contribute to the classroom textbooks by creating "textbooks of their lives" (Style, 1998).

Much of the research on gender in schools involves the study of boys and girls as separate entities and does not sufficiently explain how changes in the educational settings for one gender may affect the learning or experiences of the other. Moreover, the multiethnic and diverse social environments that are increasingly represented in schools compromise generalizations about expectations within gender groups. For example, can we describe girls' learning patterns, academic successes, self-esteem, and body image concepts without accounting for the differences influenced by their race, socioeconomic status, and other traits? The more recent educational discussion challenges us to acknowledge that there are fewer differences between males and females than among individuals or other groups.

Significantly, people still tend to assert that "boys will be boys" or "girls will be girls" in moments when their behavior matches a traditional stereotype about masculinity or femininity—for example, when a girl plays with dolls or a boy plays with guns. People rarely invoke the phrase in response to the myriad and more typical moments when children act more alike than dissimilar in their basic human qualities. Hence, when schools acknowledge that boys will be boys when they are nurturing or crying and girls will be girls when they are aggressive and assertive, they will be more reinforcing of their nongender-stereotypical behaviors. They will thus indicate one way that teachers in gender-equitable schools are both informed by and seek to deconstruct the socialized ways children mature into adulthood.

What Does the Gender Equity Research in Education Say?

The central question remains, To what extent do classroom teachers, school administrators, counselors, and peers limit the development of young people through promoting gender stereotyping and gender-biased classroom practices and school policies? How do these biases and limitations influence young people's gender identity and in turn their sexuality?

Beginning in the 1970s and continuing through the early 1990s, the gender-equity research consistently revealed differential treatment of girls and boys in the same classrooms with the same teacher, experiencing the same curriculum (Koch, 2002). This was because classrooms continued to be microcosms of society mirroring the gender roles that teachers and students developed through their own socialization patterns. Both ingrained in our individual identity and mediated by social class and ethnicity, gender roles informed much of the behavior we observed in classrooms and then, by extrapolation, in society at large. Gender-equitable schools, then, are those where there is equal access and the outcomes of education would not be predictable based on sex or, for that matter, race, ethnicity, or socioeconomic status (L. Phillips, cited in AAUW, 2001). Moreover, programs that were established to benefit one sex or another would be decreased and their characteristics recognized to be helpful to both sexes.

Common Gender Issues for Teachers

Although teaching environments are moving toward more equitable classrooms, one may still observe classroom practices that support or classify children's learning styles and behaviors by sex or gender. Here are some examples:

- Classroom teachers who engage boys in question-and-answer periods more frequently than girls. Involving boys more actively in the classroom dialogue has been seen as a way to control male behavior in the classroom and has often been a response to male aggressiveness.

- Classroom discourse in which boys who frequently raise their hands, sometimes impulsively, sometimes without even knowing the answer, are given preference over girls, who tend not to raise their hand as often or are overlooked frequently when they do
- Teachers who call on boys more frequently for responses and coach boys for correct responses more frequently than they do girls
- Teachers who tend to praise young girls for how they dress and wear their hair
- Teachers who tend to ask boys more open-ended, thought-provoking questions than they might ask girls, with the underlying expectation that boys are capable of greater abstract thinking
- Teachers who reprimand girls exhibiting boisterous behavior and impulsively calling out responses while not reprimanding boys who routinely exhibit the same behaviors
- Teachers who interpret girls' silence and fear of asking questions as not understanding some aspect of what is being taught
- Teachers who tend to give boys more of all types of teacher's attention in classrooms and who are given more time to talk in class
- Teachers who tend to offer more praise, criticism, remediation, and acceptance to boys than they do to girls
- Teachers who give boys harsher punishment than girls for the same offense and who unduly punish girls when exhibiting more stereotypical male social behavior
- Teachers who are invested in the silence of the girls, believing that girls who call attention to themselves, who are not quiet, social, and well behaved in classrooms, are not acting appropriately
- Teachers who sanction "good girl" behavior in elementary classrooms as a way of maintaining their vision of proper classroom management
- Teachers who tend to offer different types of praise, rewarding girls for their appearance or the appearance of their work, while praising boys for the ways in which they solve a problem or accomplish a task. This approach can support girls learning that their appearance matters in ways that are not valid for boys. Being pretty, cute, thin, charming, alluring, well dressed, or sexy are attributes that some girls aspire to because those qualities are valued for them by adults and media messages.
- Teachers who tend to exhibit longer wait times for boys to answer questions than for girls. (*Wait time* refers to the period of time between asking a question and calling on a student for a response.) Although the use of longer wait times may happen as a means of keeping interest and managing boys' classroom behavior, it supports higher-order and more critical thinking and is often more expected of boys than of girls.
- Teachers who tend to coach boys for the correct answers through prodding and cajoling but go on to the next student when a girl has an incorrect response (Sadker & Sadker, 1995)

Teachers often believe that they treat girls and boys in the same way; research still reveals that they frequently do not. The teacher's gender has little bearing on the treatment; it is the gender of the student that determines the differential behavior. Several researchers have noted that consistent gender-biased practices ultimately contribute to lowered self-esteem especially for girls, but these can be remedied by intervention strategies (Sadker & Sadker, 1995; Chapman, 1997). However, awareness of gender-stereotyped behavior alone is not sufficient to change behavior because well-intended teacher behaviors have been ingrained and practiced for so many years that teachers automatically respond in certain ways to boys differently than they do to girls (Orenstein, 1994). These school experiences can either enhance or detract from the more gender-stereotypical behavior patterns that children develop and maintain into adulthood.

FAMILY, COMMUNITY, AND PEER INFLUENCES ON GENDER

Bandura's (1977) social learning theory explains the influence of behaviors that are modeled and how they will shape the future behavior of individuals. Behavioral theorists explain the influence of reinforcement on the maintenance of behavior. It is believed that reinforcement of gender identity, gender roles, and individual notions of masculinity and femininity are influenced by what children observe in their family, community, and peer group, as they develop.

Family

From the time one is classified as male or female, the parental interactions, the manner in which the young child observes significant other's behavior, and the treatment the child receives in the earliest gender roles and gender-related behaviors formulate that person's gender identity. The linear modeling of the same-sex parent is thought to have the greatest impact on what young children expect of themselves.

Where the family encourages aggressiveness, strength, financial acumen, and the like, among its males, and compliance, attractive appearance, and peacemaker roles among its females, children will adopt these stereotypical behavior patterns. On the other hand, if the observed family behaviors follow a less gender-defined example, then the children will exhibit less gender-defined behaviors.

Community

It is only recently that late childhood/preadolescent sports, particularly organized sports, are encouraged for girls in the same way as for boys. Even so, boys who are competitive and aggressive in their sport activities are still more powerfully reinforced as successful than are aggressive and competitive girls. Aggressiveness has become less acceptable today than in the past, but any weakness, fear, or gentle behavior still labels a young boy a "wimp" and compromises his position among his peers. Boys whose interests do not include sports or those who are less athletic during these earlier years experience challenges to their self-esteem and gender identity. Girls' disinterest in sports, however, is more readily accepted.

As the need for recognition and acceptance grows during adolescence, worth is reinforced by physical appearance. Although culture plays an important role in stereotypical notions of masculinity, a well-defined muscular appearance seems to be a desirable trait across many cultures. Short, skinny, or overweight young men, negatively reinforced by peer and community messages about their appearance, become dissatisfied with their body image and in turn with their self-concept. This dissatisfaction is similar in character in young heterosexual as well as homosexual boys (Westheimer & Lopater, 2004). "How big am I?" "How strong am I?" "How aggressive at sports can I be?" These questions are asked by many young men. Puberty, marking the growth of the genitalia, is another marker for young men to assess their masculinity and sexuality. The larger the penis, the more "manly" a young male feels. This characteristic is often employed as a gauge of how well a young man will satisfy a sexual partner.

The media often portrays unrealistic images of what physical beauty is in women. These images may be somewhat different across cultures, but large, heavy women often fall outside the realm of what is defined as feminine. In similar ways as for men, women too often derive their body image and sexual worth by unrealistic measures. Large breasts and thin, shapely bodies are accepted as valuable commodities in the heterosexual marketplace. For girls, "How pretty am I?" and "What do I have to do to be popular?" reveal the messages of importance.

Girls who are encouraged to be successful are often not considered to have reached their ultimate success until they find a man who will marry them. The expression "having it all" used to be having a husband and children for whom she is the primary caretaker. Today it is more a description of the woman who can hold down an impressive job and have a husband and children whose primary responsibility remains largely hers.

How do these considerations affect sexuality? The double standard is still alive and well. We have become more accepting as a society of women's sexual needs and sexual interests, but men are still expected to be more sexually savvy. It is men who are expected to know how to please women and to be the teachers about sex to women. Sexually aggressive and sexually knowledgeable women create anxiety in men and are often labeled as "loose" or "promiscuous," terms rarely applied to men.

Peers

During adolescence, when sexual feelings are stimulated by hormones and puberty is marked by changes in the genitals, boys' sexual needs are acknowledged and girls' are discouraged. The sexual dance of heterosexual boy adolescents is less about intimacy and relationships than it is about having their first sexual experiences. It is more about having sex for the sake of the experience without much real consideration for the partner. Boys reinforce each other by affirming how often and how many times they have had sex. Parents are less apt to tell boys to abstain and more apt to encourage them "to be careful" and not "get a girl pregnant." The experience and expectations for homosexual adolescent boys is more complicated because sexual activities with same-sex partners are rarely encouraged or reinforced except with traditionally heterosexual messages, as gay boys are often still "closeted" (see Chapter 5).

Heterosexual girls are encouraged to refuse sex at least until they have established a love relationship. The catch-22 for them is that they also come to believe that their popularity and or their ability to have a relationship is based on their sexual attractiveness and their ability to be sexually flirtatious without actually "doing it" or at least not as frequently as their male counterparts. Although sex within a relationship is more acceptable than ever before, having sex during adolescence, for the sake of the experience alone, is still not widely acceptable for girls. Adolescent heterosexual girls are increasingly performing oral sex on adolescent boys, while the reverse is far less likely. Frequently the oral sex is performed in groups or between friends and not intimate partners. Some report that they feel safer from contracting HIV/AIDS (see Chapter 10) and others that they are "practicing" for their future love relationships.

If adolescents do participate in sexual intercourse, the degree to which they protect themselves against STIs or pregnancy is more directly related to the degree of pressure they are feeling to participate rather than having made a personal decision of readiness. It is acceptable for adolescent men to wear a condom, but adolescent women are often still too embarrassed to suggest its use and are still too often regarded negatively when they do. It is young women who are flirtatious, but young men who choose and act on initiating dating and sex most frequently. Hence, adolescent women are less empowered to be equal in relationships and to assertively refuse or accept sexual encounters based on their own needs and desires.

Homosexual adolescents have additional concerns. Similar to young gay men, young lesbian women often find that their "closeted" selves do not provide opportunities during adolescence to experience relationships or to be studied for their similarities or differences from the heterosexual experience (see Chapter 5).

HEALTH LITERACY, PERSONAL SKILLS, AND SEXUAL HEALTH

Health literacy is the capacity of individuals to obtain, interpret, and understand basic health information and services, and the competence to use such information and services in ways that enhance health (Joint Committee on National Health Education Standards, 1995). The health-literate person is a critical thinker and problem solver; a responsible, productive citizen; a self-directed learner; and an effective communicator (Cleveland State University, 2003). In sexuality education, health literacy is supported by building confidence and competence with personal life skills that allow people to make healthy choices about their sexual behaviors. Each gender may demonstrate differing levels of competence in personal skills development due to modeling and other socially constructed phenomena. An understanding of these potential differences and how they do or do not influence learning about sexual relationships, attitudes, behaviors, and values will make instruction more effective. Experiencing pressures to conform, to be an accepted part of a learning community, and to be competent in social relationships are qualities manifested in different ways throughout the precollege education of students across and within genders, as well as across other sociocultural groups.

With regard to gender education, the role of the teacher is in understanding and valuing differences where they exist, not limiting or calling attention to those that are covertly or overtly limiting, and helping students develop capacities that stretch the limits of gender stereotypes. Moreover, when teachers themselves exhibit deliberate and planned gender-fair practices in classrooms, the result is a more equitable learning environment and a greater likelihood of students to incorporate these practices in their life choices and interpersonal relationships.

Personal Life Skills: A Gender-Developmental Approach in Schools

As discussed in Chapter 1, schools play an important role in developing and/or reinforcing personal life skills, including communication, conflict resolution, and decision making. It is believed, for example, that expressing feelings and thoughts in a public sphere begins in school. Some research indicates that the cultural differences between men and women explain their later communication and decision-making styles. For example, when it comes to communication, some research suggests that men and women are socialized in markedly different cultures; in fact, when they communicate with one another, they do so as they would with individuals from an entirely different culture, not always understanding one another's meanings (Tannen, 1990). This research goes on to explain that women engage in "rapport talk," or talk for interaction and establishing connections, whereas men engage in "report talk," or talk, even in their private conversations, as if they were public speaking or giving a report. McGinty, Knox, and Zusman (2003) describe women as more attentive to nonverbal messages than are men. These communication styles emerge from social messages received throughout development and have implications for how people will communicate in their sexual relationships.

Conflict resolution can also be discussed through a gender lens. Research suggests that gender surfaces in the ways people interpret and give meaning to conflict and in the ways that they negotiate resolutions. Much of the research on conflict resolution emerged from workplace conflict studies (Birkoff, 2004) and is easily extrapolated to intimate relationships. Conflict resolution styles can be explained by the way women and men differ in their social construction of the conditions under which the conflict exists, such as power inequalities and a sense of vulnerability, especially in terms of aggression and violence. Some studies found that women and men differed in the ways that they talked about their conflicts. For example, women talked in depth and at length about the context of the dispute, particularly focusing on their involvement in the relationship with the other party; whereas men used more rational, linear, and legalistic language to talk about their disputes. Women talked more about fairness in a way that incorporated both their material interests and the network of relationships in a dispute (Birkoff, 2004). These differences are outgrowths of earlier learned behaviors. Teachers who are successful in addressing classroom interaction strategies that further the growth and development of both females and males are ones who are aware of the research findings about gender and equity and who employ conscious strategies on behalf of creating equitable environments.

PERSONAL LIFE SKILLS IN ELEMENTARY SCHOOL EDUCATION

The development of gender roles, behavior, and attitudes beginning as early as preschool fosters less gender-stereotypical life choices in later life. Because children come to elementary schools having already experienced biased messages about themselves and others based on gender, it behooves teachers to be cognizant of gender inequities and model more individual, non-gender-based educational strategies in their classrooms.

Communication, Decision Making, and Conflict Management. A "gender agenda" in an elementary classroom would include using gender-inclusive language and encouraging activities that deconstruct the limitations of gender-stereotypical behaviors. In early childhood classrooms, this approach could include arranging the primary classroom in a way that encourages mixed-gender play and providing children with classroom rules that discourage exclusions by gender. The rule that all children can play in all areas of the classroom—in the block corner, in the make-believe corner, in the dolls area, in the tools and crafts corner, and at the computer stations—stimulates mixed-gender play and decreases stereotyping.

Whether communication is of a verbal or nonverbal nature, some differences in early childhood experiences with communication have implications for educators. For example, frequently it is young boys who have been encouraged to use their bodies to intimidate and bully others. This bullying behavior is an expression of their feelings and also a confirmation of their masculinity. Boys' communication is often dominated by these body movements. Being overly harsh in reprimanding boys when they do exhibit these inappropriate behaviors only reinforces unspoken hostility and does not encourage boys to express their feelings verbally. From the earliest grades, anger needs to be channeled; feelings need to be talked about and emotions expressed as a model of communicating that is more socially acceptable. The outcomes of these healthy practices might be translated later in life into an increased capability for discussions about feelings, especially in intimate relationships.

Girls, on the other hand, are frequently praised for using soft voices, waiting their turn to speak, and exhibiting "good girl" behaviors in classrooms. This kind of reinforcement does not encourage the development of assertive language or refusal skills necessary for the development of a healthy sexuality, particularly in fending off peer pressure to conform or, later, coercion to participate in sexual behaviors not of their choosing.

PERSONAL LIFE SKILLS IN MIDDLE SCHOOL EDUCATION

For many years, early adolescence was identified as a time of heightened psychological risk, particularly for girls (Brown & Gilligan, 1992). Girls at this stage in their development were observed to lose their vitality, their voice, their resilience, their self-confidence, and, often, their "spunkiness" (Orenstein, 1994). These behaviors are still too often invisible in middle grade classrooms since teachers and students alike see them as "normal" for girls at this time in their development and not as behaviors influenced by culture, the hidden curriculum, or gender socialization. This view underscores the importance of defining and redefining a "gender issue" in the classroom (Koch & Irby, 2002).

The bullying of boys by boys and the fear of being called a "sissy" or "fag" profoundly affects middle school boys and reinforces their notion of maintaining gender norms (M. S. Kimmel, cited in AAUW, 2001). Kimmel suggests that being seen as a sissy or weak is really the dominant fear for boys. He goes on to explain that it is easier and more acceptable for girls to be "tomboys" than it is for boys to be "sissies," and he further suggests that it could be homophobia that is the underlying fear. Other researchers have noted that in the middle grades boys have difficulty expressing themselves, particularly in writing reflective journals (Bowman, 2001). Encouraging these skills will develop more reflective and responsive adults.

Communication and Decision Making. Practicing behaviors that increase communication and decision-making skills across gender groups is but one way to decrease learned gender stereotypes. One of the learning experiences described at the end of this chapter, inviting both girls and boys in middle school to imagine that they wake up the next day as a member of the other sex, is one way to improve communication skills and make the gender agenda overt. One middle school teacher asked the students to make a list of how their lives would be different if they were members of the other sex (Logan, 1997). Through carefully structured discussions, students come to see that they are more similar than different. This can be an important step toward mutual respect and an understanding of the power of communication.

One middle school classroom teacher approaches gender issues in the classroom by using sentence starters such as "Being a female means . . . " or "Being a male means . . . ," according to their gender. Then students respond in terms of the other sex. This gets discussion going and quickly uncovers the expectations each gender has for its own and the other gender (Mitchell, 1996, p. 77). Additionally, inviting middle school students to analyze picture books, popularly read magazines, and media presentations through the lens of gender proves powerful as students research the images and draw conclusions about the messages.

Helping girls and boys talk together is a major goal for middle school education. Yet students too rarely have programs and places where they can talk openly and critically about gender with one another. The negotiation of gender identity is a major element of boys' and girls' lives inside and outside school. Susan Bailey, who participated in a professional conversation sponsored by AAUW (2001), has remarked that "one of the things we need to do more explicitly is to talk about these [gender] issues with students of both sexes because when you can talk about gender, it isn't invisible anymore." The learning experiences included in this chapter are designed to build on this concept and listen to girls and boys as they express their conflicts and emotions. This type of open communication helps students build this skill and make decisions for themselves based on authentic dialogue and not on stereotypes.

Stress and Relationship Management

Females respond to stress differently than males. This difference has important implications for managing the classroom and for developing stress and relationship management skills in middle school and high school. Stress research has revealed that, when people experience stress, they trigger a hormonal cascade that alerts the body to stand and fight or to flee as fast as possible. Now researchers have identified the phenomenon called "tend and befriend," suggesting that friendships between women tend to counteract a considerable amount of much of the severe stress experienced daily. It appears that a female biological reaction to stress produces the hormone oxytocin, which some research suggests encourages a woman to tend to children or to gather with other women rather than to fight or flee (Taylor, Klein, Lewis, Gruenewald, Gurung, & Updegraff, 2003). Testosterone, however, seems to reduce the effects of oxytocin, while estrogen enhances them. Keeping abreast of the research is important as we help adolescents express themselves and engage in conflict resolution and stress and relationship management.

Segregation by gender, a common occurrence in elementary school activities, has implications for how communication occurs between girls and boys in middle school and how they behave with one another. Moreover, when boys in middle school want to develop friendships with girls, adults tend to explain the friendships in sexualized relationship terms, and boys, embarrassed, feel they need to hide their friendships or discontinue them

(W. Pollack, cited in AAUW, 2001). It is important for teachers to intervene and promote times of cooperation and acceptance of friend-to-friend relationships across the sexes that are not always interpreted as more intimate connections (B. Thorne, cited in AAUW, 2001).

PERSONAL LIFE SKILLS AND SECONDARY SCHOOL EDUCATION

Secondary students are at risk in many areas of relationship management, stress management, and conflict resolution that have roots in gender identity. Some risks for secondary students, through the lens of gender, include those discussed in the following paragraphs.

Girls in secondary schools are more vulnerable to sexual violence and harassment. One out of every five girls says she has been sexually or physically abused; one in four girls shows signs of depression (AAUW, 1998). Girls are often underdiagnosed with attention deficit disorder (ADD), resulting in less intervention at early ages. Their early symptoms go unnoticed because, although they are inattentive and lack focus, they do not usually exhibit hyperactive or disruptive behaviors. Thus, by the time they reach middle and high school, girls with ADD have an increased incidence of school anxiety and depression. This condition has unfortunate implications for their development through high school.

Secondary-level boys repeat grades and drop out of school at considerably higher rates than do girls. However, girls who repeat a grade are more likely to drop out than boys who are held back. Not only is being held back more harmful to girls, so is dropping out. Girls who drop out are less likely to return and complete school and are also correlated strongly with lower-income families and higher rates of unintended pregnancy. Dropout rates are especially high among Hispanic girls.

Boys are more likely than girls to engage in high-risk behavior, experimenting with drugs and alcohol, and they are more prone to accidents caused by violence. Girls and young women, however, become addicted to cigarettes, alcohol, and drugs more quickly and for different reasons than boys. Teen girls often begin smoking and drinking to relieve stress or alleviate depression, whereas boys do it for thrills or heightened social status. Girls' addiction is faster, on lesser amounts, and they suffer the consequences faster and more severely (National Center for Addiction and Substance Abuse [NCASA], 2003).

In secondary school, boys' misbehavior is more frequently punished than is girls. More than 70 percent of school suspensions involve boys. As they enter high school, girls are likelier than boys to compare themselves physically and academically to their new peers, increasing doubts about how they feel about themselves.

Although we have made considerable progress in increasing career and academic pursuits for both men and women, interesting negative results still abound. Young women today are encouraged, more equally with men, to pursue their interest in math, science, and technology than in the past. They are no longer viewed as less competent in these academic disciplines.

Yet, although more women are encouraged to select medicine or early childhood teaching as a career choice, it does not appear that men are equally as encouraged to choose nursing or, for that matter, elementary education as their profession. We speak about valuing family and the caretaking of children in our society, but we do not value caretaking equally for both genders. Women are still encouraged to be primary caregivers, and when men choose to be home parents, they are not as valued as much as are women.

Relationship, Stress, and Conflict Management.   Gender identity and notions of masculinity and femininity are solidified during the high school years, especially as they relate to practices in interpersonal relationships. High school students can be encouraged to reflect on the relationships that they have experienced in their family and how they are reflected in their own notions of the roles and behaviors that they will exhibit in their intimate relationships. What sexual behaviors they will participate in, who will initiate, how they will talk about their sexual interests with one another, and so forth, have gender-related considerations. Whether the couple is same-sex or other-sex, the roles and behavior choices do not have to be restricted by gender stereotypes.

Teaching human sexuality at the secondary level requires that teachers (1) examine gendered classroom and social interactions, (2) search for teaching practices that encourage people to express their emotions and demonstrate their competence, (3) and explore their own internal landscapes for an understanding of their gendered selves that could inform their teaching behavior. The following checklist may be useful:

Whose voices are most dominant in your classroom?
Who are the best students in your health class?
How are students grouped in cooperative activities?
What are the strengths that the boys bring to the classroom?
What are the strengths that the girls bring to the classroom?
In what ways, if any, do you deconstruct gender stereotypes?
Are the boys and girls in your class more similar than different? In what way(s)?
How often do you notice girl–boy friendships?
What's wrong with the expression "Boys will be boys"?
Why is the consideration of gender issues important in developing personal life skills?
What are some of the gender issues in relationships?

SUMMARY

This chapter on gender has explored the biopsychosocial influences on students as they mature into adulthood. Acknowledging the impact of familial, community, and school behaviors and expectations on young people's gender identity development requires understanding the power of modeled behaviors and the social construction of gender-related phenomena. The roles and behaviors that parents exhibit at home, the roles and behaviors that teachers display in schools, and the messages in the popular media all have powerful implications for students' learning about gender. Young people exploring gender roles, gender identity, and gender stereotypes will come with a variety of ethnocultural and personal values and experiences that influence their personal gender identity.

Discussing the limitations of gender role stereotyping on the range of human possibilities is a challenge for sexuality educators. It benefits students to reflect on their own future careers, relationships, and personal goals and how these may be impacted by self- or other-imposed limitations associated with gender.

What men want and need and what women want and need from one another in a same- or other-sex relationship has been steeped in stereotypical limitations that have become accepted as facts and sometimes self-fulfilling prophecies. For example, many people still believe that women have less sexual desire and fewer sexual needs than men. This notion has limited women's freedom to express their needs and in some cases to feel them at all, particularly in heterosexual relationships. One can only extrapolate these unequal gender influences to other relationships involving men and women. Hence, the way gender-specific expectations in a sexual relationship can imbalance the relationship is important to discuss.

WEBSITES

Gender Change: www.genderhealth.org

Gender and Law: www.academic.udayton.edu/gender

Gender and Sexism Ethics Updates: www.ethics.acusd.edu/gender.html

Gender and Society: www.gas.sagepub.com

Gender Education and Advocacy: www.gender.org

Gender Equity in Education: www.ed.gov/offices/ODS/g-equity.html

Gender Equity Introduction: www.genderequity.org

Gender Identity Disorder and Transgenderism: www.genderpsychology.org

Gender Issues Research Center: www.gendercenter.org

International Foundation for Gender Education: www.ifge.org

Kinsey Institute: www.kinseyinstitute.org/about

National Center for Gender Physiology: www.genderphysiology.org

UN Information and Resources on Gender Equality: www.un.org/womenwatch

Women and Gender Studies: www.libr.org/wss/WSSLinks/index.html

REFERENCES

American Association of University Women (AAUW). (1992). *How schools shortchange girls: A study of major findings on girls and education.* Researched by the Wellesley College Center for Research on Women. Washington, DC: American Association of University Women Educational Foundation.

AAUW. (1995). *How schools shortchange girls: The AAUW report.* Washington, DC: American Association of University Women Educational Foundation.

AAUW. (1998). *Gender gaps: Where schools still fail on children.* Washington, DC: American Association of University Women Educational Foundation.

AAUW. (2001). *Beyond the gender wars: A conversation about girls, boys, and education.* Washington, DC: American Association of University Women Educational Foundation.

Bandura, A. (1977). *Social learning theory.* New York: General Learning.

Birkoff, J. E. (2004). *Gender, conflict and conflict resolution.* Toronto: International Academy of Mediators.

Bowman, B. (Ed.). (2001). *Eager to learn: Educating our preschoolers.* Washington, DC: National Academy Press.

Brown, L. M., & Gilligan, C. (1992). *Meeting at the crossroads: Women's psychology and girls' development.* Cambridge, MA: Harvard University Press.

Chapman, A. (1997). *A great balancing act: Equitable education for girls and boys.* Washington, DC: National Association of Independent Schools.

Cleveland State University, Department of Health Education. (2003, May 15). *Why national health education standards?* Available online: www.csuohio.edu/healthed/standard.htm.

Joint Committee on National Health Education Standards. (1995). *National health education standards.* Reston, VA: Association for the Advancement of Health Education (1900 Association Drive, Reston, VA 22091).

Klein, S., Ortman, P., & Friedman, B. (2002). What is the field of gender equity in education? Questions & answers. In J. Koch & B. Irby (Eds.), *Defining and redefining gender equity in education.* Greenwich, CT: Infoage.

Koch, J. (2002). Gender issues in the classroom. In W. R. Reynolds & G. E. Miller (Eds.), *Educational psychology,* Vol. 7 of the *Comprehensive handbook of psychology,* I. B. Weiner, Editor in Chief. New York: Wiley.

Koch, J., & Irby, B. (Eds.). (2002). *Defining and redefining gender equity in education.* Greenwich, CT: Infoage.

Logan, J. (1997). *Teaching stories.* New York: Kodansha.

Logan, J. (1998). Guess what, Ms. Logan? In C. L. Nelson & K. A. Wilson (Eds.), *Seeding the process of multicultural education* (pp. 213–226). Plymouth, MN: Minnesota Inclusiveness Program.

McGinty, K., Knox, D., & Zusman, M. E. (2003). Nonverbal and verbal communication in "involved" and "casual" relationships among college students. *College Student Journal, 37,* 68–71.

McIntosh, P. (2000, May 25). *A learning community with feminist values.* Address at Ewha Woman's University, Seoul, Korea.

Mitchell, D. (1996). Approaching race and gender issues in the context of the language arts classroom. *English Journal, 85*(8), 77–81.

National Center for Addiction and Substance Abuse (NCASA). (2003). *The formative years: Pathways to substance abuse among girls and young women at 8–22.* New York: Columbia University National Center for Addiction and Substance Abuse.

Orenstein, P. (1994). *School girls: Young women, self-esteem and the confidence gap.* New York: Doubleday.

Sadker, M., & Sadker, D. (1995). *Failing at fairness: How America's schools cheat girls.* New York: Scribner's.

Style, E. (1998). Curriculum as a window and mirror. In C. L. Nelson & K. A. Wilson (Eds.), *Seeding the process of multicultural education* (pp. 149–156). Plymouth, MN: Minnesota Inclusiveness Program.

Tannen, D. (1990). *You just don't understand: Women and men in conversation.* New York: Ballantine.

Taylor, S. E., Klein, L. C., Lewis, B. P., Gruenewald, T. L., Gurung, R. A. R., & Updegraff, J. (2000). Female responses to stress: Tend and befriend, not fight or flight. *Psychological Review, 107*(3), 41.

Westheimer, R. K., & Lopater, S. (2004). *Human sexuality: A psychosocial perspective* (2nd ed.). Baltimore, MD: Lippincott, Williams & Wilkins.

LEARNING EXPERIENCES

After the learning experiences described here, early elementary school students will be able to

- Explain similarities between boys and girls.
- Recognize common gender stereotypes and gender-biased language.
- Describe roles in the family and deconstruct gender limitations associated with roles.

By later elementary school, they will be able to

- Recognize gender-stereotypical language.
- Deconstruct gender stereotypes associated with sports and career choices.
- Identify cultural factors associated with gender.

During middle school, they will be able to

- Recognize the influence of culture and media on gender roles.
- Evaluate their notions of masculinity and femininity.
- Recognize their gender biases.
- Advocate for gender equity.
- Explain the limitations of gender stereotypes on life choices.

The learning experiences will provide high school students with skills to

- Describe the meaning of *gender, gender role, gender identity,* and *sex role stereotypes.*
- Identify gender biases and how they limit or affect relationships.
- Explain the concept of gender equity.
- Recognize personal gender bias and associated limitations on their personal career and relationship choices.

LEARNING EXPERIENCE 1

TITLE: Something Special about Me

GRADE LEVELS: K–3

TIME REQUIREMENT: 1 hour, once a week (number of weeks determined by the curriculum sequence)

LEARNING CONTEXT

This learning experience can be used at any point in establishing classroom community and validating the importance of each individual student, female and male. The purpose of this activity is to provide a structured time when each student can be the center of the whole class's attention and to encourage appreciation of one another in ways not based on gender or class status. It is also designed to encourage the group to create a "gift" for one person. This experience encourages communication and decision making and introduces relationship management as the group reaches consensus about the contents of the final product.

NATIONAL LEARNING STANDARDS

4:   Students will analyze the influence of culture, media, technology, and other factors on health.

5:   Students will demonstrate the ability to use interpersonal communication skills to enhance health.

7:   Students will demonstrate the ability to advocate for personal, family, and community health.

PROCEDURE

Similar to show-and-tell, this experience invites only one student per week at an appointed time (usually the same day) when the selected student may, for 15 minutes, share something special with the class. The student may bring in something he or she made, something someone made for him or her, something the student found, or something from a public place. The student may read a poem, a favorite story, teach about her or his cultural background, or teach a song. The class focuses attention on the one student and asks questions about the presentation. Afterward, the class works together to make an affirmation poster, using paper or poster board, markers, or crayons. This poster for the focus student contains his or her profile (simply shine a flashlight to cast the student's shadow and trace it on to the paper). Students write affirmations of the student on the poster. You may also draw the student's name in large letters outlined and connected together. The affirmations that the group writes are usually based on the presentation.

INSTRUCTIONAL/ENVIRONMENTAL MODIFICATION

Students with difficulty with fine-motor skills and language proficiency will need extra assistance.

RESOURCES

Paper or poster board; markers or crayons; flashlight

ASSESSMENT PLAN

Ask the following questions of each focus student:

1. How did it feel when you were the focus? In what ways was it fun? Frightening? Why?
2. What did you learn about your classmates in this activity?
3. What did you learn about yourself when you read what your classmates wrote about you?
4. How did you feel when you read your poster? How do you feel when you look at it in your room?

REFLECTION

Giving each child a time to feel special provides a good foundation for a gender-equitable classroom while encouraging communication skills and building self-esteem. Often, in classrooms boys dominate discussions; however, this activity gives each student in the class an opportunity to feel special.

REFERENCE

This activity is adapted and modified from *Cooperative Learning, Cooperative Lives* (pp. 53–54), by N. Schniedewind and E. Davidson, 1987, Dubuque, IA: Brown.

LEARNING EXPERIENCE 2

TITLE: Rebecca's Always Crying

GRADE LEVELS: 4–6

TIME REQUIREMENT: 1.5 hours

LEARNING CONTEXT
This activity is designed to help students distinguish between constructive and destructive ways to change another student's behavior. It encourages cross-gender communication and helps to confront stereotypes. This experience can be used to introduce gender issues in your own classroom context or as part of a larger unit on stereotypes.

NATIONAL LEARNING STANDARD
> 5:   Students will demonstrate the ability to use interpersonal communication skills to enhance health.

PROCEDURE
Working in pairs, students read the story "Rebecca's Always Crying" (which follows) to each other and then work together to complete the questions. With younger students, the teacher can read the story. Students consider the discussion questions on the handout among themselves.

As part of a teacher-facilitated discussion, discuss the answers that students have placed on their worksheets, and gather behavior-changing ideas and ideas about gender from each of the working pairs. Ask, "Are there other problems in our class that we could work together to solve?"

RESOURCE
"Rebecca's Always Crying" handout

ASSESSMENT PLAN
Have students become involved in their own assessment of this activity by asking them to rate its success using the scoring guide included on the handout.

REFLECTION
This lesson is important because it engages the class, as a learning community, in problem solving and in problem generation. It gives the students permission to express their own feelings and engage in conflict resolution, first about a fictional situation and then about their own context. Issues of gender arise when crying is considered solely "girl" behavior.

REFERENCE
This activity is adapted and modified from *Cooperative Learning, Cooperative Lives* (pp. 65, 78), by N. Schniedewind and E. Davidson, 1987, Dubuque, IA: Brown.

Rebecca's Always Crying

"I didn't do anything to her, and she is crying again," moans Ben.

"Yeah, all I did was stretch and maybe touch her arm and she starts crying," adds Evan.

Jason says, "I don't see why we always have to be so careful of her. You can't even get near her."

"What do you usually do when Rebecca starts crying?" asks Ms. Bauer, the teacher.

"Tell her to stop, and tell her it is stupid and that she is a crybaby girl" said Evan and Jason.

"And does that help?" asks Ms. Bauer.

"No, she starts crying again because she says we are mean to her," says Jason.

Ben adds, "Yeah, and then the whole class has to wait until she stops in order to do something. You won't explain stuff to us or let us go anywhere while she's crying, and we are always late."

"Could you do something that would work better?" Ms. Bauer asks.

Discussion Questions

1. Why do some children cry more easily than others?

2. In what ways are Rebecca's classmates making her cry even when they do not mean to?

3. What could Rebecca's classmates do to help her to cry less often?

4. If they do cause her to cry, what could they do to make her stop?

5. What are some behaviors besides crying that we might want others to stop?

6. What could we do to help change those behaviors?

7. Why do most girls cry more easily than most boys?

8. When do *you* feel like crying?

Self-Assessment

This discussion made me think about things I had not thought of (circle one).
not at all   a little   a lot

We collected good ideas about what girls do and what boys do.
not at all   a little   a lot

We explored new ways to help people change their behaviors.
not at all   a little   a lot

The problem I did not get to discuss is _____

LEANING EXPERIENCE 3

TITLE: Draw a Scientist

GRADE LEVELS: 4–6

TIME REQUIREMENT: 45 minutes

LEARNING CONTEXT

This activity is designed to deconstruct stereotypes about gender, ability, and careers while emphasizing the importance of both males and females feeling socially entitled to many types of careers. It relates to the importance of scientists and health care workers creating environments where cures for diseases may flourish. The more diverse the scientific workforce becomes, the more probable that many points of view will be considered. This produces good science.

NATIONAL LEARNING STANDARD

4: Students will analyze the influence of culture, media, technology, and other factors on health.

PROCEDURE

At this point in your reading, you need to close this book. But first get a piece of paper and a pencil and find a firm writing surface. Close the book, and sketch a picture of what you think a scientist might look like. When you have completed the drawing, open the book again to this spot.

If you are like most other people, your scientist drawing will show a white male with one or more of the following characteristics: wild hair, eyeglasses, a white lab coat, a pocket protector, and some bubbling flasks. Both students and teachers frequently draw this popular image of the scientist. Of course, this image is a stereotype because it exaggerates what real scientists look like. The stereotype is reinforced by the scientist images we see in cartoons, movies, magazines, and the popular press. Such stereotypes become part of our belief systems and influence our future behavior. All too often, they limit what we do and think.

Provide your students with paper and crayons, pencils, or markers. Ask them to draw a picture of what they think a scientist might look like, and place a caption on their drawing. Ask the students to hold their pictures up as they form a horizontal line in front of the class. Ask those holding females to step forward; then ask those holding males to step forward; then those with wild hair, with test tubes, with explosions; and then explore other images. Students should be encouraged to talk about their pictures.

RESOURCES

Paper; crayons, pencils, or markers

ASSESSMENT PLAN

Ask students to respond to these questions in writing, working with a partner:

1. Who is omitted in this stereotype?
2. Does the type of person represented in the stereotype reflect the makeup of any elementary school class you have recently seen?
3. If the children in a typical classroom were omitted by the stereotype, how would that make them feel about science?
4. What other careers are gender stereotypes? What is an argument against "women only" and "men only" jobs? An argument for?

REFLECTION

You may suppose that stereotypes about scientists diminish as children mature. In fact, however, a study of more than 1,500 students in Grades K–8 revealed that the students' drawings of scientists became more stereotypical as the children got older. These students drew mostly white male scientists, suggesting that the stereotype persists despite recent changes in curriculum materials. It is important to note that scientists work in teams, and the more diverse the teams, the greater the possibility for varied observations and inferences and, in fact, better science. While promoting discussion of gender stereotypes, this learning experience helps to further communication about gender in the classroom.

REFERENCE

This activity is adapted from Janice Koch, *Science Stories: A Science Methods Book for Elementary School Teachers* (Boston: Houghton Mifflin, 2002).

LEARNING EXPERIENCE 4

TITLE: What If? A Gendered Journey

GRADE LEVELS: 7–9

TIME REQUIREMENT: 45 minutes

LEARNING CONTEXT

This experience promotes overt discussion about gender roles among students and about each gender's view of the other gender. It facilitates understanding by "outing" differences and similarities and promoting a nonjudgmental discussion of the lives of adolescent girls and boys. It has implications for introducing a unit on gender issues and stereotypes during middle and high school. Respecting privacy of students is important and students must know that they are offering their stories only as volunteers. They may also decline to participate by using the "pass" option established at the beginning of the semester.

NATIONAL LEARNING STANDARD

5: Students will demonstrate the ability to use interpersonal communication skills to enhance health. Performance indicators relate to interpersonal communication, refusal and negotiation skills, and conflict resolution.

PROCEDURE

Ask the students to clear everything off their desks except for a pen or pencil and a piece of blank paper. Ask them to put their heads down and close their eyes and take a journey back through time in their imagination, and then read this passage aloud:

"To begin, step out of your body and see yourself at your desk with your head down. Now, travel back in time until you are in fifth grade, then third grade. What are you wearing? Who is your teacher? What are you doing? See yourself at home; what does your room look like? Who are your friends? What do you do after school? Now, see yourself as a kindergartener; see how you are playing. What do you love to do? Travel back again until you are a baby. Look around your room. Notice things around you. Now travel back again and here you are, ready to be born! Everyone is excited and happy, waiting for your birth. Now here you are but this time imagine you are born as the other sex. Hence, if you are a boy, pretend you are born a girl. If you are a girl, pretend you are born a boy. See yourself as a baby, coming home, learning to walk, starting school, going through elementary school. Look at your room and your friends and your activities. Without talking to anybody, create a list of how your life seems different since you were born a person of the other sex."

Tape large sheets of paper labeled "MALES" and "FEMALES" onto the blackboard, and ask the students to write one thing from their list onto the sheets of paper. In this way, they come up and share their thoughts about the other sex and the lists get created. The important ground rule is that neither girls nor boys can judge what is being placed on the list even when it doesn't feel true for their gender. This activity is about getting to know what boys think being female is all about and what girls think being male is all about. When the lists are complete, the teacher facilitates the discussion of the items. When girls and boys in class have the opportunity to state what is true for them about being female and male, the students come to see that they are more alike than different. Very few pink and blue bedrooms abound; most are white, for example. Other more troubling items emerge, such as "If I were born a girl, I'd kill myself" or "If I were a boy, I would have more freedom." Help the class to analyze their beliefs and deconstruct the extreme stereotyping.

RESOURCES

Large sheets of paper or poster board; tape

ASSESSMENT PLAN

Ask students to reflect on the following questions in writing:

1. What did you think about this activity?
2. What, if anything, did you learn about members of the other sex?
3. What belief(s) surprised you the most? Why?
4. How would you like your life to be different?

REFLECTION

To keep classroom teaching about gender from falling into a war of the sexes, you must begin by allowing students to focus on their own attitudes, beliefs and feelings about their own and the other sex. Students need to recognize their own habits of sexual stereotyping before they can see them at work in the larger world. Gender work is about bringing a critical self-awareness into every corner of our lives. The important outcome of this activity is that students shift from a personal view of the other sex to an awareness that certain pressures and expectations are exerted on the other sex that may not fit who they are.

REFERENCE

This learning experience is adapted from Judy Logan, *Teaching Stories* (pp. 34–36) (New York: Kodansha, 1997).

LEARNING EXPERIENCE 5

TITLE: Carving Mount Rushmore

GRADE LEVELS: 10–12

TIME REQUIREMENTS: Two 45-minute periods

LEARNING CONTEXT

This exercise helps secondary students to focus on heroes and heroines and to share those images in a group setting. It helps students to see the gender issues implicit in who gets remembered in history and makes them aware that *greatness* is a term loaded with political and social implications. The idea of who defines "greatness" and who that definition serves is at the heart of this experience. Students are encouraged to think of greatness in terms of those currently contributing to furthering the social welfare of humanity, in a public or private way. This learning experience fosters communication and refusal skill building while improving relationship management.

NATIONAL LEARNING STANDARDS

4:   Students will analyze the influence of culture, media, technology, and other factors on health.

6:   Students will demonstrate the ability to use goal-setting and decision-making skills to enhance health.

PROCEDURE

Session 1

Form the class into groups of four. Ask the students whether they are familiar with the faces on Mount Rushmore (Thomas Jefferson, Abraham Lincoln, Theodore Roosevelt, and George Washington). Their first task is to recarve the faces of Mount Rushmore so that all the images are female. Ask, "Who would you select?" Students may choose either a public figure or a private figure known only to the student. Each name requires an explicit, written rationale. On poster board taped around the room, the student groups share their results. Each group discusses their choices and the rationale.

Session 2

The next part of the experience is a private part. Each student is asked to create his or her own personal Mount Rushmore, with public or private figures, male or female. Discussion of the personal Mount Rushmore is on a voluntary basis, with students sharing their selections with their group initially and then the class if they choose.

RESOURCES

Poster board; tape

ASSESSMENT PLAN

Invite students to indicate, in writing, what the most difficult part of the assignment was for each of them, considering the following points:

> Did you struggle with females to carve on Mount Rushmore?
>
> What were the decisions you had to make as a group to decide on four women?
>
> How did you reach consensus for posting the names to your group's paper? What skills did you use in the group to reach agreement?
>
> What did you learn from this activity? About yourself? About others?

REFLECTION

This is an important exercise for understanding what each gender knows about famous women. It is very significant for defining personal heroes/heroines and, in this process, defining personal values. These are essential skills for developing a healthy sexuality.

REFERENCE

This activity is from the National SEED Project (Seeking Educational Equity and Diversity), directed by Peggy McIntosh at the Wellesley Centers for Research on Women in Wellesley, Massachusetts (see www.wcwonline.org).

LEARNING EXPERIENCE 6

TITLE: My Favorite Childhood Fairytale Characters

GRADE LEVELS: 10–12

TIME REQUIREMENT: 45 minutes

LEARNING CONTEXT

This activity can be used as an ice breaker in an initial session in this unit. It promotes an understanding of how early childhood experiences have affected students' gender identity and gender roles. Students will learn to recognize gender role stereotypes and be able to identify gender bias as it relates to masculinity and femininity.

NATIONAL LEARNING STANDARDS

4: Students will analyze the influence of culture, media, technology, and other factors on health.

5: Students will demonstrate the ability to use interpersonal communication skills to enhance health.

7: Students will demonstrate the ability to advocate for personal, family, and community health.

PROCEDURE

Arrange the class in a U so that all students can see and hear one another. If it is an especially large class, break the class up into several smaller groups. Ask the students to brainstorm a list of favorite childhood characters (fairytale, sports, or media) from their early childhood. Then instruct them to go around the room and introduce themselves to the rest of the class as their own favorite childhood fairytale character and describe a little about themselves as if they were that character. For example: "I am Sylvester the Cat. I am slick and fast and clever. I . . . ."

Now put the students into small groups of five or six in a circle. Each student will then describe what qualities this character has and how they were significant as a child and which of those qualities may have affected the student as an adolescent. The group will then be asked to reflect on how childhood learning about gender roles may affect adults in their decision making, communication patterns, and other ways. The class will summarize the groups' reflections.

ASSESSMENT PLAN

Assess the students on the following assignment: Ask the students to pose the same questions to their parents individually. Then they will reflect on their parents' responses in their journals.

LEARNING EXPERIENCE 7

TITLE: Raising Elizabeth and Raphael

GRADE LEVELS: 10–12

TIME REQUIREMENT: One 45-minute session

LEARNING CONTEXT
This experience will promote student's understanding of how people learn about gender roles. They will recognize gender bias behaviors and attitudes in themselves and others. Students will be better prepared to advocate for a more gender-equitable family and community.

NATIONAL LEARNING STANDARDS
    4:   Students will analyze the influence of culture, media, technology, and other factors on health.

    5:   Students will demonstrate the ability to use interpersonal communication skills to enhance health.

    6:   Students will demonstrate the ability to use goal-setting and decision-making skills to enhance health.

    7:   Students will demonstrate the ability to advocate for personal, family, and community health.

PROCEDURE
Arrange the students in four groups with a mix of males and females. Tell the groups that it will be their responsibility to develop a plan for raising their child to have the following characteristics that will be assigned to their group:

    Group 1: Raise Elizabeth to be a stereotypically feminine girl.

    Group 2: Raise Elizabeth to be a gender-neutral or androgynous girl.

    Group 3: Raise Raphael to be a stereotypically masculine boy.

    Group 4: Raise Raphael to be a gender-neutral or androgynous boy.

Provide the worksheet of factors to consider (included later), suggesting, "Think about what experiences, activities and conversations, rules and regulations you might have your character experience while he or she is growing up." Then the students will share their activities with the whole class.

RESOURCE
"Raising Elizabeth and Raphael" worksheet

ASSESSMENT PLAN
The following rubric can be used to assess the group's activities:

A: The students covered each of the factors on the worksheet, and their work indicated an understanding of the concepts of gender bias, gender neutrality, and androgyny.

B: The students covered all but three of the factors on the worksheet and their work indicated that they understood the concepts of gender bias, gender neutrality, and androgyny.

C: The students covered only half of the factors on the worksheet, and they were not clear about the concepts of gender bias, gender neutrality, and androgyny.

D: The students covered only a few of the factors, and they were not clear about the concepts of gender bias, gender neutrality, and androgyny.

E: The students did not do the assignment properly, and they do not understand the concepts of gender bias, gender neutrality, and androgyny.

REFLECTION
This activity can also be incorporated in the parenting unit. It can also be done in a more simplistic manner in seventh through ninth grades.

"Raising Elizabeth and Raphael" Worksheet

1. What occupations would the parents of your pretend family have?

2. What roles will be assigned to the mother, father, brother, and sister?

3. What would your character see in the extended family (aunts, uncles, grandparents, and so forth)?

4. What toys would you have your character play with when he or she is very young?

5. What books would you read to the character or have the character read as he or she gets older?

6. What activities or sports would you have your character participate in?

7. What would you tell Elizabeth or Raphael about dating and intimate relationships?

8. What expectations would you have for your character in school?

9. What careers would you encourage?

10. What rules would you make as your character is growing up?

11. What kinds of jobs would you have your character do while he or she is growing up?

LEARNING EXPERIENCE 8

TITLE: Is It a Man's Role or a Woman's Role?

GRADE LEVELS: 10–12

TIME REQUIREMENTS: Two 45-minute sessions

LEARNING CONTEXT
The students will be able to recognize stereotypical gender roles, determine their personal gender biases, and evaluate their notions of masculinity and femininity.

NATIONAL LEARNING STANDARDS
4: Students will analyze the influence of culture, media, technology, and other factors on health.

5: Students will demonstrate the ability to use interpersonal communication skills to enhance health.

7: Students will demonstrate the ability to advocate for personal, family, and community health.

PROCEDURE

Session 1

Tape three large pieces of paper on three different walls in the room with the following comments: "I least agree," "I am neutral/don't care," and "I most agree." Have the students stand in the middle of the room. When each of the following statements are read, have the students move under the sign that best explains their position. Then call on students in each position to explain why they chose that particular position.

1. A career for a married woman is most appropriate after her children are in school.
2. Women are better suited to work for men than men are suited to work for women.
3. The world would be more efficiently managed by women than by men.
4. Alimony should be abolished.
5. Women are instinctively more nurturing than men.
6. Running the home and the family is primarily a married woman's responsibility, and she should expect help from her husband.
7. Sex roles are obsolete, and we should be moving toward a time when there are no female or male roles.
8. One parent should stay at home rearing the children. The couple should decide which person should be the stay-at-home parent.
9. Men have more inherent logical thinking ability than do women.
10. Women and men should be equally liable for military service. but men should be the ones to fight.
11. Women should be equally free to ask for a date and to initiate sexual relationships.
12. Men have the advantage in our society because they have the more powerful and higher-status jobs.
13. Most women want to find a man who will be able to take care of them and their children.
14. Women have the advantage in our society because they do not have the same pressure to achieve.
15. Most men aren't interested in a strong, competent woman.
16. Men and women simply have different inherent traits linked to their gender.
17. A man can best achieve self-development by being a good provider.
18. Men and women should be equally ready to move if the spouse's job requires it.
19. The father should have the final decision about financial matters.
20. Women who bring condoms to dates are promiscuous.
21. Women should be totally responsible for birth control.

Session 2

Ask students to bring in their homework assignment (see assessment), in a blind copy with no self-identification, in a sealed envelope. Collect the responses, shuffle them, and hand them out. Place the students in small groups and ask them to read the answers given to them, one question at a time. Tell them not to divulge whether they happen to have their own copy. They will then discuss their answers as they relate to their own attitudes and values. Groups will share any surprises they found from their discussions.

INSTRUCTIONAL/ENVIRONMENTAL MODIFICATION
For students who are not mobile, provide three sheets with the same categories and have them hold up their response from wherever they are seated.

RESOURCES
Tape; three signs: "I least agree," "I am neutral/don't care," and "I most agree"

ASSESSMENT PLAN
Ask students to reflect on this experience as a homework assignment by answering the following questions:
1. What did you learn about gender roles from this activity?
2. What did you learn about the values and attitudes of your peers?
3. What did you learn about your own gender biases?
4. What factors contribute people's gender-stereotypical values and attitudes?
5. What do you think we can do to change this?

REFLECTION
This activity provides the teacher with some understanding of what students are thinking and how well they have been introduced to gender-equitable thinking.

LEARNING EXPERIENCE 9

TITLE: Is It Better to Be a Man or a Woman?

GRADE LEVELS: 10–12

TIME REQUIREMENTS: 45 minutes

LEARNING CONTEXT

This experience will develop an ability to recognize stereotypical gender roles. Students will be able to recognize their personal gender biases and reflect on their notions of masculinity and femininity.

NATIONAL LEARNING STANDARDS

4: Students will analyze the influence of culture, media, technology, and other factors on health.

5: Students will demonstrate the ability to use interpersonal communication skills to enhance health.

7: Students will demonstrate the ability to advocate for personal, family, and community health.

PROCEDURE

Distribute the handouts included here, and have the students brainstorm in writing their first responses to the statements provided. Then ask the students to share some of their answers with the class. Discuss how they learned these notions of masculinity and femininity. By highlighting the differences in thinking among the students, have them discuss how different cultures, ethnicities, and the media may influence notions of masculinity and femininity.

RESOURCES

Handouts 1 and 2

ASSESSMENT PLAN

The students will be asked to interview a parent or other adult relative with the same handout and reflect on their answers in their journals. Then have them discuss, in their journal, how their own answers were the same as or different from those of their interviewee.

REFLECTION

This activity can be done early in the unit and then repeated toward the end of the unit to determine whether students have shifted to more gender-equitable thinking.

Handout 1

Complete the following sentences:

1. Responsible men are _____, _____, _____.

2. Aggressive women are _____, _____, _____.

3. Nice guys are _____, _____, _____.

4. Nice girls are _____, _____, _____.

5. The little boy(or girl) in me _____.

6. The more grown up man or woman in me _____.

7. The worst thing a woman can call a man is _____.

8. The worst thing a man can call a woman is _____.

9. Men are superior to women in _____.

10. Women are superior to men in _____.

11. It is more advantageous to be a woman professionally because _____.

12. It is more advantageous to be a man professionally because _____.

13. It is more advantageous to be a woman personally because _____.

14. It is more advantageous to be a man personally _____.

Handout 2

Free association: Write down the first two thoughts that come to your mind.

1. Stay-at-home moms _____ _____

2. Single women _____ _____

3. Successful women _____ _____

4. Married women _____ _____

5. Divorced women _____ _____

6. Women in education _____ _____

7. Stay-at-home dads _____ _____

8. Single men _____ _____

9. Successful men _____ _____

10. Married men _____ _____

11. Divorced men _____ _____

12. Men in education _____ _____

SEXUAL ORIENTATION: GAY, LESBIAN, BISEXUAL, AND TRANSGENDER PEOPLE

DAVID KILMNICK

CHAPTER OUTLINE

OBJECTIVES

After reading this chapter, students will be able to

1. Describe the sexual orientations.
2. Discuss the development of sexual orientation.
3. Identify the difference between a person's sexual orientation and his or her gender identity.
4. Decrease misconceptions and the negative notions that underlie prejudices about orientations other than heterosexual.
5. Explain the coming-out process.
6. Explain transsexualism and transgenderism.
7. Create safe and effective learning environments for gay, lesbian, bisexual, and transgender (GLBT) youth.

REFLECTIVE QUESTIONS

1. What challenges might seventh or eighth grade students who are aware that their sexual orientation differs from that of their heterosexual peers be feeling or experiencing?
2. What are the concerns of those who are considering coming out, or disclosing their sexual orientation?
3. What is the responsibility of a human sexuality educator regarding the teaching of sexual orientation?
4. What is the teacher's or school's responsibility to intervene when negative verbal and physical expressions are used toward gay and lesbian youth?
5. How does a homophobic environment affect all students?
6. What is your attitude about the legalization of same-sex marriage?
7. What is your attitude about gay and lesbian parenting?

SCENARIO

It is May of Jim's senior year in high school and time to think about the senior prom. In about his sophomore year, Jim acknowledged that he was gay. He came out only to his family and a few very close friends in his junior year. In the local gay and lesbian youth center, he met Alec, who is also gay and having a hard time telling anybody about his sexual orientation. For almost a year, Jim and Alec have been a couple, but except for the times they are alone, they only see one another at the center's programs once each week. Alec lives in a neighboring town, and his parents don't want anyone to know that he is gay. They are afraid he will have to deal with the terrible discrimination that they have heard from the parents of other gay kids. Alec plays on the school soccer team and is a great student. He won a scholarship to the college of his choosing. Jim will be going to the same college.

Jim asked Alec to go with him to the school prom. Alec thinks Jim has lost his mind. Not only would the school probably not permit them to attend as a couple, they certainly couldn't dance together in front of everyone. Jim says, "It's about time I am able to be who I am. I don't care what they think. High school is over, and I don't want to pretend anymore." Alec says, "I just can't do it."

What do you think you would do if you were Jim?
What would you do if you were Alec?
What are some of the fears that Alec has?
Should the school have rules about gay and lesbian couples attending school-sponsored social functions? If so, what should those rules be?
How might your school overcome some of the discrimination that gay and lesbian youth experience so that they could come to a school prom, or any other school function, without the fears described in this scenario?

INTRODUCTION

Sexual orientation is a person's enduring emotional, romantic, and sexual attraction to individuals of a particular gender, and it is only one of four aspects of sexuality. The other three aspects of sexuality are *biological* (identification of male or female depending on genitalia at birth), *gender identity* (a person's psychological sense of being a man or a woman), and *social gender role* (composed of traditional cultural norms for feminine and masculine behavior).

Sexual orientation is probably the most misunderstood, misinterpreted, and undertaught aspect of human sexuality, though a growing amount of literature is helping to increase our understanding of this phenomenon. However, the most significant shortcoming of research and supporting literature about sexual orientation is the belief that heterosexuality is the only normal and accepted sexual orientation that exists. This view only compounds the issue: Sexual orientation is not a structured listing of categories, as most people have come to believe and accept, but rather a more complex array of feelings and emotions, behaviors, and experiences.

Most people identify their sexual orientation as being *homosexual* (attraction to individuals of the same gender), *heterosexual* (attraction to individuals of the opposite gender), or *bisexual* (attraction to individuals of both genders). Sexual orientation is often thought of as a dichotomous classification—you're either straight (heterosexual) or gay (homosexual). However, an individual's sexual orientation can fall anywhere along a broad spectrum ranging from exclusive homosexuality to exclusive heterosexuality, which includes various forms of bisexuality. A person's sexual orientation involves his or her self-concept and feelings and cannot be defined by behavior alone.

Additionally, gender identity and expression are part of the discussion about GLBT people. Transgender people in particular are widely misunderstood and stigmatized, even more so than gay, lesbian, and bisexual people. A key part of this chapter lies in understanding the difference between people's sexual orientation and their gender identity. Often, people assume that being gay or lesbian means that someone wants to "be" the other sex. This is not true! Moreover, such a belief undermines a complete understanding of human sexuality.

This chapter will explore sexual orientation from sociological, physiological, and psychosocial perspectives, with a focus on GLBT people. GLBT people are members of a stigmatized community because of a general lack of understanding about sexual orientation in the larger society. Hence, a full understanding of sexual orientation must include GLBT people and the resulting challenges they face.

UNDERSTANDING TERMINOLOGY

Teaching about GLBT people requires a clear understanding of the more common terms associated with sexual orientation. The following list briefly describes the terms as they are referred to throughout this chapter:

- *Transgender:* An umbrella term encompassing various forms of gender identities; a person whose outward gender presentation (feminine or masculine) does not conform with his or her biological sex (being male or female). Transgender persons may identify as transsexual, transvestites, drag queens, female/male impersonators, or intersexed.
- *Sexual orientation:* The object of our emotional, romantic, and sexual attractions
- *Sexual preference:* A belief by some people that we choose the sex to whom we are attracted. This term is often used politically to

oppose the belief that sexual orientation exists or to defend one's constitutional right to control what happens in the privacy of one's home.

- *Heterosexuality:* Primary emotional, romantic, and sexual attraction and/or behavior with the opposite sex
- *Homosexuality:* Primary emotional, romantic, and sexual attraction and/or behavior with the same sex
- *Bisexuality:* Emotional, romantic, and sexual attraction and/or behavior with both sexes
- *Transsexuals:* People who feel different from the biological or anatomical sex with which they were born; males or females who feel they are one sex trapped in the body of the other sex and do not fit their inner convictions of who they are
- *Transvestites:* People who receive sexual gratification from wearing the clothes of and/or appearing as the other sex. Most are heterosexual.
- *Homophobia:* The fear of others based on the perception (or fact) that they are homosexual; often includes bigotry and prejudice directed toward gays and lesbians
- *Heterosexism:* The institutional response to homophobia that assumes that all people are, or should be, heterosexual, thereby excluding the needs, concern, and life experiences of GLBT people

WHAT DETERMINES SEXUAL ORIENTATION?

It is not known what makes people gay, lesbian, or bisexual, just as it is not known what makes people heterosexual. Theories abound about the origins of a person's sexual orientation; most agree that sexual orientation is likely the result of a complex interaction of environmental, cognitive, and biological factors. None of these factors alone is responsible for determining sexual orientation. In most people, sexual orientation is shaped at an early age, established well before puberty and sexual activity (Troiden, 1989). More than likely, sexual orientation is determined before birth in much the same way that a person's anatomical and genetic sex is determined. Research suggests that the homosexual orientation, like the heterosexual orientation, is in place very early in the life cycle, possibly sometime in fetal development (American Psychological Association, 1994).

Psychological and social influences alone cannot create homosexuality (Bodde, 1988). There is no evidence that certain childhood experiences or a particular type of parent determines someone's sexual orientation. In fact, evidence indicates that parents have very little influence on the outcome of their children's sexual orientation under normal upbringing conditions (Reinisch, cited in Bodde, 1988). Similarly, "family fears that their children can catch or be recruited into homosexuality in school or any other setting is without scientific foundation" (Weinberg, 1977).

It is unclear whether or how genetics, prenatal influences, or other biological factors influence the development of sexual orientation, but biology evidently does play a role. Recent research has uncovered medical evidence that people seem to be born with a predisposition, or a leaning, toward a sexual orientation. Biological differences between male heterosexuals and gay men have been found to exist in certain areas of the brain. Research has found that when two sisters or two brothers both have a homosexual orientation, they are much more likely to be identical twins and share genetic makeup than to be fraternal twins (each having her or his own genetic makeup) or siblings (American Psychological Association, 1994).

Sexual orientation, whether heterosexual, homosexual, or bisexual, does not appear to be something that one chooses. It is a deep-seated phenomenon that a person knows about him- or herself and not one that the person decides to be or not to be (Bell, Weinberg, & Hammersmith, 1981; Troiden, 1989). Like heterosexuals, gay, lesbian, and bisexual people discover their sexuality as a process of maturing; they are not recruited, seduced, or taught to become homosexual (Bell et al., 1981). The only choice most gay, lesbian, and bisexual people have is whether to live their lives honestly in a heterosexual culture.

GENDER IDENTITY: TRANSGENDER

A discussion about sexual orientation would be incomplete without discussing the issue of gender and, specifically, transgender people. Often, sexual orientation and gender are grouped into one category when in fact they are two distinctly different aspects of human sexuality.

Transgender is an umbrella term used to describe a person whose gender presentation either sometimes or always runs contrary to the traditional definitions of "man" or "woman" in society. Transgender encompasses various forms of gender identities and expressions. Most often, though, *transgender* is used to define someone whose gender identity is different from the biological sex to which he or she was assigned at birth. However, use of the term *transgender* in this way is not fully accurate.

Transsexual is the correct term to describe people who feel this way—their anatomical sex and corresponding biological identification (male or female) are incongruent with their inner convictions of who they are and how they feel (man or woman). Transsexuals are often interested in permanently changing their gender through cross-gender hormones and various surgeries. Feelings of being "trapped" in the wrong body are often cited by transsexuals. This condition is referred to as *gender dysphoria.* Sex reassignment surgery (SRS) can be used to change the anatomy of transsexual persons, in order for their genitals to "match" their gender identity. In terms of the sexual orientation of transsexuals, approximately 35 percent identify as gay or lesbian (Israel & Tarver, 1997).

A *cross dresser,* commonly referred to as a *transvestite,* is a person interested in wearing clothing of the opposite gender privately and/or socially as an opportunity to explore masculinity or femininity. This person is content with his or her biological sex. Most often cross dressers are heterosexual males. This term is not to be confused with *drag queen,* which is used to describe gay men or transsexual women who dress as the opposite sex for the sole purpose of entertainment in traditionally gay venues. Impersonators also dress as the other sex for the sole purpose of entertainment, but they do so on a professional level and in some cases as a serious, long-term profession. One example of a famous impersonator is Dame Edna (seen on *Ally McBeal*), who is a heterosexual man impersonating a woman.

Also associated with transgender is the term *intersexed* or *hermaphrodite*. Intersexed individuals are people born with ambiguous or contradictory sex characteristics, either fully or partially developed.

Are transgender and intersexed people a part of the gay community? Many people tend to group transgender people with gays, lesbians, and bisexuals. However, although transgender people are part of a sexually stigmatized community, they do not always associate themselves with gays, lesbians, and bisexuals. Simply put, gender identity and sexual orientation are two different things; being gay, bisexual, or heterosexual constitutes a sexual orientation, and being transgendered constitutes a gender identity.

BECOMING VISIBLE—COMING OUT

Coming out and *coming out of the closet* are terms used to describe the process of GLBT people disclosing their homosexual or bisexual orientation. The process of coming out is not just one discrete experience but rather a set of experiences that occur over time. Most often, *coming out* refers to the first time that a GLBT person discloses his or her sexual orientation to someone else, but the overall coming-out process is initiated when a GLBT person acknowledges to him- or herself a sexual orientation, a vital and most difficult component of the coming-out process.

Why come out? The concept of a need for a GLBT person to disclose a sexual orientation is important to understand. GLBT people come out because of cultural and institutional heterosexism. *Heterosexism* is the assumption that heterosexuality is normal and right, and that other forms of sexuality are abnormal and wrong. Coming out allows the person to develop fully, allows for greater empowerment, and is a necessary part of developing a healthy and positive identity. Once "out," the person is more able to share with others who he or she is and what is important to him or her, as well as to develop close and mutually satisfying relationships. This context is more honest and real, and it ends the stress of hiding or keeping a secret and living a double life. It reduces isolation and alienation, allowing for increased interaction with, and support from, other GLBT individuals.

Why are some people afraid to come out? Rejection and loss of relationships from family, friends, and peers, and discrimination are barriers to coming out for GLBT people. They are often unsure of how important people in their own lives will react to them when they come out. The real possibility of harassment and abuse from others, ranging from verbal insults to physical violence against them or their possessions, inhibits GLBT people from coming out. Institutionalized discrimination and prejudice are tools in heterosexism, creating a sense of fear for the GLBT person. For example, losing a job, being denied opportunities for military service, and being denied housing and other equal opportunity rights silences GLBT people who remain closeted, especially when they perceive little or no support from others in their lives.

The Cass Model: A Theoretical Model Explaining the Coming-Out Process

Cass (1979) developed a theoretical model of coming out for gay, lesbian, and bisexual (GLB) people that consists of six stages, incorporating several developmental milestones. It is important to note that the coming-out process varies from person to person and depends on a multitude of factors. This model is useful in understanding the coming-out process conceptually and to understand developmentally what GLB people may be experiencing.

Although the Cass model can also be applied to transgender people with a homosexual or bisexual orientation, it probably does not accurately reflect the complete scope of experiences for transgender people, especially transsexuals. Transsexuals frequently report confusion at very young ages when differentiating between coming to terms with their sexual orientation and an incongruity between their biological sex and their gender identity. For this reason, transgender people are not specifically cited in this process due to a more complex set of factors associated with coming out.

STAGE 1: IDENTITY CONFUSION

This first stage of the Cass model is the "Who am I?" stage, associated with feelings of difference and personal alienation. The person begins to be conscious of the same-sex feelings or behaviors and labels them as such. This stage also brings uncertainty because GLB people will question how they feel in the context of a heterosexist world. This can catapult them into the next stage.

STAGE 2: IDENTITY COMPARISON

This is the rationalizing and bargaining stage. It includes questioning what these feelings mean and a great deal of isolation. Identity comparison is the point at which GLB people rationalize their feelings and begin considering the possibility that it is just a "phase." This stage sometimes includes feeling as though same-sex attractions are "bad" or "wrong." They are comparing themselves to heterosexual people and considering the normality and acceptance of being heterosexual versus being homosexual or bisexual.

STAGE 3: IDENTITY TOLERANCE

In this stage, GLB people begin to say, "I am probably a gay [or lesbian or bisexual] person." They begin to meet other GLB individuals to counter loneliness but merely tolerate, rather than accept, the identity. Identity tolerance brings a major milestone to the coming-out process. GLB people begin to accept the notion that their sexual orientation is different from the perceived societal norm of being heterosexual. This stage is also marked by the first contact with other openly GLB people.

STAGE 4: IDENTITY ACCEPTANCE

As contact with other GLB people grows, whether on a platonic, casual, or intimate level, GLB people will enter identity acceptance in which a more positive view of GLB people develops. A greater sense of belonging and identity occurs, as does a more positive view of other gays and lesbians. This stage is also associated with the development of identity with the greater GLBT community.

STAGE 5: IDENTITY PRIDE

This fifth stage of the Cass model includes the development of a positive GLB identity. This identity evolves to include feeling pride about homosexuality, identifying strongly with other homosexuals, and experiencing anger about the way society treats GLB people as a whole. During this stage, involvement with the greater GLBT community also occurs. This activity results in a greater feeling that "these are my people." One begins to see incongruity between pride in identity and societal rejection. More involvement and immersion into culture and lifestyle are observed, and often an intense anger at heterosexuals is experienced—a "them versus us" attitude.

STAGE 6: IDENTITY SYNTHESIS

The Cass model culminates with identity synthesis, in which GLB people develop a complete understanding of heterosexism, identify with heterosexual allies, and experience less anger. The GLBT community becomes an integral part of GLB people's lives, and they have fully integrated their identity with other parts of their life. They begin to see less of a dichotomy between heterosexual and homosexual worlds. Less anger is experienced, and the gay/lesbian identity becomes an integral part of their complete personality structure.

SEXUAL ORIENTATION, IDENTITY, AND BEHAVIOR

Sometimes GLB people don't come out and instead remain closeted. Some follow a specified path of heterosexual marriage as dictated by society, family, culture, and/or religion. Thus, a person's behavior does not necessarily indicate a sexual orientation. Take the example of the 45-year-old man, married with children, who comes out of the closet as gay. This man has always known he was gay and has always dealt with those feelings, but he chose to repress them due to fear of rejection, living in a heterosexist world. He did not "turn" gay.

Many often question a person's sexual orientation in similar situations. The significant element to be learned here is understanding that a person's intimate sexual relations are not necessarily an indicator of a sexual orientation. Someone can identify as bisexual and never have a same-sex experience, whereas someone else can self-identify as homosexual (gay or lesbian), outwardly and publicly identify as heterosexual, and maintain heterosexual intimacy. Sexual orientation; the individual's identity, whether inward or outward; and behavior in terms of who the person is intimate with are all exclusive of each other. Each area is independent of the other, and neither identity nor behavior could accurately be reflective of the individual's sexual orientation.

The "Lifestyle" Myth

Just as there is no such thing as a single heterosexual lifestyle, there is no such thing as a single gay lifestyle. Antigay activists have attempted to promote the idea that the lives of homosexuals revolve around sex and the pursuit of sexual encounters and that the only identity homosexuals have is with being gay. To antigay organizations, this is the only gay lifestyle that exists, and they do their best to promote this misconception.

In reality, the lifestyles of gays and lesbians are as varied as the lifestyles of heterosexuals (Garnets & Kimmel, 1993). Some choose to live in long-term committed relationships; others decide to remain single. Some individuals or couples choose to raise children, whereas others do not. Hobbies, occupations, and activities are just as varied as within the heterosexual population.

Gay and lesbian people are just as capable of being good parents as are heterosexual parents. Children who are raised in gay or lesbian homes are no different in any aspects of psychological, social, or sexual development from children in heterosexual families (Patterson, 1992). Multiple studies have shown that children of gay and lesbian parents are no more likely to become homosexuals than children of heterosexuals, and they are just as well adjusted.

Gay men and lesbian women are rarely involved in child sexual abuse. In the United States, 90 percent of all sexual child abuse is committed by heterosexual men. The molesters are almost always family members, close family friends, or the mother's boyfriend (Koss, 1994).

Contributions by GLBT People

The identity of well-known GLBT people often remains invisible either by choice or sometimes simply by lack of acknowledgment by the society. Providing students with the names and range of contributions made by

GLBT people who have helped to shape our world and continue to enrich our lives serves to decrease myths, misconceptions, and stereotypical notions. Such a list might also help young people to recognize that someone they know, respect, and admire is GLBT.

Susan B. Anthony, human rights activist
James Baldwin, writer (*Go Tell It on the Mountain; Giovanni's Room; Another Country*)
Chastity Bono, activist and daughter of Sonny Bono and Cher
Rita Mae Brown, novelist
Leonardo da Vinci
James Dean, actor
Ellen DeGeneres, actress/comedian
Emily Dickinson, poet
Brian Epstein, first manager for the Beatles
Melissa Etheridge, musician
Rock Hudson, actor
Elton John, musician
David Kopay, retired NFL football player
Audre Lorde, African American poet and activist
Greg Louganis, three-time Olympic gold medalist in diving
Michelangelo
Dave Pallone, ex–Major League baseball umpire
Cole Porter, songwriter
Eleanor Roosevelt, former first lady
RuPaul, entertainer
Bessie Smith, singer
Gertrude Stein, writer
Michael Stipe, lead singer of REM
Lily Tomlin, actress/comedian
Walt Whitman, poet (*Leaves of Grass*)
Oscar Wilde, playwright/novelist (*The Portrait of Dorian Gray*)
Tennessee Williams, playwright (*The Glass Menagerie; A Streetcar Named Desire*)
Virginia Woolf, writer

SOCIOPOLITICAL ISSUES

Curricula about sexual orientation that acknowledge the psychological, social, physical, and spiritual aspects of sexuality should include discussions of sociopolitical issues that have implications for GLBT people. Some of these issues reflect a society that lacks information and understanding of the diversity of human sexuality and tends to discriminate or isolate that which lacks familiarity. Moreover, familiarity and understanding of the range of sexual orientations provide for more comfort and acceptance not only of the issues but also of the individual.

Heterosexism/Homophobia

Heterosexism, or the assumption that heterosexuality is normal and right and that other forms of sexuality are abnormal and wrong, is a persistent social problem for GLBT persons. Heterosexist attitudes, consciously held or not, prevent GLBT people from obtaining good health care, feeling safe as they pursue their education, attaining full property rights, and living daily life without fear of harassment and violence. Though attitudes toward GLBT persons have changed for the better in recent decades, discrimination remains, and the cost of this discrimination—economically, socially, and personally—is high.

Many people continue to have an irrational fear of homosexuality. This fear, homophobia, results in dislike or even hatred of homosexuals. Such people are prejudiced and often are hostile toward the GLBT community.

Hate/Bias Crimes: An American Epidemic

Hate crimes or *bias crimes* are criminal actions intended to harm or intimidate people because of their race, ethnicity, sexual orientation, religion, or other minority group status. Hate crimes often encompass not only violence against individuals or groups but also crimes against property, such as arson or vandalism. Such crimes send a threatening message to the entire community that is targeted. The key difference between hate crimes and other crimes is that the offender is motivated by the victim's personal characteristics.

In 2001, hate crimes against gay, lesbian, and bisexual Americans constituted about 14.3 percent of all reported hate crimes, with 1,393 cases reported. After those targeting race and religion, hate crimes based on sexual orientation make up the third highest category. It is estimated that 70 percent of all hate crimes against gays and lesbians go unreported.

One of the more notable and publicized hate crimes was the brutal murder of Matthew Shepard. Matthew had been lured from a campus bar in Laramie, Wyoming, shortly after midnight, on October 7, 1998, by two men who told him they were gay. He was driven to a remote area nearby, tied to a split-rail fence, and was tortured, beaten, and pistol-whipped by his attackers while he begged for his life. He was left for dead in near-freezing temperatures. A cyclist who found him on a snowy mountain road some 18 hours after the attack at first mistook him for a scarecrow. He was unconscious and suffering from hypothermia. His face was caked with blood, except where it had been partially washed clean by tears. Matthew died a few days later, with his family at his bedside. He never regained consciousness after being found and remained on full life support until his death. A message to the public offered by his mother summed it up so succinctly: "Matt is no longer with us today because the men who killed him learned to hate. Somehow and somewhere they received the message that the lives of gay people are not as worthy of respect, dignity, and honor as the lives of other people." The president of Wyoming University, Philip Dubois (1998), said, "We must use Matt's example in life to work against hatred, bigotry, and violence."

What is even more telling is what happened nearby: While Matthew lay dying in the hospital, a group of students from Colorado State University thought it would be funny to ride atop a homecoming float that featured a scarecrow figure designed to resemble Matthew's battered body. The figure was wearing a sign that said, "I'm gay." An obscene message was painted across the back of the scarecrow's shirt.

While Matthew's case is among the more notorious ones, other hate crimes continue to occur. Teena Brandon was born and raised as a girl but was living as a man known as Brandon Teena in Falls City, Nebraska, when he was murdered at age 21. In December 1993, two men who discovered his gender raped him. His attackers later shot and killed him after learning Brandon had reported the rape and was to help police in the investigation.

On the Fourth of July, 2000, J. R. Warren, 26, who was black and gay, was beaten to death by three men in West Virginia, and then run over by a car to make it look like a hit and run. Pfc. Barry Winchell, 21, was beaten to death by fellow service members in 1999 while sleeping in his cot at Fort Campbell, Kentucky. His army colleagues thought (correctly) that he was gay, so they killed him. On May 8, 1995, Bill Clayton, 17, committed suicide after having been brutally assaulted for being bisexual.

We can go on and on in documenting these despicable acts of violence, but suffice to say that they are a result of a society immersed in hatred and discrimination that must be ended.

Civil Rights

Civil rights issues are important to the GLBT community because in many circumstances homosexuals do not have the same basic rights as other U.S. citizens. In most states and cities, a gay person can legally be denied housing, employment, and public accommodation simply because of sexual orientation. Organizations opposed to gay rights claim homosexuals have some hidden plan to tear apart the moral fabric of U.S. society and often refer to gay communities' efforts to obtain equal rights as the "gay agenda." To the contrary, gay and lesbian people are seeking equal rights and equal protection of those rights with regard to housing, employment, public accommodation, and the ability to offer financial and legal security to their families. The invention of the "gay agenda" is nothing more than a scare tactic employed by antigay organizations in an effort to place fear in the minds of the American public.

Gays in the Military

For nearly 50 years, it had been the U.S. military's official policy to exclude homosexuals from service. In November 1992, President-elect Bill Clinton (D) told Americans that he planned to lift the military's long-standing ban on gays and lesbians. Homosexual men and women, he said, should not be prevented from serving their country based solely on their sexual orientation. Soon after taking office in 1993, Clinton faced powerful military and congressional opposition to lifting the ban. General Colin Powell, then-chairman of the Joint Chiefs of Staff, and Senator Sam Nunn (D-Georgia), who was chair of the Senate Armed Services Committee between 1987 and 1994 and left Congress in 1996, announced that they would seek to block his attempts to lift the ban.

For the next 6 months, debate raged over what to do about the military's ban on gays and lesbians. Clinton's liberal supporters wanted him to follow through on his promise to lift the ban, emphasizing the need to end discrimination against gays and lesbians. Conservatives, military leaders and some lawmakers of both parties argued that the presence of declared homosexuals in the armed forces would be detrimental to military readiness. They said that letting gays and lesbians serve would destroy overall morale and erode good discipline and order. Ban opponents maintained that gay people were capable men and women who should be allowed to serve their country.

In July 1993, a compromise policy was struck between supporters and opponents of the ban. The compromise, known as "don't ask, don't tell," allowed gays and lesbians to serve in the military as long as they did not proclaim their homosexuality or engage in homosexual conduct. Under the policy, military commanders would not try to find out the sexual orientation of personnel, and gays and lesbians would not disclose their sexual orientation. The policy marked a change from past practice in that simply being homosexual was no longer a disqualifier for military service. Conservatives saw the change as a regrettable relaxation of the absolute ban on gay people. Liberals were dissatisfied because the new policy still allowed the military to oust gays and lesbians if they revealed their orientation.

Recent debates have centered on whether the policy is working. When the compromise was struck, Clinton declared that it would mean "an end to witch-hunts to ferret out individuals who have served their country well." However, gay advocacy and civil rights military investigators routinely question personnel about their sexual orientation, in violation of the policy. Not only is the policy not being followed, they say, but persecution of gays and lesbians has actually gotten worse since it took effect in 1994. The Service Members Legal Defense Network (SLDN), a group representing gay military personnel, documented 563 violations of the policy in 1997. The following list documents evidence of the results of the violations:

- At least $500 million has been spent over the past decade replacing men and women who were forced from military service because of their homosexual orientation.
- Military service branches discharge an average of 1,500 people each year for being gay.
- The Pentagon's policy against homosexuality appears to fall disproportionately on women (at almost a 10:1 ratio).

- Since the implementation of the "don't ask, don't tell" policy in 1994 by President Clinton, the number of gays and lesbians dismissed from military has increased 42 percent (*Los Angeles Times,* 1992).

Same-Sex Marriage

The institution of marriage has been in a state of flux for centuries. It was only after the Civil War that African Americans were allowed to marry in all areas of the United States. And, after a U.S. Supreme Court decision in 1967, mixed-race couples could marry anywhere in the country as well. But, until recently, same-sex couples could not marry anywhere in the United States or in the world.

Gay couples desire to marry for the same reasons heterosexual couples do: love, companionship, shared interests, common goals, emotional and financial security, and, in some cases, desire to raise a family. Yet, the institution of marriage is still limited to heterosexual couples in 49 of 50 states.

The Defense of Marriage Act, which President Clinton signed into law in 1996, stipulated that although the states could decide for themselves what they recognize as marriage, the federal government would only recognize a marriage between a man and a woman. So far, no state has passed legislation allowing same-sex unions to be recognized as legal marriages. However in a historic decision on February 4, 2004, the Supreme Judicial Court of the State of Massachusetts ruled that same-sex couples must have the right to marry and be afforded the same rights that married heterosexual couples receive. The court declared that another system to accommodate same-sex couples, such as civil unions, would be "considered choice of language that reflects a demonstrable assigning of same-sex, largely homosexual, couples to second-class status." The opinion added:

> For no rational reason the marriage laws of the Commonwealth discriminate against a defined class; no amount of tinkering with language will eradicate that stain. . . . Barred access to the protections, benefits and obligations of civil marriage, a person who enters into an intimate, exclusive union with another of the same sex is arbitrarily deprived of membership in one of our community's most rewarding and cherished institutions.

On May 17, 2004, Massachusetts become the first and only state where same-sex couples could marry legally.

Yet, millions of gay men and lesbians across the United States are living in long-term committed relationships despite the fact that homosexual unions lack many financial, legal, and social benefits that are automatically provided for heterosexual couples upon marriage. The typical married couple in the United States receives more than 1,500 benefits and rights by virtue of their union. It seems ironic that a heterosexual couple married for 1 hour has more rights and benefits than a same-sex couple that has been together for 30 years.

Currently, gay couples do not have the automatic right to make medical, legal, or financial decisions on behalf of their partner should the need arise. They may be denied access to visit their partner in intensive care units and other hospital departments. Gay and lesbian couples do not have the automatic right to make funeral arrangements or to assume ownership of property (even jointly owned property) when a partner dies.

Gay couples also lack many of the financial benefits of marriage. They may not have access to their partners' employee health insurance, retirement, or death benefits. They are not eligible for the tax breaks that heterosexual couples receive, nor are they eligible for insurance discounts that are frequently provided for married couples.

Before the Massachusetts Supreme Judicial Court 2004 ruling, several attempts by other states to provide some minimal benefits to same-sex couples were taken:

- On April 26, 2000, Vermont governor Howard Dean signed a landmark bill allowing same-sex unions in his state. The bill, which was given final approval the day before by the state legislature with a vote of 79–68, allows gay couples to form "civil unions" that provide them with a wide range of benefits previously available only to heterosexual married couples. While an amendment to the bill defines marriage as a union between a man and a woman, the civil union legislation is viewed as a breakthrough for gay rights. The legislation was precipitated by the Vermont Supreme Court's December 1999 ruling that homosexual couples must be granted the same protection under the law as married heterosexual couples.
- On March 7, 2000, California voters passed Proposition 22, proposed by State Senator Pete Knight, which mandates, "Only marriage between a man and a woman is valid or recognized in California." The proposition, known as the Protection of Marriage Act, passed by a margin of 63 percent to 37 percent.
- In 2001, the Netherlands enlarged its definition of marriage to include both other-sex and same-sex couples. Belgium followed suit during 2003. Next came Ontario, Canada. Finally, on July 9, 2003, same-sex marriage also became permitted in the Canadian province of British Columbia. Any adult couple—same-sex or other-sex—from any country can come to one of these two provinces, buy a marriage license, and get married. Same-sex marriages are expected to be legal and available across Canada sometime soon.

Gays and lesbians would like to see same-sex marriages legalized so that they could provide the same type of legal, financial, and emotional security for their loved ones that heterosexual couples currently enjoy. More and more people believe that same-sex marriage—or its equivalent under another name—will eventually become available to all loving, committed adult couples throughout North America and Western Europe, whether they be same-sex or other-sex spouses. The same-sex marriage debate will most likely play out like the one for interracial marriage did. In 1948, California was the first state to make it legal for a couple of mixed race to be married, and it wasn't until 17 years later that the entire nation followed suit. Today, interracial marriage is a nonissue; a decade from now, we will hopefully be saying the same for same-sex marriage.

GLBT YOUTH

Earlier, we explained sexual orientation and discussed the issues associated with it. Now let's look at information that pertains particularly to adolescents.

Adolescence can be difficult enough at times, but for GLBT youth, the differences often leave them feeling isolated and confused. Born into a culture that assumes everyone to be heterosexual, GLBT youth often lack the acceptance, understanding, and support that their heterosexual peers receive. Society's ignorance and negative views of homosexuality leave many gay and lesbian youth feeling confused, ashamed, guilty, afraid, and alone, placing them at greater risk for suicide, drug and alcohol abuse, homelessness, and sexually transmitted diseases.

Compared to students who were not harassed, students harassed based on actual or perceived sexual orientation are more than twice as likely to report seriously considering suicide and more than twice as likely to report making a plan for suicide, three times as likely to report missing school, more than three times as likely to carry a weapon to school, and more than twice as likely to report depression (feeling so sad and hopeless that they stopped normal activities for 2 weeks) (California Safe Schools Coalition & 4-H Center for Youth Development, 2004). Moreover, 91 percent of students reported hearing students make negative comments based on sexual orientation, 46 percent said their schools were not safe for GLBT students, and two out of every three students who identified as GLBT reported harassment based on actual or perceived sexual orientation (California Safe Schools Coalition & 4-H Center for Youth Development, 2004).

Other research indicates similarly disturbing trends among GLBT youth. For example, 19 percent of gay men and 25 percent of lesbians report suffering physical violence at the hands of a family member as a result of their sexual orientation (Philadelphia Lesbian and Gay Task Force, 1992). Another study notes that 42 percent of homeless youth identify as gay or lesbian (Safe Horizon Victims Services, 1991).

Some families recognize the dilemma their children are experiencing regarding their sexuality, whereas others are unaware. The peer pressure to socialize in socially acceptable ways is enormous for all teens but especially for GLBT teens. Rarely are models of behavior available for these young people, who are sometimes dealing with their differences for the first time.

Creating Safer Schools for GLBT Youth

Because a considerable amount of the time young people spend with each other is in the school environment, it is an ideal place for learning about sexual orientation and becoming tolerant of feelings and behaviors different from their own. It is essential that school communities begin to provide a safe environment for learning while simultaneously supporting and nurturing the growth of GLBT youth. Every school has GLBT students or students whose families have someone who is a GLBT person. Schools should be learning communities where differences are acknowledged and respected rather than hostile environments of harassment, verbal abuse, discrimination, and violence. Here are some suggestions for making schools safe and supportive places for GLBT youth:

- *Create and enforce policies.* Add sexual orientation to existing nondiscrimination policies. This will provide legal protection from discrimination against GLBT students, teachers, and school staff and create a safe and supportive learning environment. Enforcement of policies must treat all students equally. All students, regardless of sexual orientation, should be held to the same standards of conduct, behavior, and appearance.
- *Confront violence and harassment.* Making schools a safer place requires school staff to confront harassment, discrimination, and violence immediately each and every time it occurs. Identify the act of violence or harassment as the problem, not the victim's appearance, behavior, or sexual orientation. Send a clear message that there is zero tolerance for harassment, violence, and discrimination of all kinds, including those based on sexual orientation.
- *Talk about GLBT issues in the classroom.* In elementary schools, include issues about gay and lesbian people in discussions of different families, different communities, and acceptance and respect of differences. In middle and high schools, incorporate GLBT issues in discussions of communities, diversity, health, bias, and discrimination in classes such as English, social studies, health, and political science. Include content on sexual orientation, suicide prevention, and ways to help a person who tells you he or she is GLBT.
- *Support gay-straight alliances (GSAs).* GSAs can be formed for GLBT and heterosexual students to address anti-GLBT harassment, discrimination, and violence by increasing awareness through educational school activities and programs.
- *Be mindful of heterosexism.* Heterosexism, that belief that being heterosexual is superior to being homosexual or bisexual, comes across in the assumption that students are heterosexual. Be sure to include both other- and same-sex couples in discussions.
- *Address incorrect use of language and derogatory words* (Long Island Gay and Lesbian Youth, 2003). This measure is discussed more fully in the next section.

Strategies for Addressing Anti-GLBT and Hate Language in Schools

To create safe and supportive schools, anti-GLBT language must be addressed each and every time it is heard. Anti-GLBT language includes a number of words and terms often overlooked by both students and staff or unrecognized as antigay. For example, the word *gay* in a person- or object-directed comment is not meant to describe an individual's orientation but is perceived as a put-down by GLBT adolescents overhearing it. The following are common incidents, with suggested responses:

In a person-directed comment: "You're so gay!" occurs when a student calls another student gay. Address the harmful nature of name-calling. Avoid responding with "Don't call anyone gay!" because it sends a message that being gay is a bad thing. Instead, explain, "It is offensive to myself and others to use the word *gay* to mean something negative." Talk privately to the target of the harassment to make sure that he or she is okay. Ask students how GLBT students might feel when hearing this statement and explain why it may make GLBT students feel uncomfortable.

In an object-directed comment: "That's so gay!" occurs when a student calls an object (such as a book, clothing, or activity) gay. Ask the student, "What do you mean when you use the word *gay*?" Many students will reply that they use *gay* to indicate something negative, like the words *dumb* or *stupid*. Respond to these incidents by stating, "Being gay is not a bad thing, and using the word *gay* to mean something negative is offensive to myself and others."

Words such as *faggot, dyke, homo, queer,* and *lesbo* also need to be addressed when used in a derogatory way. Address these words the same way that you would other offensive words and terms addressing other communities of people. Take advantage of opportunities to teach about the impact of using these words. When students use such language, ask, "Do you know the origins of these words?" Often, students think that they know but often don't know the older, deeper origins of most words. You might ask students to reflect on why they use those particular words and how the words may be affecting others around them (Long Island Gay and Lesbian Youth, 2003).

Antigay language affects most students; it is offensive to the GLBT students and those students who have a friend or family member who is GLBT. It is also offensive to anyone who respects and supports diversity. Not intervening when the language is used sends an approval message and suggests the language is acceptable.

SUMMARY

A discussion of sexual orientation as a significant component of human sexuality is essential in a sexual education class. Using a developmental model, one can describe and explain the various sexual orientations as part of the normal development of human sexual beings.

It is important that sexual orientation not be seen as an absolutely dichotomous model but rather as a place somewhere on a continuum between the heterosexual and gay (Kinsey, Pomeroy, & Martin, 1948). One of the goals of sexuality education is to help students to recognize that the human sexual experience embraces enormous variability beyond the traditional homosexual/heterosexual models, to include bisexuality, transgenderism, and more. Moreover, students can learn that one's sexual or other behaviors do not necessarily match or explain their classification. Also, the notion of lifestyle cannot be boxed into a strictly dichotomous model. There is as much lifestyle variability in the homosexual community as there is in the heterosexual community.

When sexuality education acknowledges and addresses the phenomena associated with sexual orientation effectively, it will normalize the information and decrease the myths and misconceptions that abound. The ultimate outcome is that students achieve a better understanding and acceptance of the range of human sexual identities and intimate expressions as part of the human condition. One should attempt to help people accept themselves and support and nurture all sexual orientations and gender identities.

WEBSITES

Parents, Families, and Friends of Lesbians and Gays (PFLAG): www.pflag.org

National Journal of Sexual Orientation Law: www.ibiblio.org/gaylaw

Lambda Legal Defense and Education Fund: www.lambdalegal.org

National Gay and Lesbian Task Force: www.ngltf.org

Gay and Lesbian Alliance against Defamation: www.glaad.org

Freedom to Marry: www.freedomtomarry.org

Children of Lesbians and Gays Everywhere (COLAGE): www.colage.org

Family Pride Coalition: www.familypride.org

My Child Is Gay: www.mentalhelp.net/poc/view_doc.php/type/doc/id

OutProud! The National Coalition for Gay, Lesbian, and Bisexual Youth: www.outproud.org

P.E.R.S.O.N. Project: www.youth.org/loco/PERSONProject

Gay and Bisexual Male Youth Suicide Studies: www.virtualcity.com/youthsuicide/suicide.htm

Long Island Gay and Lesbian Youth (LIGALY): www.ligaly.com

Lavender Youth Recreation and Information Center (LYRIC): www.lyric.org

REFERENCES

American Psychological Association. (1994). *Statement on sexual orientation.* Washington, DC: Author.

Bell, A. P., Weinberg, M. S., & Hammersmith, S. K. (1981). *Sexual preference: Its development in men and women.* Bloomington: Indiana University Press.

Bodde, T. (1988). *Why is my child gay?* Washington, DC: Federation of Parents and Friends of Lesbians and Gays.

California Safe Schools Coalition & 4-H Center for Youth Development. (2004). *Consequences of harassment based on actual or perceived sexual orientation and gender non-conformity and steps for making schools safer.* Davis: University of California.

Cass, V. C. (1979) Homosexuality identity formation: A theoretical model. *Journal of Homosexuality, 4*(3), 219–235.

Dubois, P. (1998, October 12). Statement at vigil for Matthew Shepard.

Garnets, L. D., & Kimmel, D. C. (1993). *Psychological perspectives on lesbian and gay male experiences.* New York: Columbia University Press.

Israel, G. E., & Tarver, D. E. (1997). *Transgender care.* Philadelphia: Temple University Press.

Kinsey, A. C., Pomeroy, W. B., & Martin, C. E. (1948). *Sexual behavior in the human male.* Philadelphia: Saunders.

Koss, M. (1994). *No safe haven: Male violence against women at home, at work and in the community.* Washington, DC: American Psychological Association.

Long Island Gay and Lesbian Youth. (2003). Training handouts. Bay Shore, NY: Author.

Los Angeles Times. (1992, June 19). Pentagon cost of discharging gays put at $500 million. P. A14.

Patterson, C. J. (1992). Children of lesbian and gay parents. *Child Development, 63.*

Philadelphia Lesbian and Gay Task Force. (1992). *Discrimination and violence toward lesbian women and gay men in the Philadelphia and the Commonwealth of Pennsylvania.* Philadelphia: Author.

Safe Horizon Victims Services. (1991). *Streetwork Project study, New York City, 1987–1990.* New York: Author.

Troiden, R. R. (1989). The formation of homosexual identities. *Journal of Homosexuality, 17,* 43–73.

Weinberg, J. (1977). *American Psychiatric Association, public statement.* Washington, DC: American Psychiatric Association.

LEARNING EXPERIENCES

The following learning experiences are geared toward providing students with the content and skills enabling them to be able to

- Recognize family structures with same-sex parents as no different than those with other-sex parents.
- Define the terminology: *heterosexuality, homosexuality, bisexuality, gay, lesbian, transsexual,* and *transgender.*
- Explain that some people have sexual feelings for people of the other sex and some for people of the same sex.
- Recognize how language can be prejudicial and painful to gay and lesbian peers.
- Advocate for decreasing biased language and behaviors exhibited by their peers.
- Understand the true meaning of friendship and how it is accepting of difference.
- Understand that early sexual experimentation is not necessarily a determinant of sexual orientation.
- Clarify their personal values about issues associated with homosexuality.
- Challenge the myths and misconceptions associated with homosexuality.
- Explain stereotypes and how they are perpetrated in society.
- Understand the process of coming out and the difficulty people have in coming out.
- Understand the political issues associated with sexual orientation.

LEARNING EXPERIENCE 1

TITLE: So? What Do You Think?

GRADE LEVELS: 7–9

TIME REQUIREMENTS: 10 minutes for introduction and background; 30–35 minutes for reading, writing, and class discussion

LEARNING CONTEXT

This value clarification activity provides students with a variety of questions surrounding controversial issues that deal with homosexuality. It asks and challenges students to take a deeper personal look at these issues, and also helps to identify areas in which knowledge needs to be acquired.

NATIONAL LEARNING STANDARDS

1: Students will comprehend concepts related to health promotion and disease prevention.
2: Students will demonstrate the ability to access valid health information and health-promoting products and services.
3: Students will demonstrate the ability to practice health-enhancing behaviors and reduce health risks.
4: Students will analyze the influence of culture, media, technology, and other factors on health.
5: Students will demonstrate the ability to use interpersonal communication skills to enhance health.
6: Students will demonstrate the ability to use goal-setting and decision-making skills to enhance health.
7: Students will demonstrate the ability to advocate for personal, family, and community health.

PROCEDURE

This lesson follows a discussion of the basic concepts of sexual orientation. Distribute the "Self-Assessment Worksheet: Personal Opinions Related to Sexual Orientation" (included later). Have the students fill out the questionnaire individually and anonymously. When they have completed the questionnaire, discuss each of the questions with the class. Immediately following the discussion, have the students write in their journals what they learned about their attitudes and knowledge regarding sexual orientation. Collect the anonymous questionnaires, and review them as part of the assessment of the unit.

RESOURCES

"Self-Assessment Worksheet"; student journals

ASSESSMENT PLAN

The "Self-Assessment Worksheet" acts as an assessment tool following discussion about sexual orientation. It provides the students with a self-assessment of their content knowledge and attitudes and the teacher with an understanding of what the students have achieved.

Self-Assessment Worksheet: Personal Opinions Related to Sexual Orientation

Instructions: Please indicate how you feel about the following statements by circling the number that best describes your attitudes or knowledge, on the following scale:

Strongly Agree	Agree	Disagree	Strongly Disagree	Not Sure
1	2	3	4	5

1. I would attend a bar or party where I knew most of the guests would be gay, lesbian, or bisexual.

Strongly Agree	Agree	Disagree	Strongly Disagree	Not Sure
1	2	3	4	5

2. I would feel comfortable to learn that a person of my same gender found me attractive.

Strongly Agree	Agree	Disagree	Strongly Disagree	Not Sure
1	2	3	4	5

3. If my son or daughter told me that he or she was gay, lesbian, or bisexual, I would be supportive.

Strongly Agree	Agree	Disagree	Strongly Disagree	Not Sure
1	2	3	4	5

4. Elementary schools should teach children that gay, lesbian, bisexual, and straight people all have normal, natural, healthy, and equally valid sexual orientations and should be accorded the same respect.

Strongly Agree	Agree	Disagree	Strongly Disagree	Not Sure
1	2	3	4	5

5. Gay, lesbian, and bisexual people should be allowed to be teachers or counselors of children of any age.

Strongly Agree	Agree	Disagree	Strongly Disagree	Not Sure
1	2	3	4	5

6. I would feel comfortable going to a doctor of my same gender who is openly gay, lesbian, or bisexual.

Strongly Agree	Agree	Disagree	Strongly Disagree	Not Sure
1	2	3	4	5

7. Gay, lesbian, and bisexual people should be allowed to serve openly in the U.S. military.

Strongly Agree	Agree	Disagree	Strongly Disagree	Not Sure
1	2	3	4	5

8. It's fine if same-sex couples hold hands, hug, and kiss in public.

Strongly Agree	Agree	Disagree	Strongly Disagree	Not Sure
1	2	3	4	5

9. The atmosphere in my workplace or school is supportive of gay, lesbian, and bisexual people.

Strongly Agree	Agree	Disagree	Strongly Disagree	Not Sure
1	2	3	4	5

10. The atmosphere in my synagogue, church, or house of worship is supportive of gay, lesbian, and bisexual people.

Strongly Agree	Agree	Disagree	Strongly Disagree	Not Sure
1	2	3	4	5

11. Same-sex couples should be allowed to have legally sanctioned marriages.

Strongly Agree	Agree	Disagree	Strongly Disagree	Not Sure
1	2	3	4	5

12. Gay, lesbian, and bisexual people should be allowed to legally adopt children.

Strongly Agree	Agree	Disagree	Strongly Disagree	Not Sure
1	2	3	4	5

13. I would vote for an openly gay, lesbian, or bisexual person running for any public office.

Strongly Agree	Agree	Disagree	Strongly Disagree	Not Sure
1	2	3	4	5

14. I would become friends with someone who I knew was gay, lesbian, or bisexual.

Strongly Agree	Agree	Disagree	Strongly Disagree	Not Sure
1	2	3	4	5

15. I would actively support a gay, lesbian, or bisexual coworker who was experiencing harassment because of his or her sexual orientation.

Strongly Agree	Agree	Disagree	Strongly Disagree	Not Sure
1	2	3	4	5

Please complete the following two sentences with as many responses that come to your mind:

1. It's important to talk about homophobia and heterosexism because _____ .

2. It's difficult to talk about homophobia and heterosexism because _____ .

LEARNING EXPERIENCE 2

TITLE: Am I Really So "Different"?

GRADE LEVELS: 7–9

TIME REQUIREMENTS: 10 minutes for introduction and background; 30 minutes for reading, writing and class discussion on questionnaire.

LEARNING CONTEXT

This activity should be administered toward the beginning of the unit of sexual orientation. Communication skills and self-management skills are developed. Specifically, students will

- Be able to recognize the heterosexual frame of reference of questions frequently asked of gay, lesbian, and bisexual people.
- Be able to explain how these questions are frequently based on unfounded stereotypes and are discriminatory and oppressive.
- Acknowledge how difficult or impossible stereotypical questions are to answer.

NATIONAL LEARNING STANDARDS

2: Students will demonstrate the ability to access valid health information and health-promoting products and services.

4: Students will analyze the influence of culture, media, technology, and other factors on health.

5: Students will demonstrate the ability to use interpersonal communication skills to enhance health.

6: Students will demonstrate the ability to use goal-setting and decision-making skills to enhance health.

7: Students will demonstrate the ability to advocate for personal, family, and community health.

PROCEDURE

The students will work individually. (If one of the students is GLBT, he or she can feel very threatened working with someone else. This approach can also stir individual critical thinking.)

Answer the "Heterosexual Questionnaire." After the activity, the students will discuss their answers with the class. They will then write a personal reflection of the experience in their journals.

RESOURCES

"Heterosexual Questionnaire"; journals

ASSESSMENT PLAN

Assess student performance through the class discussion as well as a review of entries in students' journals.

REFERENCE

Developed by Martin Rochlin (1972).

Heterosexual Questionnaire

1. What do you think caused your heterosexuality?

2. When and how did you first decide you were heterosexual?

3. Is it possible your heterosexuality is just a phase you may grow out of?

4. Is it possible your heterosexuality stems from a neurotic fear of others of the same sex?

5. If you have never slept with a person of the same sex, is it possible that all you need is a good gay lover?

6. To whom have you disclosed your heterosexual tendencies?

7. Why do heterosexuals feel compelled to seduce others into their lifestyle?

8. Why do you insist on flaunting your heterosexuality? Can't you just be what you are and keep it quiet?

9. Would you want your children to be heterosexual knowing the problems heterosexuals face?

10. A disproportionate majority of child molesters are heterosexuals. Do you consider it safe to expose your children to heterosexual teachers?

11. With all the societal support marriage receives, the divorce rate is spiraling. Why are there so few stable relationships among heterosexuals?

12. Why do heterosexuals place so much emphasis on sex?

13. Considering the menace of overpopulation, how could the human race survive if everyone was heterosexual like you?

LEARNING EXPERIENCE 3

TITLE: Addressing Harassment of Gay and Lesbian People: What's Wrong with What I Am Saying?

GRADE LEVELS: 7–9

TIME REQUIREMENTS: Two sessions of 40 minutes (10 minutes for ice-breaker activity, 20 minutes for discussion, and 10 minutes for arts-and-crafts activity)

LEARNING CONTEXT

The students will become aware of language that they or their peers use that negatively affects gay and lesbian people, as well as students who have gay or lesbian parents, family members, or friends. They will make a personal commitment to discontinue antigay language and to intervene in its use in their school and community.

NATIONAL LEARNING STANDARDS

2: Students will demonstrate the ability to access valid health information and health promoting products and services.

4: Students will analyze the influence of culture, media, technology, and other factors on health.

5: Students will demonstrate the ability to use interpersonal communication skills to enhance health.

6: Students will demonstrate the ability to use goal-setting and decision-making skills to enhance health.

7: Students will demonstrate the ability to advocate for personal, family, and community health.

PROCEDURE

This lesson is a means of defining terms associated with sexual orientation following basic definitions and as an introduction to discussions about bias.

Session 1: Brainstorming Activity

1. Organize students into groups of four or five, giving each group paper and a pencil or pen. Ask them to select one person to record group answers.
2. Ask students to brainstorm any words that come to mind relating to food. Give them 2 minutes.
3. Ask each group to read some of their answers while you write them on the board.
4. Review the list with the group, using the following facilitation questions:
   - What do you think of this list that you made?
   - What do you think about when you look at the list?
   - Did we all think of the same things?
   - Why do you think we all made different lists?
   - How come some people didn't like some of the things on the list?

   Take the time to point out to students that "we all came up with different lists because we're all different, and that's OK."
5. Repeat the brainstorming activity, but this time use the words *gay and lesbian* instead of *food*. Give them 2 minutes to brainstorm. Emphasize that "there are no right or wrong answers in brainstorming" and to "write down anything that comes to mind."
6. Ask each group to read some of their answers while you write them on the board.
7. Review the list with the group as before using the aforementioned facilitation questions. Here is an additional list of questions and talking points for the discussion about gay and lesbian people:
   - What does the word *gay* really mean?
   - Where did you get your brainstormed words?
   - How do people use the word *gay*?
   - What do people mean when they say, "That's so *gay*"?
   - How might you feel if you were a gay person hearing the words in the ways expressed here?
   - The word *gay* means happy or homosexual—it doesn't mean bad, wrong, not normal, freak, or weird.
   - The word *gay* does mean when two men or two women love each other just like when a man and a woman love each other.

Session 2

1. Have the students reflect aloud on the following questions:
   - How many of you have ever been teased?
   - How did it feel to be teased?
   - What did you or anyone standing by do?
   - How many people know a gay person? What can you tell us about that person?
   - How do you think someone who is gay or lesbian, or has two mothers or two fathers would feel in situations where the words we discussed yesterday were used?
   - What can you do if someone is being teased by being called "gay"?
   - What can you do or say when you hear words that might offend a gay person?
2. Distribute colored pieces of construction paper.
3. Write on the board the following: "When I hear someone use the words gay or lesbian to tease someone, I will _____." Ask students to write this statement on their paper but to fill in the blank with something they feel comfortable doing—something they are willing to make a commitment to. Review their answers from the previous section.
4. Have the students make a paper chain with the pieces of paper. Ask them whether they know why they are using the colors of the rainbow, and discuss with the class how the rainbow is used to represent the gay and lesbian community.
5. Hang the paper chain in the classroom, and ask students to use the chain as a reminder of their commitment to addressing harassment in school.

RESOURCES

Paper and pens or pencils for each group of students; 3″ × 11″ pieces of construction paper in colors of the rainbow (red, orange, yellow, green, blue, and purple); tape

LEARNING EXPERIENCE 4

TITLE: Deciding for Myself!

GRADE LEVELS: 10–12

TIME REQUIREMENTS: Two 35-minute sessions

LEARNING CONTEXT

This learning experience can be either an initial activity to determine what students know or think or a conclusion statement after a unit on sexual orientation. After this activity, the students will be aware of the myths and misconceptions they have about sexual orientation. They will also be able to identify concepts about sexual orientation for which they need more information.

NATIONAL LEARNING STANDARDS

1: Students will comprehend concepts related to health promotion and disease prevention.
2: Students will demonstrate the ability to access valid health information and health-promoting products and services.
4: Students will analyze the influence of culture, media, technology, and other factors on health.
5: Students will demonstrate the ability to use interpersonal communication skills to enhance health.
6: Students will demonstrate the ability to use goal-setting and decision-making skills to enhance health.
7: Students will demonstrate the ability to advocate for personal, family, and community health.

PROCEDURE

Tape three signs on three different walls in the room: "Agree-Disagree," "Need More Informa-tion," and "Don't Know." Read one statement at a time from those provided here. Ask the stu-dents to stand and move to the sign that best describes their position. When the students are un-der the sign, ask them to explain their position (for example, the students under the sign "Need More Information" will ask for clarification). Have the other students respond if possible. Then the students can stay or change their mind and move. Follow this same procedure for all state-ments. Add more sophisticated questions if they are developmentally appropriate.

Statements

A person is either heterosexual or homosexual.

You can tell people's sexual orientation by the way they behave.

At puberty one decides what sexual orientation one will be.

A bisexual person is usually a person who is confused about his or her sexual orientation.

A child of a homosexual parent is more likely to become homosexual.

A transgendered person is really gay.

Homosexuals live a very different lifestyle than do heterosexuals.

Lesbians are usually good athletes.

Homosexual couples cannot have children.

In most homosexual relationships, one person acts like the man and one acts like the woman.

AIDS is a gay disease.

It is against the law for homosexuals to marry.

Homosexuals are more sexually active than heterosexuals.

RESOURCES

Paper signs reading, "Agree-Disagree," "Need More Information," and "Don't Know"; tape

ASSESSMENT PLAN

The activity itself can act as an assessment of what students know at the beginning of the unit or what they have learned at the end of the unit.

LEARNING EXPERIENCE 5

TITLE: What Are Friends For?

GRADE LEVELS: 10–12

TIME REQUIREMENT: One 45-minute session

LEARNING CONTEXT

This exercise may follow a discussion about the coming-out process as part of the sexual orientation unit. It involves no formal assessment. After this activity, students will

- Understand the difficulty associated with the coming-out process.
- Recognize the different meanings for friendship.
- Identify some of the myths and misconceptions associated with sexual orientation.

NATIONAL LEARNING STANDARDS

4:   Students will analyze the influence of culture, media, technology, and other factors on health.

5:   Students will demonstrate the ability to use interpersonal communication skills to enhance health.

6:   Students will demonstrate the ability to use goal-setting and decision-making skills to enhance health.

7:   Students will demonstrate the ability to advocate for personal, family, and community health.

PROCEDURE

This exercise is conducted as a fishbowl role play. Arrange the class in a circle, and place five chairs in the center of the circle. Choose four students to begin the role play in the center of the circle. Give each of the students an index card with the information described later. The students are to leave the index card on their desk and play the role as assigned to them in the description on the index card. The students in the outer circle will observe the role play, and at any time that they wish to make a point, they will stand behind the person whose role they wish to take and tap them on the shoulder and change seats. The new person will be given a minute to read the role and continue the dialogue. The teacher may choose to put someone from the outer circle into the role at any time. When the role play is complete, ask the students to reflect on their experiences in the role and what they observed, writing their impressions in their journals.

The Roles

Explain to the students that these are four best friends since childhood. They played sports together, went to camp together, and hang out together all the time. They are getting ready to go away to college right after the summer. They're planning to room together after their freshman year in the dorms. Person 1 begins the discussion.

> *Person 1:* You are a gay person, and these are your best friends since childhood, but they don't know that you are gay (or you think they don't know). You feel bad because you have not been truthful with them about yourself; now that you are all getting ready to go to college, you want to come out to them. You have recently come out to your parents and are very nervous about what will happen.

> *Person 2:* After you hear Person 1 tell you why he or she wanted to have this "summit" together, you are stunned. After a few minutes to think about it, you want to be supportive, but you also want to let Person 1 know that you are so disappointed that he or she never told you.

> *Person 3:* You are totally horrified. You think that homosexuality is a sin and surely is unnatural. You can't believe the whole thing, and it changes everything about your friendship.

> *Person 4:* You just can't believe it. You think maybe your friend made a mistake. You want to help him or her get better because you are sure it is something else. Maybe it is that Person 1 doesn't trust anyone because someone hurt him or her in the past.

RESOURCES

Ample room for a circle of chairs; moveable chairs

LEARNING EXPERIENCE 6

TITLE: The Big Debate!

GRADE LEVELS: 10–12

TIME REQUIREMENTS: Two sessions for each debate (depending on how many debates are chosen)

LEARNING CONTEXT

After this learning experience, students will be able to

- Identify various current political issues about sexual orientation being discussed.
- Clarify their values and positions regarding the political issues.
- Understand the issues' impact on the society and the individuals involved.

NATIONAL LEARNING STANDARDS

1: Students will comprehend concepts related to health promotion and disease prevention.
2: Students will demonstrate the ability to access valid health information and health-promoting products and services.
4: Students will analyze the influence of culture, media, technology, and other factors on health.
5: Students will demonstrate the ability to use interpersonal communication skills to enhance health.
6: Students will demonstrate the ability to use goal-setting and decision-making skills to enhance health.
7: Students will demonstrate the ability to advocate for personal, family, and community health.

PROCEDURE

Put students in two different groups to prepare a debate. One way to select the groups is to pose a question and have the students who agree move to one side of the room and those who disagree move to the other side. (Debates are sometimes useful if a student gets an opportunity to debate the alternate side to their belief system. You can choose to organize the groups in that way or in support of their belief system.)

Instruct the groups to develop their arguments using the Internet and the library of resources about sexual orientation in the library and classroom. Then ask the students to line up their chairs opposite one another for the debate. Each group selects a person to make the initial position statement by the group. The rules are that each person gets a chance to speak by raising his or her hand either to make a point or to debate a point made by the opposite side. At the end of the debate, the student will reflect on the various positions.

Present the class with a rubric measuring the quality of the debate (included later). The class will use it to determine which group presented a more substantial debate. The following points can be debated:

1. Homosexual couples should be permitted to legally marry one another in this country and be afforded the same rights that heterosexual couples get with civil marriage.
2. "Out" homosexual people should be permitted to serve in the military with the same privileges and responsibilities as heterosexual people.
3. Homosexual couples should be permitted to adopt children in the same way that heterosexual people adopt.
4. "Out" homosexual people should be able to teach in elementary schools in the same manner as do heterosexual people.

RESOURCES

Computers with Internet access; pertinent journal and newspaper articles; other information sources

ASSESSMENT PLAN

A grade will be chosen by the class for each group worth 50 percent of the assignment grade. Using the rubric, the teacher will assign a grade worth the other 50 percent.

For an A:

- The group presented their position clearly and succinctly.
- The group had supporting information for their position.
- The group refuted all of the opponent's positions with documented information.
- The group showed evidence that they understood the controversy.
- Each member of the group participated.

For a B:

- The group presented their position clearly and succinctly.
- The group had supporting information for most of their position.
- The group refuted most of the opponents' positions with documented information.
- The group showed evidence that they understood the controversy.
- Almost all members of the group participated.

For a C:

- The group did not present their position clearly.
- The group had some supporting information for their position.
- The group refuted some of the opponents' positions with documented information.
- The group showed evidence that they understood some of the controversy.
- Only half of all members of the group participated.

For a D:

- The group did not present their position clearly.
- The group had little supporting information for their position.
- The group refuted only a few of the opponents' positions with documented information.
- The group showed little evidence that they understood the controversy.
- Only a few of the members of the group participated.

LEARNING EXPERIENCE 7

TITLE: It's the News, Nothing but the News!

GRADE LEVELS: 10–12

TIME REQUIREMENTS: Two sessions

LEARNING CONTEXT
After this learning experience, students will
- Be able to advocate against bias crimes.
- Be able to express their feelings against violence.
- Be sensitive to the dangers of discrimination.
- Be able to identify with the fears and persecution of people with different orientations than heterosexual.

NATIONAL LEARNING STANDARDS
2: Students will demonstrate the ability to access valid health information and health-promoting products and services.
4: Students will analyze the influence of culture, media, technology, and other factors on health.
5: Students will demonstrate the ability to use interpersonal communication skills to enhance health.
6: Students will demonstrate the ability to use goal-setting and decision-making skills to enhance health.
7: Students will demonstrate the ability to advocate for personal, family, and community health.

PROCEDURE
Working in groups of four, the students will pretend that they are reporters for the local newspaper and have been asked to write an essay about a crime and what it means to the neighborhood. The crime: A bias crime has occurred in this neighborhood in which a group of teens attacked, taunted, and physically assaulted a gay teen couple. It is the job of the group to write the article and to educate the public. The group will then develop a rubric that they would use to determine how effective the article is. The various rubrics will be combined until there is one class rubric. Then each group will present their article to the class. Using the rubric, the class will choose the most effective article, and the students who prepared it will get an extra-credit A.

RESOURCES
Paper and pens/pencils

ASSESSMENT PLAN
The rubric developed in class as part of the lesson can be used as the assessment instrument.

RELATIONSHIPS

ESTELLE WEINSTEIN

OBJECTIVES

After reading this chapter, students will

1. Identify the factors that contribute to a healthy relationship.
2. Describe the various relationships in which human beings participate.
3. Identify relationships associated with various developmental levels such as family, friends, dates, and mate selection.
4. Develop skills for maintaining healthy relationships, including communication, decision making, and goal setting.
5. Describe the characteristics of unhealthy relationships.
6. Explain the relationship issues commonly associated with setting boundaries, feeling jealousy, ending relationships, and so forth.
7. Identify resources in the community for helping people with relationship problems.

REFLECTIVE QUESTIONS

Elementary School Students
1. Who are the members of your family?
2. How does your family differ from other families that you know?
3. What are the characteristics of your close friends?
4. What makes you a good friend?

Middle School Students
1. Who are the members of your family?
2. What are the important functions of your family?
3. What are your expectations for a "best friend"?
4. What do your close friends say about you as a friend?
5. What does dating mean to you?
6. What does it mean to be a couple?
7. What are some of the expectations of being in a couple relationship?
8. What are the advantages and disadvantages of being in a couple relationship?

Senior High School Students
1. What are the advantages and disadvantages of being identified with one peer group?
2. What are the expectations of you as part of your group of close friends?
3. What characteristics do you look for in your closest friends?
4. What characteristics do you look for in a dating/partnering relationship?
5. What do you look for in a couple relationship?
6. What are the boundaries and expectations of people in couple relationships (particularly sexually intimate ones)? How do you establish those boundaries?
7. What characteristics would you find important in a long-term/permanent relationship?
8. How will having sexual intercourse with your partner affect the relationship and your future goals?

SCENARIO (FOR UPPER-LEVEL STUDENTS, 10TH–12TH GRADES)

(Note: This scenario can be presented using the names Sebastian and James, making it equally comfortable for gay and lesbian couples in your classes and for normalizing gay and lesbian relationships.)

It is almost the end of summer, and Sebastian and Anna are getting ready to go to college for the first time. They have both been accepted to the colleges of their choice. Sebastian is going upstate, and Anna is going to a college on the West Coast. They have been a couple for more than 2 years and have often talked about "someday" when they will be together always, but they have not always agreed. Their parents have been concerned about their relationship and have told them they need to have experiences with other people. They have been avoiding a discussion about the boundaries of their relationship when they are away at college primarily because they know they do not have the same ideas. Anna has lofty career goals and isn't sure that a permanent relationship is what she wants. Sebastian also has big career goals, but he wants to be married and have children after he graduates from college. Sebastian has had experiences with other women, but he is Anna's first boyfriend. Anna does not want an exclusive relationship during her college years and believes that if they are meant to be together in the future, it will happen. He thinks she is right but is just not sure.

What would you want if you were Sebastian?
What would you want if you were Anna?
What are some of the rules and boundaries that can be established between them?
What are the advantages and disadvantages of staying as an exclusive couple?
What are the advantages and disadvantages of changing the relationship?

INTRODUCTION

Searching for your "ideal" love, creating your "ideal" family, and developing your "ideal" friendships are the lifetime quests of individuals across cultures. These special connections that people make with one another constitute personal relationships. Yet, the characteristics and expectations that make up each of the ideal relationships are different within and across cultures and individuals. Through them, individuals experience love and respect and learn to love and respect others in return. Healthy relationships nurture self-esteem, raise self-confidence, and contribute to one's ability to trust, know intimacy, and feel safer in what is sometimes a frightening world.

As you no doubt realize, there is considerable distance between "ideal" relationships and generally healthy relationships. Early childhood and adolescent relationships are training grounds where the personal life skills necessary to create future adult, personally enriching relationships are learned. Thus, this chapter is devoted to these early parenting, initial, and subsequent friendships, dating, lifetime partnering, and other such important relationships. Exploring the factors that make for healthy interactions, and the personal life skills necessary to maintain them, will be presented.

LOVE

One cannot discuss relationships without some mention of love. Love, that magical ingredient that poets, storytellers, philosophers, sociologists, and ordinary folk have been trying to explain for centuries, is the stuff of which "dreams are made." Humans search for love and need it from the very beginning of their existence. Yet, exactly what love is eludes us when trying to explain it. How love is experienced and described is different for people in different kinds of relationships (family, friends, partners), different cultures, and different ages, and there is also considerable difference by gender. Although it is beyond the scope of this chapter to describe each of these differences at length, we will consider concepts about love that commonly exist in relationships.

Hatfield and Rapson (1993) explain two different types of love. *Passionate* love they describe as a "state of intense longing for union with another" (p. 5). This state of love is one of volatility filled with powerful emotions that usually involve a desire for sexual union. *Companionate* love, they say, is the "affection and tenderness we feel for those with whom our lives are deeply entwined" (p. 9). These researchers explain "companionate" love is that love sometimes called "true love" or "marital love." When compared to passionate love, companionate love "is a warm, far less intense emotion. It combines feelings of deep attachment, commitment, and intimacy" (p. 10).

How people experience love is associated with their early experiences with nurturance, trust, independence, dependence, and intimacy, in addition to cultural and gender differences. The more secure individuals feel about love, the more likely they are to experience companionate love, the more likely they are able to commit to their partner, and the more intimate the relationship (Hatfield & Rapson, 1993).

Sternberg (1986) describes love as three components that constitute a triangle. *Intimacy* is the emotional component of love that includes a feeling of connectedness found in family, friendship, and love relationships. *Passion* is the motivational component of love that consists of the physical needs and attractions for one another, the chemistry that leads to desire, arousal, and sexual relations. *Decision and commitment,* the cognitive component of love that maintains the relationship, exists in permanent partner relationships and child–parent relationships. According to Sternberg, a relationship that does not contain the three components is not a complete love relationship and does not achieve "consummate or complete love." Moreover, although people who experience what Sternberg calls "friendship love" have enormous and sometimes overwhelming feelings for one another and for their well-being, it is not "consummate or complete love." Nor is what Sternberg calls "infatuated or romantically in love" whereby there is only an intense physical attraction and a desire to be sexual with the other. Hence, Sternberg suggests that to develop into complete or consummate love, these relationships must occur in the context of a conscious commitment. Furthermore, people who have commitment without intimacy or passion have what Sternberg refers to as an "empty love." Thus, beginning with any one component, it is the development and ultimate existence of all three components of love (intimacy as the emotional component; passion as the motivational component; decision and commitment as the cognitive components) that constitutes the "completeness of love."

Boundaries get established by the people in a relationship. These boundaries are often expectations and limitations defined by society and accepted by the participants. One of the boundaries is sexual intimacy. American society, similar to other societies across the globe, acknowledge some differences in where sexual behavior fits into relationships. Those that include love are not always sexual, and those that include sex are not always love.

In U.S. society, sexual relationships are inappropriate among immediate family members (see Chapter 11 on sexual violence) and sometimes confusing in friendships. Some friendships change to become passionate and sexually intimate, whereas others are distinctly sexual and passionate from the onset, having friendship as a component. The decision to permit a passionate, or any other love relationship, to include sexual intimacy should be a conscious decision even when the passion feels overwhelming. It should be one that is agreed on by two mature adults in a noncoercive agreement that defines the type of relationship that it will be.

RELATIONSHIPS

The following section discusses the various relationships that people create with each other and their inherent boundaries and limitations.

Families

A *family* is a recognizable institution or group of people with specific roles, tasks, boundaries, and personalities that affect each member and the group as a whole. The specific functions and expectations of a family may differ from one culture to another. The family is influenced by and influences the larger society in which it exists. Hence, it is a dynamic institution that is constantly changing as society changes.

As the definition of family changes over time, so do those individuals believed to constitute family membership. Families are usually made up of people (two or more) related to one another by blood, marriage/long-term committed relationships, or adoption. Yet, groups of people who do not fit these criteria also function as and are considered family units—among them unmarried same- or other-sex couples with or without children; one-parent families including never married, widowed, or single-parent households of divorced or separated spouses; reconstituted families or stepfamilies consisting of children from multiple marriages; and blended families in which either or both partners bring children to the family, and they may also have additional children together. Beyond the "nuclear" family is the extended family of grandparents, aunts, uncles, cousins, and other relatives. These extended family members also affect the way a family functions in any given society.

The central focus of families is to care for, protect, love, and socialize one another. Families are responsible for economic maintenance and the provision of material resources. They foster a sense of security and a feeling of belonging. They provide for healthy physical and psychological growth and development throughout the life cycle. These roles and responsibilities of family members to each other, and how successful they are in meeting the needs of one another, are not more or less effective in any particular family constellation. Conservative views of the mother, father, children, dog, and white picket fence as the "best" family type have not been substantiated by the literature. Single-parent families, families without children, and gay and lesbian families can and do meet each other's needs equally as well. (See Chapter 7 for a further discussion of families as they relate to child rearing.)

Although many families decide at some point to have children, some families choose to remain childless. Some people recognize that they are not "cut out to be parents" or have interests or responsibilities such as careers that require long working hours or travel that might compromise their vision of effective parenting. Still others define parenthood in terms of genetics. When they cannot achieve a pregnancy, they also may choose to remain childless (see Chapter 7 on parenting). Having or not having children should be a free choice, yet in the United States, a still somewhat traditional society, couples who decide not to have children are sometimes viewed with disdain or pity.

Children initially learn about love, intimacy, feelings, problem solving, gender roles, and behaviors from their family of origin. How the family disseminates information to one another and who has access to that information are constructs of family dynamics that are the earliest lessons in negotiating relationships. Healthy families provide an opportunity for children to learn to communicate effectively; influence values, attitudes, and behaviors; and cultivate religious and spiritual belief systems. From this list of tasks for healthy families, one can understand the overwhelming job and important dynamics families provide in society. When children are launched into relationships outside the family, they use the initial behaviors and skills modeled by their family of origin.

In some situations, families can be the cause of pain and suffering, a diminished self-esteem, and poor communication and coping styles. Framo (1992) describes some of the problems associated with unhealthy families that potentially damage family members: scapegoating, humiliation, shaming, parentification, crazy-making, physical, sexual and verbal abuse, cruel rejection, lies, deceit, and general outrage against the human spirit. (Additional discussion about the impact of child abuse on children appears in Chapter 12.)

Children coming to the school setting with limited experiences and knowledge about family constellations can learn about family life and families different from their own, expanding their ability to negotiate successful relationships in the future, developing a tolerance for the uniqueness of culture and ethnicity as they influence families, and creating greater possibilities for living happily in this diverse world. Students can develop a better understanding of the roles and responsibilities exhibited by their family and those family scripts that are possible for them. They then will be better able to recognize patterns that are not healthy and the resources available for assistance.

Friendships

Friendships are relationships between two or more people involving mutual trust, support, respect, and intimacy that may or may not include sexual intimacy. Friendships, like families, have boundaries that are specific to those in the friendship and require that each person communicate his or her understandings, needs, expectations, limitations, and affections.

EARLY TO MIDDLE CHILDHOOD FRIENDSHIPS

The initial friendships children develop are but extensions of messages and styles exhibited within their family. The definitions of friendships and how families respond to their members' friendships vary, and they can influence with whom friendships are made. Young children create friendships that involve play and learning to share (initially with reluctance) that does not initially involve bonding or commitment; they are often referred to as play dates, usually planned by adults. It is not until about the 6th or 7th year that friendships actually involve some reciprocity. Children at this age begin to share feelings as well as toys and play, and they in turn experience the rudiments of trust, comfort, and acceptance. As they share themselves with others, they deepen the meaning of their friendships.

Throughout the remaining elementary school years, children begin to formulate their own perceptions about the characteristics they will cherish in others and the styles of relationships they are likely to embrace. During these later childhood friendship experiences, children come to recognize that friendships take on different meanings and people in friendships take on different roles. Some friendships are limited to sharing recreational or sport interests, some are restricting of independence ("I can't do anything without him [or her]"), whereas others are nurturing of it ("Let's ask Miguel to come along with us!"). Some friendships support leaders, and others support followers. Some friendships develop and are maintained because of family or peer pressure. They occur when children are limited to play with and befriend people whom their family or peers think are "right" for them.

Children begin to learn that they can barter things for friendship such as popularity, acceptance, and approval. If they experience early friendships that are not safe or comfortable and ultimately disappointing, they may grow to be reluctant about friendships later in their life.

PREADOLESCENT TO ADOLESCENT FRIENDSHIPS

Friendships that include strong connections have their roots in preadolescence. These friendships, when they are healthy, tend to validate each person's self-worth and recognize and embrace their individual needs. They are mutually satisfying. Preadolescents' closest friendships are commonly of the same gender. As individuals begin to emerge as adolescents, their relationships include both genders and develop into more serious attachments. These "special" friendships are training grounds for the commitment, permanency, and dependability associated with more mature long-term relationships.

Early adolescents often create their friendships somewhat haphazardly. Their friends are people who are in their class, live on their street, play on their team, or are generally easily accessible. By middle adolescence, teens are searching for a personal identity, separate and distinct from their family, at the same time as they are attempting to feel included, attached, and accepted by their peer group. They begin to find friends that are not necessarily associated with their very immediate surroundings and friends who are not always approved of by their family. Although some twosomes may begin at this stage, adolescents are usually part of a larger group. The outcome of these friendships are still a matter of "luck" rather than "skill" because they are meeting developmental needs that are not yet associated with the particular individual's higher-order needs.

Later in adolescence, if maturity is within reach, ego identity is established, and the relationships begin to represent independent choices. When young people choose healthy relationships, they experience support, their sense of self is nourished, their independence is appreciated, they feel relaxed, they can communicate, and their decisions are accepted, all of which empowers them to trust their ability to relate to others in connected ways. On the other hand, if they have had unsuccessful attempts at friendships, they may feel isolated and lonely.

The school environment is one that can foster learning about the functions of friendships, ways to seek out and evaluate friendships, and how to set boundaries and adopt roles that complement them such that adolescents are less likely to succumb to negative peer pressure. Discussions about how to develop mutually acceptable expectations of friends and how to maintain the friendship through the various developmental changes are part of the learning process.

DATING/EARLY PARTNERING RELATIONSHIPS

As children move into adolescence, they tend to add a "dating" dimension to their relationships. What that means is that in addition to the group activities, they begin to seek a partner with whom they will spend couple time.

In Chapters 2 and 4, we discussed the theory of social scripting (Gagnon & Simon, 1984). *Dating* is an interpersonal relationship involving social scripting that suggests that we each have a predetermined notion about what role we will play and what behaviors constitute that role in couple relationships. In dating relationships, that can mean who will initiate the first encounter, who will plan the way time is spent, how conversations will occur and what will be talked about, how sexually intimate the relationship will become, and who will initiate sex and how. Individual social scripts will impact how these roles are played out. Sometimes the scripts are very different for each participant; those differences represent sociocultural influences, gender, age, sexual orientation, family values, and so forth. Early partnering styles also emerge from the peer group with which young people are associated. A pecking order exists in these groups, and partners are often chosen because they are acceptable to their peer group.

The expected behaviors of these early dating relationships are representative of the heterosexual experiences and group norms, values, attitudes, and behaviors. The rules or social scripts begin to operate as the mechanics of dating are attempted: "How do I ask someone to go out?" "Where should we go, and what should we do?" "How do I refuse an invitation without insulting, rejecting, or demeaning the other person?" Armed with early dating skills helps a teen to feel more secure and less vulnerable. These initial romantic interests may also include their initial sexually intimate experiences or they may not. They also provide opportunities to practice behaviors that may lead toward selecting a permanent partner later in their lives.

For youth who are interested in same-sex connections, the opportunities are far less available. In the social milieu as it exists today, homosexual teens are not yet likely to have come out to their peers. Unless they have made connections through concerned organizations, homosexual young people often do not have the opportunity to practice their initial partnering skills in same-sex situations until much later in adolescence or early adulthood (see Chapter 5 for a more extensive discussion). Often their first experiences, then, are with other-sex partners.

As pre- and early adolescents mature, more individual characteristics of the partners they choose become important but still within the cultural and acceptable norms established by the peer group. Such things as sense of humor, interests, outgoingness, and intelligence factor into the partnering. The couple also begins to practice the more serious characteristics that they will embrace later in their lives, including the ability to communicate, self-disclose, care, and trust.

Courtship, dating, or hooking up—or whatever the most current terminology is—is an important process for young people. Essentially it is the experience of moving a relationship through a series of phases that result in sexual intimacy. Freund and Blanchard (1986) describe a useful four-phase process that is still applicable today:

1. Location and the initial appraisal of a potential partner
2. Pretactile interaction (for example, smiling at, posturing for, or talking to a prospective partner)

3. Tactile interaction (for example, touching, embracing)
4. Effecting genital union

The authors explain that the power of the drive to sexual union is determined by the degree to which each of the partners responds to the other's initiations. They discuss various problems in the process that include rejection or misinterpretation of the signals of courtship that may lead to disappointment and embarrassment.

Adolescents' personal notions of physical attractiveness, how to behave when out with someone new, and what sexual behaviors will be transacted are rooted in culture, gender roles, messages from the popular media, and early childhood fantasy stories such as "Snow White" or "Cinderella." These factors strongly influence the roles and scripts that they will play in their relationships and are often stereotypically gender based (see Chapter 4). A sense of physical perfectionism displayed in the media results in such things as eating disorders and self-doubt as youth desperately seek peer acceptance. Moreover, popular media biases against people with special physical challenges often restrict people who do not fit some "ideal" from getting to know one another as potential partners and friends. The more serious the dating, the more practice in developing future, successful, long-term committed/marital relationships if they choose them.

SEXUAL BEHAVIOR IN EARLY PARTNERING RELATIONSHIPS

Sexual behavior from preadolescence to early adulthood is a phenomenon that grows out of multigenerational messages, developmental tasks, family, and peer pressures. The pleasures of sexual activity abound in the messages people receive from one another and the media, but the road to achieving those pleasures is full of myths and pitfalls including emotional stigma, unintended pregnancy, sexually transmitted infections, and rejection. Yet, young people continue to participate in sexual intercourse at earlier and earlier ages.

A recent study by Ryan, Manlove, and Franzetta (2003), sponsored by the National Campaign to Prevent Teen Pregnancy, provides an interesting look at the relationships in which first sexual experiences occur. Forty-two percent of the sexually experienced adolescents in this study reported that they were already friends with their first sexual partner before they had their first sexual relationship and that they met their first partner in school or at a place of worship. Moreover, they were more likely to have participated in "couple-like" behavior before their first experience (boys somewhat less so than girls, and teens younger than 14 rather than older teens). These couple-like behaviors included not only thinking of themselves as a couple but also announcing to others that they were a couple, going out alone, meeting each other's parents, exchanging presents, and telling each other "I love you."

Because sexual intimacy is so much a part of the rules of dating and early partnering, it behooves the sexuality educator to begin discussions of it in the earliest preadolescent stage. Sexual intimacy is often defined by heterosexual teens as a measure of the quality and importance of their couple relationship. Although having sex sometimes occurs without a sense of couple, a relationship is deemed as important when it includes increasing sexual intimacy. Since adolescents often do not know how to define the "specialness" of their relationship in other than sexual ways, the sexuality educator must also offer opportunities for them to reflect on attaining these skills. Among the skills to be fostered is an ability to set personal boundaries about sexual behavior within the context of their relationships that are congruent with their personal values, their family and religious values, and so forth. Being able to communicate these boundaries with one another in effective and respectful ways can also be learned. Saying no and accepting no without feelings of rejection are additional essential communication skills to be achieved. Moreover, knowing how to tell someone you love them and are important to them, and receiving those messages in return, in other than sexual ways are also skills that may delay the onset of early sexual behaviors. The challenge to have their needs met and limitations respected is an enormously difficult concept to master when adolescents' very self-concept is determined by the acceptance of their peer group.

Progression of Sexual Behaviors

When people feel an attraction for one another, they begin to desire a physical connection or physical way to share their sexual feelings. The initial behaviors frequently include embracing and light kissing that slowly deepens. Stirrings for more intimate touching occur and progress to "petting" that includes touching the sexually arousing parts of each other's body. This sexual touching stimulates physical changes in the body, particularly the genitals (see Chapter 3 for a discussion of human sexual response). Petting leads to more intimate embraces that may include nudity and become intensely stimulating. As the intensity builds, the genitals engorge with blood, lubricate, and prepare for sexual intercourse. What is important for young people to recognize is that, when the intensity becomes great and the intimacy grows, it becomes extremely difficult to resist having sexual intercourse. Hence, sexuality education can encourage young people to limit their sexual behaviors until they have made very clear decisions about which behaviors they are willing to participate in, when, and how. Such decisions are personal; they need to be communicated, and they need to be accepted and respected by both partners. The decisions need to represent a sense of self-respect, responsibility, and maturity.

When a couple is comfortable and ready for sexual intercourse, one would expect that they are able to and have discussed the potential outcomes, the effect it will have on their sense of themselves and on their relationship, and the ways in which they will keep themselves and each other safe from disease or unintended pregnancy. Their agreement to be sexual with one another will not be for purposes of gaining an adult identity, holding on to a partner, being popular, or demonstrating manhood or womanhood. The 2003 study sponsored by the National Campaign to Prevent Teen Pregnancy reports that before having sexual intercourse for the first time, adolescents participated in several other intimate behaviors including kissing, holding hands, and intimately touching under clothing or nude. The study further indicates that the more couple-like behaviors teens had before their first sexual experience, the more likely they would be to have discussed contraception. Moreover, the more intimate behaviors they participated in before sexual intercourse, the more likely they were to have discussed contraception (Ryan et al., 2003).

Achieving mature sexually intimate relationships, those that support each partner's well-being, self-concept, and trust, also emerge out of a developmental process. The earliest sexual experiences represent a search for the answer to "Who am I as a sexual being?" During this stage, adolescents are busy comparing themselves to others, including the size of their genitals and the number and kinds of behaviors they have done. Soon they begin to explore their partner: "Who are you as a sexual being?" Then, they are interested in the other's sexual response and their own part in it. Finally, when they achieve mature sexual intimacy, they begin to experience the couple dynamic: "Who are we as sexual partners?" and "How do we achieve a mutually satisfying sexual relationship?"

While adolescents are learning and practicing their early coupling experiences, they frequently mistake them for the "one" that they will be in forever, and the rules and boundaries become somewhat foggy. Hence, education can explore the notion that one might or might not seek a permanent long-term relationship/marriage and, if they do, when in their life plans they would consider it. Also, education can help students to determine what characteristics they would seek in a permanent partner and whether and how they might differ from those they seek in other coupling relationships. Moreover, students can be encouraged to reflect on how serious attachments and sexual intimacy may enhance or create potential barriers for reaching their more long-term life goals.

Choosing to Be Single

Some people remain single by choice, and others because they have not found the right person with whom to permanently cohabit or marry. Some people make the choice to remain single after they have lost a permanent partner as a result of separation, divorce, or death. Particularly in later age, those who have had permanent partners and lose their mates to death often make the choice to remain single. Cultural beliefs and the economics of our society also influence the choice to be single. Our tax laws and pension parameters create a disincentive for heterosexual couples to remarry, particularly among the elderly. They lose the Social Security benefits of their deceased partner and sometimes their pension. On the other hand, women in some cultures do not have status unless they are married; moreover, because a great unevenness persists in income levels between men and women, women have greater incentive to marry or permanently partner even though they might prefer to remain single.

In a society where dual incomes are almost a necessity for survival of a couple (especially one with children), people who are economically able to provide for themselves are more able to remain single, if they so choose. Although the vast majority of people in the United States opt to marry (and some others are not legally able to marry), estimates have it that today approximately 10 percent of Americans plan to be single. Remaining single does not preclude having deep, important friendships and intimate partners throughout life, many of whom decide to cohabit without the legal boundaries of a marital agreement. It also does not mean that one cannot change plans at some later time. Hence, what is important for students to discuss and reflect on is what they believe about themselves and permanent relationships, what their personal view of the advantages and disadvantages of being permanently partnered or remaining single are (since what one individual may see as an advantage may be a disadvantage to the other), and how to choose a lifestyle based on their own decisions and not societal pressure.

Choosing a Long-Term Committed/Marital Relationship

For those who choose to marry or create a lifetime committed relationship, that decision requires considerable reflection. Although physical attraction is often the initial connection between people, the factors that determine who we will "like," "love," and choose for a mate are driven by a host of sociocultural factors. The immediacy of appearance does not necessarily fade, but other characteristics are sought when one begins to think about long-term commitment.

The early study by Troll and Smith (1976) of attraction and attachment provides some interesting information to contemplate today as it relates to permanent relationships. The researchers claim that attraction, early in a relationship, is powerful, whereas attachment is low. As the power of attraction diminishes, attachment increases. They go on to explain that, if the quality of a marital or long-term committed relationship is defined in terms of attraction, it will be deemed somewhat unsatisfactory over time, whereas if happiness is attachment, security, loyalty, and the like, satisfaction will increase over time.

Levine, Sato, Hashimoto, and Verma (1994) asked young people if a potential mate had all the other qualities desired including "love," but they were not "in love" with their partner, would they want to marry that person? Most of the participants responded no. The notion of being "in love" with or ultimately learning to love a prospective mate is rooted in the history of marriage agreements and gender influences.

Historically, marriage partners were chosen by the elders in their family, usually the father, based on the suitor's ability to meet many social, political, and financial obligations. Because women had little of their own to barter in the way of education or financial security, mates were sought contingent on how well they could and how willing they would be to care for the prospective bride and future children. Oftentimes the partners had never met until the selection was made, and love and attraction were expected to come later as the relationship developed. As women's conditions began to change and as they became more able to control pregnancy and achieve financial and social independence, their choice of partner became more their own. The factors that determine their choices are similar to those of men, including the search for such characteristics as appearance, romance, sexual appeal, personality, education, career, religious and cultural similarities, and "being in love" (Travis & Yaeger, 1992; Hatfeld & Rapson, 1996). Hence, learning to love a partner chosen by someone else is less appealing today. However, family acceptance and support continue to be of importance.

The relationship of sexual intimacy to committed permanent relationships/marriages is also changing as standards of sexual behavior change. The vast majority of Americans (more than 90 percent) will marry or develop long-term committed relationships at some point in their lives. The time frame for creating those relationships has changed over several generations; today many people delay this decision until well into their 30s and sometimes 40s. Nonetheless, they are not delaying their experiences with sex. People often question what impact having or delaying sexual activity will have on the likelihood of the relationship becoming permanent. There does not seem to be a correlation between initiation of sex by the couple and whether or not they will commit.

Some couples have a sexually traditional attitude that requires that sexual intercourse be delayed until the relationship is long-term committed/marital and believe that sex is an expression of the love and caring that only these two people should share. Other couples, with similar feelings, believe that sexual intercourse can be initiated when there is "true love" without a specific permanent time established for the commitment. Still others do not necessarily connect sex with love or caring and believe that sex is simply a pleasurable behavior. For most couples, marriage and permanent long-term commitment means sexual monogamy. Other couples do not define their relationships as having strict sexual boundaries. Some couples have arrangements regarding sex with a person other than their partner with the partner's prior consent and knowledge (open marriages). Hence, marriage/permanent commitments, in addition to having legal ramifications, are agreements between two people who have discussed their position with one another, respect each other's position, and are mature enough to recognize the importance of their arrangement to the relationship and to their individual lives.

Studies addressing the frequency of sex in long-term relationships have looked almost exclusively at married, heterosexual data. Moreover, they generally do not address sexual satisfaction. Much of the data suggest that the younger the people and the younger the marriage, the more the sexual activity. Sexual infrequency is sometimes a measure of sexual dissatisfaction (Westheimer & Lopater, 2002). It is also thought that a sexual relationship is a lens through which one can observe the quality of the rest of the relationship. It is thought that a couple who is happy with one another are likely to be more satisfied with their sexual activity, and the more satisfied they are with one another and the sex, the more they will be satisfied with the sexual frequency. Essentially, the frequency with which couples partici-pate in sex is a product of many variables, including age, number of years in the relationship, health status, career and other time-consuming respon-sibilities, degree of privacy, individual sexual desire patterns, and sexual scripts.

Fenell (1993) studied people married more than 20 years who define their marriages as successful and describes several specific characteristics:

1. The partners had an intellectual and emotional assumption that the person they married would be their one and only spouse.
2. They expect to give this person loyalty and friendship.
3. Both individuals had strong moral and spiritual compatibility, and both had always thought that being a parent was a very important part of being married.
4. They expressed a consistent desire to make the other person happy.
5. They thought that it was very important to forgive their partner's falli-bilities and similarly be forgiven. (cited in Westheimer & Lopater, 2002, pp. 459–460)

Minirth, Minirth, Newman, Newman, Hemfelt, and Hemfelt (1991) describe a developmental process of "passages of marriage." They envision stages occurring in marriages when couples begin in their 20s. The five stages include the first 2 years called "young love"; the next 8 years called "realistic love"; the 11th to the 25th years called "comfortable love"; the 26th through 35th years called "renewing love"; and from then on, "tran-scendent love." Each of these stages has appropriate tasks that the couple must master to maintain their relationship.

Westheimer and Lopater (2002) discuss some of the characteristics that make for long-term successful marriages, suggesting that these qualities are the same in long-term committed relationships such as those entered into by gay and lesbian couples for whom marriage is still an illegal or un-available option. These characteristics include the level of communication that supports honesty, nonjudgmental attitudes, shared and equitable decision making, domestic labor and finances, and an ability to deal with conflict and solve problems. These characteristics are developed in the marriage over time and are not necessarily present at the time of the commitment.

When people have identified the physical characteristics that they are seeking in their permanent partner and feel ready to make a commitment, they might consider discussing the following:

• The expectations each partner has of the other and of the relationship
• The roles each partner will play in the relationship and how they will deal with changes in the roles over time

- How each individual's needs and interests will be managed and supported
- Where and how religious and spiritual activities fit into the relationship
- What characteristics or behaviors may create barriers or difficulties and how they will deal with them (for example, substance use or abuse, TV watching, and sleeping habits)
- How the sexual relationship will be managed and the boundaries associated with sexual activity
- The strengths and weaknesses of the partners and how they will accommodate for them
- An agreed-on strategy for resolving differences
- How they will deal with matters of money, including investments and savings
- Decisions about parenthood
- Establishment of boundaries regarding other relationships, including family, friends (past and present), and past partners
- How they will become flexible enough to accommodate for the changes that occur throughout the relationship, including differing levels of development, experience, success in careers, readiness for parenthood, retirement, and older age.

It was not more than one or two generations ago that the life span was considerably shorter and, hence, the span of a life-long relationship was also shorter. People married at younger ages, had families rather quickly, and reached old age in what we might almost consider middle age today. It is not unusual for couples today to be married/committed to one another for more than 50 years. Maintaining such a long-term relationship is a complicated matter and beyond the abstract ability with which school-age students can identify. Rather, many are afraid that they will not be able to be with one partner for so long, and, because their experience speaks to so many marriages ending in divorce, it is sometimes a disincentive for commitment. As explained earlier, people are waiting much longer to create their permanent/marital relationships and to have their children, so one might think that this generation may not experience a 50+ anniversary. But, the number of people living into the 90th and 100th year is also increasing rapidly. What the future will hold for them is interesting. Thus, long-term relationships/marriages are expected to be really long-term. Hence, a lifelong commitment seems, on the one hand, quite ominous but is, on the other, still the predominant life script held by most Americans.

Knowing that more than three-quarters of teen marriages and half of adult marriages result in divorce, teens can be helped to master skills that will result in a more successful and happy long-term relationship. Armed with some knowledge of the complicated nature of long-term relationships, young people will be better able to delay such decisions until they have developed effective skills and had the necessary experiences to support success. The skills of communication, decision making, goal setting, and stress and self-management will need to be mastered and applied to permanent relationships to increase their likelihood of permanency.

GENDER INFLUENCES ON LONG-TERM COMMITTED/MARITAL RELATIONSHIPS

Heterosexual Couples

Culturally, common scripts for heterosexual couples idealize the provider husband and housewife/stay-at-home mother roles and associated behaviors. Yet, these roles were only normative for a very brief time in U.S. history and mostly among those privileged members of the society (Sollie, 2002). Moreover, although a verbal commitment to more egalitarian relationships may exist, the traditional values of gender-stereotypical roles are difficult to overcome.

The balance of power seems to be an important variable in how couples function. Power, particularly in relationships, is often defined by the amount of career, financial, and educational success an individual achieves. Another component of power is dependency, which is closely associated with financial independence. Economic influences resulting in the dual-career family have forced changes in women's roles more so than in men's, but the financial balance of economics is still not equal. Today, women often maintain the primary household and child care roles while they continue their careers, sometimes creating more dissatisfaction in their marital relationships.

Stereotypically, women have been expected to nurture, sustain the intimacy, and maintain the emotional connections in a relationship, whereas men are thought to be less able or invested in these roles. Yet, modern couples are seeking more emotional connections and nurturing from both partners. Research indicates that more equitably distributed power in a relationship results in more connection and satisfaction (Gottman, 1999). Hence, much is changing in heterosexual relationships, and men, socialized from childhood to maintain gender-stereotypical behaviors as a component of their sexual identity, are likely to be in relationships with less satisfied partners. Women who hold more stereotypical roles will take the greater responsibility for marital conflict and experience less personal satisfaction (Sollie, 2002). However, greater numbers of people are finding ways to define their couple within nongender-stereotypical guidelines. As less gender-defined restrictions on sexual and communication patterns emerge, satisfaction with the sexual and general relationship patterns is increasing.

Homosexual Couples

The research on long-term commitment among homosexual couples is not extensive enough to draw effective conclusions about their similarities and differences to heterosexual couples. Moreover, neither heterosexual nor homosexual couple research sufficiently accounts for within-culture, age, income, religiosity, and other phenomena. That said, some data indicate that, similar to more modern heterosexual couples, a more egalitarian relationship is highly valued by homosexual couples. Power in the relationship is associated with income, level of education, and social position in the community, and power influences equality. Among gay men, income is associated with greater power. Among lesbians, power is associated more with dependency: the more dependent one partner is, the less power she has (Sollie, 2002).

Homosexual couples, like heterosexual couples, are mostly dual-career couples. Among gay couples, responsibilities and behaviors associated with the relationship are distributed based on preferences, availability, and flexibility. Among lesbian couples, there is a more equal sharing of roles and tasks. As with heterosexual couples, closeness and emotional connection, equality, and the ability to express emotional closeness are associated with satisfaction in the relationship. Some of the difficulties experienced by homosexual couples have to do with their legal and social status as couples, and the social pressures and restrictions that often accompany an inability to communicate their relationship to family and community.

AFFAIRS OUTSIDE THE MARRIAGE/ LONG-TERM COMMITTED RELATIONSHIP

Sometimes, an infidelity or an affair causes the deconstruction of a relationship. A long-term committed/marital relationship usually expects monogamy. When an affair occurs, whether it is a one-time impulsive behavior or a long-term external relationship, it compromises the couple and their trust, comfort, and safety. Most external relationships represent a general dissatisfaction with the marital or long-term commitment.

There is a whole range of personality, cultural, and gender considerations to these couplings that are far too involved to consider in this chapter. What should be included in discussions with young people about these issues is when and how they cause the relationship to dissolve and how one goes about dissolving it. Not all relationships end as a result of an external sexual relationship, but, when it is discovered or revealed, it changes the couple's interactions, requires a new set of boundaries, and often includes getting professional and therapeutic help to reestablish the trust that has been lost.

ENDING RELATIONSHIPS

Ending a relationship is a painful experience that can damage an individual's belief in his or her ability to be a friend or a partner. It can be an embarrassing situation especially for the person not choosing to end the relationship. The models that children have experienced in ending relationships are often outcomes of a bitter and hostile divorce in their family of origin. Saying good-bye in nondestructive ways is a skill one needs to learn because it is not uncommon for young people to move about in their relationships as they change and mature.

When a relationship is losing its attachment, one partner will experience a distancing, a loss of feelings, and a disinterest in the other person's life. The characteristics that seem to create distance in relationships are anger, resentment, sadness, criticism, insensitivity, and inattention (Hatfield & Rapson, 1996). Frequently, avoidance and unavailability behaviors occur as well. Communication decreases as one person is no longer able to listen and hear the other, which sometimes leads to argumentativeness and hostility. Hostility is a distancing strategy that creates unpleasant and discomforting experiences, allowing the person who is "wanting out" to set the other person up to also "want out." Sometimes, the person who wants to dissolve the relationship seeks support from mutual friends. He or she provides their friends with biased stories about the relationship and the other person, in an attempt to create an "army" of supporters so as not to be seen as the "bad one."

When a relationship is deconstructing, one needs nondestructive strategies to dissolve it. Young people can learn to communicate a change in feelings and friendships before actions and attack behaviors are implemented. They need to be empowered to discuss with their former friend or partner the reasons why they want to change the status of the relationship without making personal insults to or about the other. They should learn to use "I" language to describe feelings and dynamics that support their need to end things. For example, "I have lost interest in the things we do together" rather than "You have become boring and not interesting" is an effective, less destructive communication style. They need to minimize rejection language and speak to change, such as "I've changed over these last few years, and I feel that the changes I've made have caused us to grow in different directions."

When people master the skills for recognizing when to dissolve a relationship, minimizing pain and destruction, they will be better able to observe an adult relationship that is running into trouble, albeit their own. This skill can prepare them to appreciate and deal with the changes that will occur in their lifetime relationships with committed partners before the relationship dies.

Divorce

A divorce or a breakup of a legally committed relationship often springs each member of the couple into a hostile situation, with each person having to re-create a new identity. Approximately two of every three first marriages are likely to end in divorce, and oftentimes the divorce occurs at a time when children are still being reared in the home. Everything about the way the family functioned changes, including the economics, trust, and calmness. Most often one person is hurt, disappointed, frightened, and angry, while the other is seeking a way to leave. These new dynamics send the family into turmoil.

Divorces can be handled in an adversarial environment or in a mediated environment depending on how well the couple can use learned skills like problem solving and communication to fairly dissolve their legal arrangement. The type of divorce will also often be determined by the preference style of the attorneys who are sought to dissolve the legal agreement.

Whichever strategy is used, where there are children, they are hurt, confused, and troubled during the divorcing process and afterward. They are usually not clear about how much responsibility they had in the breakup and how they are to behave with each parent. While the parents are divorcing legally, if they plan to remain in their children's lives, they will be involved with one another permanently as coparents. It is beyond the scope of this text to address the complicated nature of divorce other than to suggest that resources for students to talk to should be made available.

The experience of divorce in their family of origin often leaves young people with fears about their own ability to make commitment. Education can help them to recognize that marrying or making a long-term commitment is serious and requires much discipline, maturity, and careful evaluation. There are no guarantees in its permanency, but developing the skills that make for satisfactory relationships and practicing them throughout their adolescence and early adulthood will optimize their likelihood of success.

There are all sorts of data about the likelihood of remarriage after divorce and the potential success of the remarriage. When divorce occurs at a young age and early in a marriage, the likelihood is greater that the partners will remarry others. It is the more complex divorce involving children that often complicates remarriage. *Reconstituted families* are those that merge children from previous relationships into one household. Suffice to say it is difficult enough to parent a household of blood-related or adopted children (see Chapter 7 on parenting); it is a Herculean feat to master a reconstituted family with peace, respect, and happiness.

Yet, as the divorce rate continues to rise, society will see more and more of children from reconstituted families in schools. Students will be trying to negotiate new roles and responsibilities as they attempt to find their place in a new family. They may be dealing with feelings of guilt about the parent who is not present, or they may be part of two new families. A change in their grades, demeanor, and friendships are often observed as they attempt to figure out whom they can depend on and how their lives will continue. Creating an opportunity to learn about reconstituted families (especially success stories) is useful to students as they experience their present situations and plan their future.

SUMMARY

Individuals encounter various relationships throughout a lifetime. They will differ considerably in their attachments, boundaries, and styles. Some will involve intimacy that will or will not include sexual intercourse. Some will be more permanent than others. All relationships will be influenced by the various factors that are operating in the sociopolitical environment in which they exist. As the world becomes quicker to transverse and as diverse populations of people interact with one another more regularly, the way relationships occur and how they function will change.

Young people will be expected to develop and practice skills that can be implemented in relationships to increase the likelihood that they will be enriching, trusting, respectful, and developmentally appropriate. With success in developing and implementing these skills, they will be better prepared to negotiate adult, more complicated, and more long-term relationships that will support their sense of themselves, their independence, and their trust. Sexuality education can provide an arena for communication, negotiation, problem-solving, and decision-making skills to be learned, practiced, and applied to relationship situations. Students will explore their notions of gender and the ways in which those notions might affect their relationships.

Prospective teachers should be familiar and comfortable with the content information about relationships. They then can make decisions about what is developmentally appropriate to teach to their population of students and what is appropriate for their particular community culture and school district. For example, those teaching in a religious school may discuss with their students the decisions that some young people make to be sexually active, but they will be expected to provide opportunities for students to reflect on the expectations of their religion to remain celibate and marry. Also to be discussed are the students' understandings of commitment and the boundaries society places on the long-term commitments/ marriages of same-sex couples. In other situations, where student peer groups are particularly "clicky" or exclusionary, the teacher should discuss the value of friendships and expanding one's relationships. Certainly, for young students in communities where family constellations are diverse—including traditional, interracial, homosexual, and single-parent—one would want to reaffirm the effectiveness and richness of these family structures.

Several learning experiences are included here that prospective teachers can use when teaching about relationships. They should modify these activities so that they are applicable to the particular student population they are teaching.

WEBSITES

Sex, Etc.: www.sexetc.org
TeenWire: www.teenwire.org
The Runaway Game:
    www.therunawaygame.org
I Wanna Know: www.iwannknow.org
Go Ask Alice: www.columbia.edu/cu/
    healthwise/alice.html
Quia: www.quia.com/jg/211707.html

Coalition for Positive Sexuality: www.3
    .positive.org
Planned Parenthood Federation of America:
    www.plannedparenthood.org
Ask Eric: Lesson Plans for Health:
    www.askeric.org/cgi-bin/health
The Cool Spot: www.thecoolspot.gov/
    default.asp

Teen Growth: www.teengrowth.com

Kids Health: www.kidshealth.org/kid

Sexuality Information and Education Council of the United States: www.siecus.org

American Association of Sex Educators, Counselors, and Therapists: www.aasect.org

Teen Relationships: www.teenrelationships.org

Tufts University Child & Family Web Guide: www.cfw.tufts.edu/viewtopics.asp?categoryid=4&topicid=85

Teen Outreach: www.teenoutreach.com

Teen Violence: www.lfcc.on.ca/teendate.htm

National Campaign to Prevent Teen Pregnancy: www.teenpregnancy.org

ADDITIONAL RESOURCES

Conville, L., & Rogers, E. (1998). *The meaning of "relationship" in interpersonal communication.* Westport, CT: Praeger.

Erber, R., & Gilmour, R. (Eds.). (1994). *Theoretical frameworks for personal relationships.* Hillsdale, NJ: Erlbaum.

Kalbfleisch, P. J. (1993). *Interpersonal communication: Evolving interpersonal relationships.* Hillsdale, NJ: Erlbaum.

REFERENCES

Brooks, B. D., & Paull, R. C. (1991). *How to be successful in less than 10 minutes a day.* Santa Cruz, CA: Thomas Jefferson Research Center.

Fenell, D. L. (1993). Characteristics of long-term first marriages. *Journal of Mental Health Counseling, 15,* 446–460.

Fetro, J. V. (2000). *Personal & social skills: Level 3.* Santa Cruz, CA: ETR Associates.

Framo, J. (1992). *Family of origin therapy: An intergenerational approach.* New York: Brunner/Mazel.

Freund, K., & Blanchard, R. (1986). The concept of courtship disorder. *Journal of Sex and Marital/Therapy, 12,* 79–92.

Gagnon, J., & Simon, W. (1984, November–December). Sexual scripts. *Society,* 52–60.

Gottman, J. M. (1999). *The marriage clinic: A scientifically based marital therapy.* New York: Norton.

Hatfield, E., & Rapson, R. L. (1993). *Love, sex and intimacy: Their psychology, biology and history.* New York: HarperCollins.

Hatfield, E., & Rapson, R. L. (1996). *Love and sex: Cross cultural perspectives.* Newton, MA: Allyn & Bacon.

Levine, R., Sato, S. Hashimoto, T., & Verma, J. (1994). *Love and marriage in 11 cultures.* Unpublished manuscript. Fresno: California State University.

Minirth, F., Minirth, M. A., Newman, B., Newman, D., Hemfelt, R., & Hemfelt, S. (1991). *Passages of marriage.* Nashville, TN: Nelson.

Sollie, D. (2002, July/August). Couples and gender: Exploring the real issues. *Family Therapy Magazine, 1*(4), 14–21.

Sternberg, R. J. (1986). A triangular theory of love. *Psychological Review, 93,* 119–135.

Ryan, S., Manlove, J., & Franzetta, K. (2003, September 5). *Characteristics of teens' first sexual partner.* Washington, DC: Child Trends. Available online at National Campaign to Prevent Teen Pregnancy: www.teenpregnancy.org.

Travis, C. B., & Yaeger, C. P. (1992). Sexual selection, parental investment and sexism. *Journal of Social Issues, 47,* 117–129.

Troll, L. E., & Smith, J. (1976). Attachment through the life span: Some questions about dyadic bonds among adults. *Human Development, 19,* 135–182.

Westheimer, R., & Lopater, S. (2002). *Human sexuality: A psychosocial perspective.* Baltimore: Lippincott, Williams & Wilkins.

LEARNING EXPERIENCES

The following describes the content and skills that students will be expected "to know and be able to do" at the various developmental levels.

Students in early elementary grades will be able to

1. Identify various members of their family.
2. Identify families of different sizes and different members than their own.
3. Recognize some of the responsibilities associated with different roles in their family (mother, father, sibling, and so forth).
4. Recognize the differences in responsibilities associated with different roles in families other than their own.
5. Identify their own responsibilities as a member of their family.
6. Express feelings including sadness, pleasure, and anger, in developmentally appropriate ways.
7. Display signs of respect, sharing, and caring for others.

By later elementary school, students will be able to

1. Identify various family constellations (two-parent families, single-parent families, extended families, same-gender families, reconstituted families, and so on).
2. Identify roles and responsibilities of family members, including their own.
3. Identify the characteristics of meaningful friendships and family membership.
4. Be able to set developmentally appropriate boundaries and limitations associated with friendships.
5. Demonstrate the ability to make decisions, solve problems, and use refusal skills in peer-pressured situations.
6. Communicate effectively with respect, caring, and consideration of themselves and others.
7. Identify acceptable resources for information and for help with a problem.

By the end of middle school, students will be able to

1. Recognize the part that communication plays in healthy relationships.
2. Identify and be respectful of family constellations different from their own.
3. Identify their roles and responsibilities as a member of their family.
4. Recognize the relationship between goal setting for the future and self-management of high-risk behaviors.
5. Express intimacy in other than sexual ways.
6. Identify, establish, and maintain healthy friendships.
7. Identify and establish healthy dating relationships.
8. Make personal decisions about sexual intimacy and be able to communicate them.
9. Strengthen refusal skills regarding peer pressure.
10. Recognize how behaviors affect interpersonal relationships.

11. Distinguish between safe and harmful behaviors in relationships.
12. Be able to end a relationship in constructive, positive ways.

By the end of 12th grade, students will be able to

1. Differentiate between healthy and nonhealthy friendships.
2. Differentiate between healthy and unhealthy intimate relationships.
3. Identify the characteristics they value in family, friendships, and intimate relationships.
4. Demonstrate effective communication skills in building and maintaining important relationships.
5. Demonstrate respect, caring, and love in healthy ways.
6. Demonstrate the ability to resolve conflicts in important relationships.
7. Make personal decisions about sexual intimacy and be able to communicate them.
8. Apply effective decision-making skills to risky behavior choices.
9. Distinguish between safe and harmful behaviors in relationships.
10. Demonstrate the ability to participate in healthy family relationships, friendships, and significant-other relationships.
11. Make personal decisions about sexual behavior and communicate them effectively.

LEARNING EXPERIENCE 1

TITLE: Families

GRADE LEVELS: K–3

TIME REQUIREMENTS: One 45-minute session

LEARNING CONTEXT

This lesson is an initial lesson about families. It will fit into a social studies session about families around the world. Before the session, the teacher will talk about different family constellations. After this activity, students will be able to identify various members of their family and describe families of different sizes and different members than their own. The skills being developed include the following:

> Communication: They are practicing communication skills as they describe their projects to the class.

> Decision making: They will need to make decisions about what other family members they will choose for their alternate family constellations.

NATIONAL LEARNING STANDARDS

> 4: Students will analyze the influence of culture, media, technology, and other factors on health.

> 7: Students will demonstrate the ability to advocate for personal, family, and community health.

PROCEDURE

Ask the students to bring in pictures of their family, reminding them to include all of the members of their family. It can be in one picture or several pictures.

Give each student an oak tag that has lines dividing it into four parts. The students will paste their own family's pictures in the top left quadrangle. From the magazines provided by the teacher, the students will cut out pictures of various people (men, women, and children of all ages). In each of the other three quadrangles on the oak tag, they will create three families that differ from their own by pasting pictures of different family constellations. One family may be a family with a mother and children. Another family may be one with a mother, father, and several children. Another family may be a father with children. Another family may be a family made up of members of mixed cultures. Another family may be a man and a woman without children. Still another family may be a same-sex couple with or without children. The children will then be asked to describe their family and how it differs from the other families.

INSTRUCTIONAL/ENVIRONMENTAL MODIFICATIONS

Because some children will have more dexterity than others, they may need assistance with cutting and pasting. Some pictures that have already been cut out can also be used. Some children will have better writing skills than others, so the description they provide to the class may be in written communication; others may speak about the differences.

RESOURCES
Oak tags; magazines with pictures of people of varying cultures and ages; paste; scissors; crayons or markers

ASSESSMENT PLAN
The students will be graded on the following:

> Ability to create four families that are different from their own: 4 points
> Three: 3 points
> Two: 2 points
> One: 1 point
> Ability to clearly explain how the families differ: 4-3-2-1
> Totals: A = 8; B = 6; C = 4; D = 2; F = 1 or 0

REFLECTION
The purpose of this lesson is for young people to develop an open and accepting view of people who are different from themselves as well as an understanding of different family constellations.

LEARNING EXPERIENCE 2

TITLE: My Jobs

GRADE LEVELS: 4–6

TIME REQUIREMENTS: One 90-minute session or two 45-minute sessions

LEARNING CONTEXT

This activity can be part of the family life unit after students have learned about different family constellations. Students will develop skills in decision making and goal setting. Specifically, they will be able to

- Recognize their roles and responsibilities.
- Make a plan for getting their jobs and responsibilities done each day.
- Realize how setting goals and a plan to accomplish them works.

NATIONAL LEARNING STANDARDS

4:   Students will analyze the influence of culture, media, technology, and other factors on health.

7:   Students will demonstrate the ability to advocate for personal, family, and community health.

PROCEDURE

For homework, ask the students to have their parent or guardian help them to list their family responsibilities. They will also have to bring in a picture of themselves. In class, ask the students to paste a picture of themselves on the top of a poster page. (If they do not have a picture, they can draw one.) Under their picture (dependent on the writing skills of the particular class), second graders will cut out pictures of people doing jobs that they are responsible for doing (including making their bed, cleaning their room, doing their homework, cleaning or emptying the dishwasher, walking the dog, taking out the garbage, and so forth); third graders will write the name of their jobs/responsibilities.

The students will then describe the jobs or responsibilities that they have and talk about how they got that job and when and how they get the job done. The students, with the teacher's help, will write a list on the board of the usual jobs each of the students have. Then the students will make a sample daily plan for how the jobs can get done each day. The students will be put in small groups with a daily planner of morning (before school), afternoon (after school), and evening listed on the top. The students will then look at the jobs they have to get done each day and list them under the time of the day they can do the jobs. Then have the students add to their list when they will have time to play and watch TV. The students will discuss the similarities and differences in their roles from their classmates' roles and responsibilities. Look for opportunities to point out that each of the roles can be performed by either a boy or a girl.

INSTRUCTIONAL/ENVIRONMENTAL MODIFICATION

Where writing or pasting is not possible, encourage the students to help one another.

RESOURCES

Poster paper; paste; markers

ASSESSMENT PLAN

The students will hang their posters around the room, and each of the students will go around the room and give each paper a grade from A to C for appearance. The teacher will give the students a grade of

> A for being able to identify more than four roles and spell them correctly.
>
> B for being able to identify three roles and spell all of them correctly.
>
> C for being able to identify at least three roles and spell two of them correctly.
>
> D for being able to identify only one or two roles and spell at least one correctly.

The students will all receive either a plus or a check for their daily goal-setting plan. If it is not adequate, ask the students to go back to their group and discuss a more manageable plan.

REFLECTION

Students will need a great deal of help and encouragement to develop a daily goal plan. It is a good idea for the teacher to explain the time problems when he or she does the daily plan example on the board.

LEARNING EXPERIENCE 3

TITLE: How My Family Works

GRADE LEVELS: 4–6

TIME REQUIREMENT: One 45-minute session

LEARNING CONTEXT

This activity, which encourages decision-making and goal-setting skills, can occur during the family life unit after students have discussed different family constellations. Students will be able to
- Identify roles and responsibilities of members of a family.
- Explain that roles and responsibilities differ from family to family.
- Understand that family roles and responsibilities are not necessarily gender based.

NATIONAL LEARNING STANDARDS

4: Students will analyze the influence of culture, media, technology, and other factors on health.

5: Students will demonstrate the ability to use interpersonal communication skills to enhance health.

7: Students will demonstrate the ability to advocate for personal, family, and community health.

PROCEDURE

Ask the students to list each member of their family across the top of a page. They will identify at least three roles and responsibilities each member of their family has to the family. In small groups of no more than four students, the students will discuss the ways their family roles are similar to and different from the other group members'. In each group, the students will make a list headed by the following and give an example of each from their family constellation including extended family members:

Child   Adolescent   Adult   Older Adult   Male   Female

Using their own lists of "jobs" that people in their family perform, the students will put the job under the column that describes who could do that job. Any one job can be under every column. The class will then discuss those jobs (if any) that are entirely gender based. They will talk about what factors, other than gender, may determine who does what job (people with special skills, size, interest, and so on).

INSTRUCTIONAL/ENVIRONMENTAL MODIFICATIONS

It would be best to put students in groups where there is likely to be the greatest difference. Try to keep close friends from working entirely with each other, giving students a chance to experience types of people and roles that exist outside their own daily circle.

RESOURCES

Paper and pencils; moveable chairs

ASSESSMENT PLAN

No formal assessment will be made with this lesson. The teacher will be able to evaluate the accomplishment of students' objectives from the charts that they prepare in groups and their sharing of the results of developing the charts.

REFLECTION

This activity provides an excellent opportunity for students to learn about families that accomplish their tasks in different ways from their own. These kinds of experiences offer students options for their own future lives.

LEARNING EXPERIENCE 4

TITLE: My Friends and Me

GRADE LEVELS: 4–6

TIME REQUIREMENTS: Two 45-minute sessions

LEARNING CONTEXT

Students will have discussed family relationships, roles, and responsibilities before this learning experience. Encouraging communication and decision-making skills, this activity should be part of an early session in their discussion of friendships.

NATIONAL LEARNING STANDARDS

     5:   Students will demonstrate the ability to use interpersonal communication skills to enhance health.

     7:   Students will demonstrate the ability to advocate for personal, family, and community health.

PROCEDURE

In small groups of four (trying to separate close friends from one another), ask students to brainstorm

- A list of reasons why some people become friends.
- A list of the characteristics they possess that make them a good friend.
- The characteristics they expect or want their friends to have.

Each person in the group will take out a piece of paper and, from the list of characteristics that they have brainstormed, identify the five most important characteristics to them. Then they will prioritize their list. They will compare their list with the others in their group and discuss the similarities and differences recognizing that friends and expectations differ.

Instruct the students to look back at their list and put the name of one or more friends who meets each of the different characteristics in their prioritized list. Opening the discussion to the larger group, the students will discuss what friendships mean to them and how the characteristics they prioritized fit into their present-day friendships. Students will discuss how some friends have some characteristics and other friends have other characteristics. It is unusual for any one friend to have all of the characteristics. Then the students will be asked to describe which of their prioritized characteristics they possess. Would their friends agree?

INSTRUCTIONAL/ENVIRONMENTAL MODIFICATIONS

The room does not necessarily need modification except that the chairs must be moveable. Students of differing skills and ability will be able to participate equally.

RESOURCES

Pencils and paper

ASSESSMENT PLAN

The students' ability to recognize and identify the important characteristics of friendships will be an assessment of the quality of the learning experience.

REFLECTION

This activity is meant to help students to recognize that people have differing attributes and not everyone has all of the attributes, yet they can make for a good friend.

LEARNING EXPERIENCE 5

TITLE: Saying No Is Hard to Do

GRADE LEVEL: 7–9

TIME REQUIREMENTS: Two 45-minute sessions

LEARNING CONTEXT

This session is part of the family living unit. The students will have discussed what makes a good friend and how peer pressure sometimes causes students to make important mistakes. They will also have discussed decision making and patterns of communication. After this activity, students will be able to

- Evaluate and recognize high-risk situations.
- Demonstrate the ability to make decisions, solve problems, and use refusal skills in peer-pressured situations.
- Communicate effectively with respect, caring, and consideration of themselves and others.

NATIONAL LEARNING STANDARDS

1: Students will comprehend concepts related to health promotion and disease prevention.

3: Students will demonstrate the ability to practice health-enhancing behaviors and reduce health risks.

5: Students will demonstrate the ability to use interpersonal communication skills to enhance health.

7: Students will demonstrate the ability to advocate for personal, family, and community health.

PROCEDURE

This exercise is a fishbowl role play in which the characters sit in the center of the circle made by the entire class. The characters begin the role play, and the students in the circle are encouraged or selected to rotate into the part of any of the characters in the circle by standing behind them with one hand on the person's shoulder that they want to replace. When that person finishes speaking, the new person takes that person's place. At any time during the role play, the students will volunteer or be required to take part.

This role play has three characters. Each is given a card with a specific role as follows:

I am Jamie, and I have been invited to go to this party Saturday with all of the cool kids. I am going to go, and I want Jessie to tell her mother she is sleeping over at my house so we can all go (apply pressure on Loren).

I am Cindy, and I have been invited also, but I am afraid to go because the cool kids smoke, drink, and some of them have a special partner. But Jessie has convinced me to go, and I want Loren to go, too (apply pressure on Loren).

I am Loren, and I have been invited to the party, but my parents said I can't go. I am really upset and want to go.

Each student reads his or her role to the class, and then Jessie starts the role play. After each student in the class has had a chance to try at least one role in the role play, the students will open the circle to the larger group. They will be asked to list on the board the choices that Loren has in this situation. Then they will be put into small groups, and, using the steps in the STAR decision-making model (taught in the previous class), they will make a decision about going. The class will share their decision and the steps that they considered to arrive at their decision. The consequences of their decision will be discussed. Ask the students to put down on a piece of paper whether they would go or not if they were Loren's best friends Cindy and Jamie. Go around the room and ask the students to state their decision and explain or support it.

The STAR Model of Decision Making

Stop: Look and clearly identify the situation and the specific issues surrounding the decision.

Think: Identify the choices and the consequences of each choice.

Act: Select one choice, outline the steps you will take to make it successful, and do them.

Review: Look at the consequences, and evaluate whether the action was positive or negative.

Put the students back in their original groups and have them write sentences that would be supportive of Loren making up her own mind even though they know that they desperately want her to go. Have the students read their supportive statements.

INSTRUCTIONAL/ENVIRONMENTAL MODIFICATIONS

Be sure that best friends are not kept together in groups, helping students to get to know one another. The groups can be set up to accommodate for specific disabilities. Students who have difficulty with verbal expression can be asked to be the "secretary" of the group. Students who have difficulty writing can be encouraged to participate in the more verbal parts of the lesson.

RESOURCE

Brooks and Paull (1991, p. 149)

ASSESSMENT PLAN

Evaluate each group's ability to use the various steps in the decision-making model:

A = They were able to identify all of the steps and explain each.

B = They were able to identify or explain three steps.

C = They were able to identify only two steps or were unable to explain more than two.

D = They did not know the steps or were not able to explain them.

REFLECTION

Role plays are very effective ways for students to learn how to use language to express their own thoughts and feelings. This experience will help students to be more supportive of friends. It will also support their use of effective problem-solving and decision-making strategies.

LEARNING EXPERIENCE 6

TITLE: We Are Just Different Now

GRADE LEVELS: 7–9

TIME REQUIREMENT: One session

LEARNING CONTEXT

Include this experience in the family life unit. Students will have discussed how friendships develop, how people change over time, how friendships change, and how to move on. The skills being developed include communication, decision making, and conflict resolution. After this activity, students will be able to

> Recognize the part communication plays in healthy relationships.
> Identify, establish, and maintain healthy friendships.
> Recognize how behaviors affect interpersonal relationships.
> Be able to end a relationship in constructive, positive ways.

NATIONAL LEARNING STANDARDS

> 5:   Students will demonstrate the ability to use interpersonal communication skills to enhance health.
> 7:   Students will demonstrate the ability to advocate for personal, family, and community health.

PROCEDURE

In groups of three, ask the students to write several scenarios where they have a best friend since kindergarten. Because they go to middle school now, they are finding it difficult to stay friends. Have them describe the ways things have changed and what they tried to do to make the situation better. They have now decided that the "best friendship" should end and that they should be free to move into different groups without one another. After they have talked about the particular story, have them write one role play card for each of the two characters that will be in their role play, in which the two will have the discussion about ending the friendship. In their groups of three, have them role-play their scenarios, with one of the three being the recorder. The recorder will record the statements that were positive and not damaging as well as the statements that were cruel and hurtful.

At the end of the role play, the recorder will share what he or she heard from observing the discussion. Then, the recorders will share with the whole class their observations of the effectiveness of the discussion and some of the remarks that they thought were helpful and positive. The conclusion of the lesson will be a reaffirmation of the effectiveness of positive, nondestructive strategies for ending a friendship or changing its boundaries.

One would expect to hear reasons and information about the relationship status spoken from the "I" rather than the "you" point of view. Changes in the interests or activities between the two parties should be expressed rather than accusatory statements about the other. The two parties would not be stating that their behavior has been supported or approved of by friends outside the twosome. Such messages as "Everyone knows you are ___" should be avoided.

INSTRUCTIONAL/ENVIRONMENTAL MODIFICATION
If students have difficulty with writing, they would best take one of the roles other than recorder.

ASSESSMENT PLAN
During the conclusion, the teacher will be able to evaluate whether the students know and are able to perform the communication skills necessary for ending a friendship in constructive ways.

REFLECTION
This activity provides important practice for people who find themselves in situations where they no longer have the feeling or desire to continue a relationship. It also will help them to recognize when a relationship is dissolving.

LEARNING EXPERIENCE 7

TITLE: Making Decisions: Options and Consequences

GRADE LEVELS: 10–12 (The teacher can select the appropriate scenario for each grade and developmental level of his or her students.)

TIME REQUIREMENT: One 45-minute session

LEARNING CONTEXT

This session may be used after the students have discussed relationships. They will also have practiced various decision-making strategies, and they will have discussed decreasing risks with healthy choices. This activity develops the skills of stress management and conflict resolution/problem solving.

NATIONAL LEARNING STANDARDS

1:   Students will comprehend concepts related to health promotion and disease prevention.

2:   Students will demonstrate the ability to access valid health information and health-promoting products and services.

3:   Students will demonstrate the ability to practice health-enhancing behaviors and reduce.

6:   Students will demonstrate the ability to use goal-setting and decision-making skills to enhance health.

7:   Students will demonstrate the ability to advocate for personal, family, and community health.

PROCEDURE

Every day, students make decisions about their personal behavior in relationships. Some decisions are made without much thought, and some take considerable thought. Some decisions have serious consequences; others do not. Described here are brief scenarios that would best be made after careful consideration of the options and the consequences.

In small groups, ask the students to read each scenario, develop the options, discuss the consequences, and then record their decision. Ask them to report whether the decision was unanimous; if not, how many were for and how many against? When they have finished, they will report their conclusions with the full class and discuss each. Use the following schema for each scenario:

Options:
Consequences:
Decision:
The number for and the number against:

Scenario 1

Billy and Jess are going out for several months. Billy has had sex before and Jess has not, but both want to. Before she met Billy, Jess always thought she would never have sex with anyone until she is committed to that person for life.

Scenario 2

A big party is going on for Saturday night, and you have been invited by a new group of cool friends. None of you regular friends were invited except for Dominica, and she is going. Your parents have told you that you cannot go because they have heard about the sex and drinking that goes on at the parties. You can tell them that you are sleeping at Dominica's house and go to the party. They will never know.

Scenario 3

Ashley and Brady are getting ready to go off to two different colleges. They have been a couple for the last 2 years, and their parents and best friends are trying to convince them that they should make a new agreement with each other not to be exclusive and see other people when they are at school.

Scenario 4

Ramon and Sophia have just recently begun to have sex with one another, and they are afraid that there will be a pregnancy. Ramon says that Sophia should get on the pill, and Sophia says that Ramon should wear a condom.

Scenario 5

Your best friend started to hang out with this older guy. She has been going to parties with him, drinking, and using marijuana. You know she is being pressured to have sex with him. You are really worried about her.

INSTRUCTIONAL/ENVIRONMENTAL MODIFICATION
Students with diverse needs and backgrounds can participate in these scenarios.

RESOURCES
Paper and pencils for recording

ASSESSMENT PLAN
This is an opportunity for the teacher to do an authentic assessment by asking the groups to discuss how they implemented the decision-making processes discussed earlier. Also, the teacher can evaluate how well the students respect differences of opinion by observing how they handle the votes about the decisions.

REFLECTION
Encourage the students to develop their own scenarios. The developmental level of the particular class must be taken into consideration when using these scenarios.

LEARNING EXPERIENCE 8

TITLE: Where I Am and Where I Want to Go

GRADE LEVELS: 10–12

TIME REQUIREMENTS: Two 45-minute sessions

LEARNING CONTEXT

This activity should be participated in after the family life unit and discussions of serious intimate relationships. Risk taking and the various components of goal setting will have been discussed. This learning experience develops skills in communication, decision making, goal setting, and conflict resolution/problem solving.

NATIONAL LEARNING STANDARDS

3:   Students will demonstrate the ability to practice health-enhancing behaviors and reduce health risks.

5:   Students will demonstrate the ability to use interpersonal communication skills to enhance health.

6:   Students will demonstrate the ability to use goal-setting and decision-making skills to enhance health.

7:   Students will demonstrate the ability to advocate for personal, family, and community health.

PROCEDURE

Session 1

Ask students to complete individually the handout included at the end of this learning experience. The handout lists activities that have both immediate- and long-term rewards in relationships.

When the students have finished the individual activity, arrange them into groups of three or four. Ask them to answer the following questions:

- Which were their most important goals, the short-term or long-term goals?
- In what ways might the short-term goals support or be a barrier for achieving the long-term goals?

Each group will share some of their conclusions with the larger group. Instruct the students to reflect on their experience with this activity.

Session 2

During the next session, ask the students, again in small groups, to select one "very important" goal that is similar for all of them. Using the goal-setting strategies learned in previous classes (the action plan presented here), the students will develop a plan for achieving their goal. Remind them to consider the following points:

- Is the goal achievable?
- Is it important to the person?
- Is it specific and clear?
- Are there realistic time limits for achieving the goals?
- Are the goals reasonable, manageable, and in the person's control?

Action Plan

- What steps have to happen to be taken to achieve the goal?
- What are some of the barriers or pitfalls that I might encounter?
- What are some of the resources (people, places, and so on) that will help me to reach the goal?
- What strengths do I have, and what do I need to develop?
- When, and how often, will the steps be taken?
- How and when will you evaluate the progress that you are making toward the goal?
- How and when should the plan be reviewed if it is not achieving the goal?

INSTRUCTIONAL/ENVIRONMENTAL MODIFICATION

Set up the groups so that they accommodate students with special needs.

RESOURCE

"Where I Am and Where I Want to Go" Handout

ASSESSMENT PLAN

Use the following guidelines to assess the groups' performance in the activity:

A = The students included all of the components of goal setting and applied the appropriate information to each.

B = The students included most of the components and applied each that they included appropriately.

C = The students included most of the components but did not fully understand the information that needed to be applied to each.

D = The students left out most of the major components of goal setting.

F = The students were unable to do the activity.

REFLECTION

Understanding the potential impact of immediate gratification on more long-term goals in relationships is important. Sometimes students cannot associate present-day decisions and actions on their later lives. This activity ties some of these together and encourages students to look toward the future while participating presently.

REFERENCE

Fetro (2000)

"Where I Am and Where I Want to Go" Handout

Directions: Using the following scale, identify the importance of each item listed here to you personally:

4 = Extremely important
3 = Quite important
2 = Some what important
1 = Barely important
0 = Not at all important

_____To have one special partner now

_____To be in love with someone who loves me now

_____To experience a sexual relationship with someone I care about

_____To make my own decisions without feeling pressured

_____To be popular with my friends

_____To be able to say yes to sex without feeling guilty

_____To be able to say no to sex without feeling pressure

_____To delay sexual activity until I am married

_____To be able to tell my partner I will not be sexual with them without a condom

_____To be comfortable talking with my partner about our sexual likes and dislikes

_____To be comfortable and be myself in all of my relationships

_____To put off sex until I am in a permanent/marital relationship

_____To make my family proud of me

_____To be married/permanently committed someday when I am ready, with my perfect partner

_____To have children when I am ready for them

_____To get into the college of my choice

_____To graduate from college

_____To have a successful career

_____To own my own house

_____To be able to support my family

_____To like myself for who I am

_____To have good friends with whom I can be myself

PARENTING

KATHLEEN SCHMALZ AND MARY GRENZ JALLOH

"Some people seem to think that you just have children, you bring them up and that's it. But it doesn't work out that way. It's hard."
A MOTHER IN THE AVON LONGITUDINAL STUDY OF PARENTS AND CHILDREN

OBJECTIVES

After reading this chapter, students will be able to

1. Explore and clarify attitudes and expectations about parenting.
2. Examine the roles and responsibilities involved in parenting in historical and changing cultural contexts.
3. Define and describe the skills that are essential to effective parenting.
4. Explore and appreciate the unique strengths of different family structures.
5. Understand human growth and development from an ecological perspective.

REFLECTIVE QUESTIONS

Elementary Grades
1. What does it mean to be a parent?
2. What kind of things does a parent do?
3. What is the most important thing for a parent to do?
4. Do you think it is hard to be a parent? Why or why not?
5. What do you think you need to know before you become a parent?
6. Do you think everyone should be a parent? Why or why not?
7. How do parents solve problems?
8. How do they find people to help them?
9. How can you help your parents?

Middle School
1. What differences and similarities do you see between parents of your friends?
2. What might contribute to the differences?
3. What do you think a parent needs to know in order to be a good parent?
4. Do you think students of your age are ready to be parents? Why or why not?
5. How can parents find help if they are having problems?
6. How can you help your parents?

Senior High School
1. What is your idea of an "ideal" parent?
2. What might keep someone from being that "ideal" parent?
3. Do you think you are ready to be a parent? Why or why not?
4. What does someone need to know before they become a parent?
5. How do parents manage the financial, medical, social, and emotional needs of their families?
6. Where can parents go to get help when they need it?
7. How can you help your parents?

SCENARIO

Jen and Madison had been friends since third grade when Jen moved next door to Madison's family with her mom and younger brother. That was 9 years ago, just after the divorce. It was spring, and the girls spent the summer playing together, sharing their secrets, hopes, and fears. Since that time, they had been nearly inseparable. Jen knew something was wrong when it seemed Madison was avoiding her at school and at home. She decided to get to the bottom of it. Nine years of friendship gave her that right! That evening, she approached Madison and asked her if anything was wrong. Madison tried to be casual, but Jen knew her well enough to tell that wasn't how she was feeling. Both were seniors this year and were waiting for that April date when they would be hearing from the colleges they applied to for admission. But Madison had an even greater concern that she finally shared with Jen. She had missed her period and thought she might be pregnant. Pregnant! After all they had been working for, thinking about in terms of their futures. This would really change all that.

If you were Madison, what decisions would you need to think about?
What would you suggest Madison do at this point?
How would you help Madison if you were Jen?
What would be involved with being a parent at her age?
How might parenting change Madison's plans for her future?
If Madison is pregnant and decides to be a parent, how will she support the financial, medical, emotional, and social needs for both herself and her child?
How might Madison bring up the subject with her partner?
If she is pregnant, how might that change her relationship with her partner?
How might it change her relationship with her partner if she is not pregnant?
How might a pregnancy change Madison's relationship with her parents?
How might Madison's parents respond to the news?
What might be some of their concerns?

[Thinking about being a parent can be exciting, and scary. With parenting come great responsibility and challenges. Consider with Jen and Madison what some of those challenges may be. For younger students, the teacher may want to revise the scenario to be a discussion of a family member about to be a parent. For older students, allow them to rewrite the scenario based on their experiences and that of others in their peer group. Encourage students to consider the differences and similarities to be considered for parents who are, for example, the same gender, of different racial and/or ethnic groups, or different ages.]

INTRODUCTION

A recent article entitled "The Good Old Days Are Now: What Today's Families Are Doing Right" highlights an interesting paradox in attitudes toward parenting by young parents of today and the "grandparent generation" (Curran, 2002). While members of the generation, whose parental role models were Ozzie and Harriet and Donna Reed, often state emphatically that "I'm glad I'm not raising kids today," their own kids are just as emphatic stating that they would rather be parenting now than a generation or two ago. If helping children to deal with such issues as substance abuse, media images of sex and violence, school shootings, changing work and family roles, and economic uncertainty seems challenging, parents who feel comfortable with the shift away from rigidly prescribed family roles generally feel up to the challenge.

Many parents today feel that they are much more adept at communication and conflict resolution skills than their own parents were (Curran, 2002). Some of this change comes from formal skills training. Attending parenting workshops has become more commonplace, especially for fathers who were a rarity in such programs a generation or two ago. Introspection is another key factor in parents' efforts to communicate with their children. Honest discussion may have been lacking in their family. Controversial issues were avoided at all costs and conflicts may have been "resolved" when someone stormed out of the room. Many men describe fathers, and sometimes mothers, who were cold and distant, which compelled them to show their children the warmth and affection that they wish they had received (Curran, 2002; Riesch, Kuester, Brost, & McCarthy, 1996). Conversely, mothers seek to present their daughters with role models for independence and achievement.

In short, "cultural shifts demand new attitudes and skills" (Curran, 2002, p. 20). It may be difficult to project the attitudes and skills that will be demanded of parents in a world dominated by cybertechnologies. Young children can begin to learn what is really involved in being a parent so they will make wise decisions about the place of parenting in their adult lives.

ATTITUDES AND EXPECTATIONS

One way of exploring children's (and adult's) future conceptions of what they may become is by constructing *possible selves* (Knox, 1998; Morfei, Hooker, Fiese, & Cordeiro, 2001). Possible selves fall into the "hoped-for" and "feared" categories—that is, one's hopes and fears for the future. Parents of infants typically report hoped-for parenting selves; most maintain hoped-for possible selves even through the "terrible twos" (Morei et al., 2001). However, mothers seem to express more feared parenting selves, which may reflect the reality that they are still typically the primary caregivers, combined with cultural attitudes that hold mothers more responsible than fathers for their children's development.

Fathers, on the other hand, show less continuity in their hoped-for and feared parenting selves. A possible explanation for this erratic picture may lie in the "cultural confusion" that surrounds the father's role as nurturer versus provider (Morfei et al., 2001, p. 222). Yet the possible selves of adolescent girls suggest that there may be equal confusion, especially if they are faced with child care responsibilities before they are ready to assume a parenting role. For adolescent girls, self-esteem is intrinsically linked with high educational and occupational aspirations (Knox, 1998).

Children, both girls and boys, may have unrealistic attitudes and expectations about combining parenting with educational and professional goals. Adolescent mothers often try to portray themselves as financially independent, even when they are actually living with parents or receiving financial aid (Higgenson, 1998). This is not surprising given that financial independence is a prominent theme in the hoped-for possible selves of young girls (Knox, 1998). Teenage fathers and young adult fathers with adolescent partners are both more likely than older parents to have financial problems due to lower educational and vocational skills and subsequent lower wages or unemployment (Elsters, Lamb, & Kimmerly, 1989). Additionally, adolescent parents tend to have more traditional attitudes about male and female parenting roles than adults. Adolescent fathers may assume that they will be allotting minimal time to caregiving responsibilities. Their attitude may be reinforced by young mothers who sometimes take inordinate pride in their parenting abilities to the extent of exaggerating their parenting competence and their babies' developmental achievements (Higgenson, 1998).

Parent education programs emerged out of recognition that new parents often embark on the venture of parenthood lacking critical information and skills and thus, understandably, lacking confidence in their ability to fulfill their new role (Zoline & Jason, 1985). At the same time, adolescents often perceive themselves as invulnerable (which increases the risk of negative outcomes such as unplanned or unwanted pregnancies) and exaggerate their abilities to succeed. Some teenage parents succeed simply out of determination to prove that they do not fit the stereotype of the "welfare-dependent teenage mother" (Higgenson, 1998, p. 139). Still, they must overcome difficult odds to do so and frequently seem to be engaged in a balancing act between the reality of their lives and a fantasy ideal.

The concept of possible selves offers a medium for exploring children's and adolescents' attitudes and expectations toward parenting with the goal of correcting unrealistic beliefs. As an exercise in which participants are asked to generate various parenting selves, it can also be used as an aid in decision making and goal setting. For example, a hoped-for parenting self might be to see a child enter college, a goal that involves financial planning as well as academic encouragement. Other hoped-for parenting selves might be less positive, such as wanting a "perfect" child or a child who conforms to parents' prescribed aspirations. Alternately, feared parenting selves might include not being able to provide for a child or being forced to sacrifice personal educational or career goals due to unplanned parenthood. Having a group generate a number of possible selves is a form of brainstorming that can act as a springboard for discussing attitudes and expectations toward parenting.

A parenting program designed for high school students showed that although male students initially had less knowledge about child care and parenting than their female classmates, the skills training program quickly diminished the gap (Zoline & Jason, 1985). In the first session, the students watched a film that encompassed the various factors that should be considered in deciding to become a parent, such as age, maturity, financial situation, lifestyle, and attitudes toward children. A lively discussion about parenting followed the film. In another session, two couples brought their small children to class and discussed the joys, and constraints, of being parents. The topics included the demands of time imposed by a baby and the impact of caring for a baby on parents' relationship and lifestyle. The students were given opportunities to question the parents on the topics and interact with other children as well.

The complete intervention juxtaposed film, guest participants, handout sheets with data and other factual information, and hands-on activities (Zoline & Jason, 1985). The guest parents provided an authentic learning experience, and the format appealed to a variety of learning styles. Over time, the participants displayed a significant increase in parenting expectations. In particular, the researchers emphasize that the program was especially effective in engaging the interest of male participants in the parenting role.

Teenage mothers, determined to combat negative cultural stereotypes, often compare themselves favorably to mothers in their 20s, 30s, and older, as well as their own peers (Higgenson, 1998). While they may exaggerate their own competence, they are not unjustly angry at the assumption that age or marital status determines whether one is a good parent. Many single parents succeed in balancing the dual responsibilities of work and parenting without a partner's support (Curran, 2002). Similarly, many teenage parents do remarkably well. A critical factor is "whether young people are actively choosing parenting as a worthwhile endeavor, or drifting into a situation which requires a commitment that they have neither the resources nor the desire to keep" (Bignell, 1980, p. 277). The same condition can be extended to parents of any age. By helping children learn decision-making and planning skills, as well as what is involved in being a parent, it is less likely that they will find themselves drifting into a serious situation for which they are unprepared.

ROLES AND RESPONSIBILITIES

Popular humor has long been used by social scientists as a tool for examining cultural trends. Note that the chapter began by evoking two TV comedies of the 1950s, *Ozzie and Harriet* and *Donna Reed,* whose title characters were depicted as the ideal parents. The two-parent, middle-class families were inevitably white, and usually so was the fence surrounding the suburban home. In some situations, father always knew best; in others, he was hopelessly incompetent when it came to children or anything that smacked of domestic skills, though he might be good at handling the dog.

Situation comedies say a lot about cultural trends, but they have been around little more than half a century. On the other hand, comic strips allow researchers to explore portrayals of parenting roles since the first wave of feminism in the early 20th century. The "American father" seems to be a particular point of interest (LaRossa, Jaret, Gadgil, & Wynn, 2000). According to a study of *Saturday Evening Post* cartoons dating from 1922, fathers were much more likely than mothers to be depicted as "awkward," "unhandy," or "gawky" until the 1970s, which marked a "paradigmatic shift in the culture of fatherhood" (LaRossa et al., 2000, p. 376). The researchers concluded that the rise in working mothers, the decline in birthrates, and powerful advocacy for gender equality brought on by the second wave of feminism had driven cartoonists to reduce the barbs aimed at fathers. In essence, "a new, improved version of fatherhood had come on the scene" (p. 376).

Without denying the radical social changes that took place in the 1960s and 1970s, LaRossa et al. (2000) view the apparent disappearance of the incompetent father image as less of a paradigm shift and more of a gradual process that began with the concept of the "New Father" (or more involved father) in the Baby Boom era. Their exploration took the form of examining the relative attention given to Mother's Day and Father's Day in a myriad of popular comic strips ranging from *Gasoline Alley* and *Blondie* to *Cathy* and *For Better or Worse* (both created by women). They did find an increase in the attention given to Father's Day in the 1970s, although there was still a significant gap (with Father's Day lagging behind) in the 1990s. At the same time, LaRossa et al. (2000) acknowledge that by the 20th century's end, fewer comic strips alluded to either family holiday.

Two questions emerge from the research. The first is, Why does Mother's Day still generate more attention? Is it because mothers are still assumed to hold the primary caregiving role? Or might it be a subtle message suggesting that mothers *should* pay more attention to their parenting role? The second question is, Why are more cartoonists ignoring both Mother's and Father's Day? In answer to this, LaRossa et al. (2000) propose three explanations. The first is that cartoonists might be more adept at conveying their ideas about parenthood without framing it as a holiday message. Another possibility is that they are sensitive to the number of single-parent and blended families and parents estranged or separated from their families. A third, related possibility is that the cartoonists of the 1990s found it difficult to reconcile the concept of the New Father with its antithesis, the "Absentee Dad."

If cartoons represent a handy tool for social scientists examining parental roles, they can easily be adapted for exercises involving children and adolescents. In fact, students growing up with *Garfield* and *Doonesbury* (not to mention *The Simpsons*) might be amused to see some of the comics that entertained their parents and grandparents. How would they perceive the parenting roles of Blondie and Dagwood or Hi and Lois? Students can also be asked to create their own cartoons illustrating their own interpretations of mothers' and fathers' roles.

Television advertisements have also been used as vehicles for analyzing cultural trends. In *The Feminine Mystique,* Betty Friedan (1963) decried the ads of the 1950s in which most women were homemakers whose self-worth depended on squeaky-clean kitchens where, paradoxically, they spent most of their time. Friedan wasn't far off; a study of television ads found that during the 1950s, men were six times more likely to be depicted as workers than parents, whereas women were twice as often depicted as parents (LaRossa et al., 2000). By the 1980s, the portrayals were converging. Men were almost four times as likely and women twice as likely to be depicted as workers than parents, although men were still more often depicted in workplace roles.

Despite irrevocable changes in gender roles, many adolescent and young adult males still believe that mothers should be responsible for more than 50 percent of parenting tasks (Elsters et al., 1989). This attitude is especially prominent among adolescent fathers or men with adolescent partners. In fact, they often do not get much opposition from teenage mothers who sometimes transform the competitiveness of American youth culture into a drive to prove themselves the "best" mother with the "best" child (Higgenson, 1998). Within the context of a parenting program, the competitive drive can have a positive impact, motivating young mothers to learn all they can in order to be good parents.

Parenting programs can have a similarly positive impact on teenage fathers. After completing a parenting program, 90 percent of a group of young urban fathers described "being a man" as being responsible (Mazza, 2002). The young men also became far more goal oriented, self-directed, and self-confident. They came to believe in their strengths and were able to make long-range plans. Noting that far fewer services are available for teenage fathers than mothers, who are still perceived as primary caregivers, Mazza states that "there is a great difference between 'primary' and 'only' parent" (p. 692).

Of course, a key purpose of introducing parenting education into schools is to minimize the need for services for adolescents who unexpectedly become parents. However, the success of parenting programs in instilling confidence and self-efficacy in teenage parents, who had often been alienated from school and had poor role models for effective parenting, highlights the potential of a well-designed program to transform existing attitudes and facilitate the development of positive living skills. In the program described by Mazza (2002), young African American fathers were able to overcome their self-doubts (at least in part the result of negative cultural images) and view themselves as capable of providing emotional and financial support for their families.

In examining students' attitudes toward parental roles and responsibilities, it is wise to expect gender and perhaps class differences. In adult circles, men who assume nurturing parenting roles are well respected and frequently envied by women in more traditional marriages (Curran, 2002).

Girls, regardless of whether their mothers are employed or whether they aspire to college or are preparing to enter the workforce, may be similarly impressed and inclined to seek out mates of their own with egalitarian gender role attitudes (Curran, 2002). College-bound adolescent boys and younger boys (ages 12–14) with employed mothers also tended to hold egalitarian attitudes. However, older adolescent boys, especially if they intended to work or marry after finishing high school and, ironically, especially if their mothers were employed, displayed more traditional gender attitudes. Despite the media images of the New Father, they considered it socially acceptable or "role-legitimate" for men to award priority to their careers over family tasks, while their attitude for women's roles was the reverse.

Findings like these suggest that teachers might need to sharpen their conflict resolution skills when the topic of parenting roles and responsibilities comes up. If it is true that some boys consider career-oriented women to be less attractive partners and less competent mothers when their own mothers work (a finding that contradicts much of the research on working mothers; Jackson, 1998), the first question that comes to mind is "Why?" Is it because they felt that their mothers neglected them? Or is it because the fathers of the boys (who tended to come from working-class families) maintained traditional attitudes, which would have left them with little emotional nurturance and support?

Many men, who felt their fathers, and sometimes mothers, were distant, desire to be nurturing parents who display warmth, support, and affection (Riesch et al., 1996). In Riesch and colleagues' study of fathers' perceptions of how they were parented, some respondents described how traditional gender roles enabled their parents to accomplish tasks that needed to be done. Through clearly delineated responsibilities, the children were ensured food, clothing, and shelter; received help with homework; and learned how to do things like riding a bicycle or fixing things around the house. Several narratives reflected Curran's (2002) perspective that parents today should credit their parents for fulfilling the roles that were demanded of them at the time, while being glad that they have more flexibility in the parenting tasks they assume today. However, there was an underlying sense of emptiness in their stories. The parents fulfilled the tasks that were necessary to keep the family together, but even where recreational activities were involved, neither they nor their children seemed to derive any real joy or meaning from them. There was no room in the prescribed roles for creativity or exploration.

A major impediment to creative decision-making in management is overestimating the degree to which others share one's beliefs (Cross & Brodt, 2001). Part of this belief is due to the desire for social acceptance; assuming that one holds the predominant view, it can boost self-esteem. The flip side of this pervasive practice is that challenges to their assumptions put people on the defensive rather than encouraging them to examine the situation from different perspectives. Does anyone really want to be locked into rigid roles? What are the advantages of having flexible roles and responsibilities? What disadvantages might there be? How do perceptions of fairness and equity come into play in a relationship where partners might have complementary strengths? Do the strengths of mothers and fathers tend to conform to traditional expectations or do they often run counter to them? Exercises that involve role playing and encouraging students to generate arguments from different perspectives can be valuable for challenging rigid assumptions and helping students to recognize the multiple roles and tasks involved in effective parenting.

ESSENTIAL PARENTING SKILLS

Children and even adolescents often see things in concrete terms. Thus, "parenting skills" may be viewed in terms of such things as cooking, helping with homework, providing a paycheck, or driving children to music lessons or soccer games. Although these are undoubtedly valuable parenting skills, essential skills encompass the "soft" skills or interpersonal skills that are central to all human relationships.

A very prominent theme in parenting literature is *boundary setting*. The fathers surveyed by Riesch et al. (1996) expressed the most favorable attitudes toward parents who set boundaries that were structured but flexible. For example:

> "They provided love, caring, and guidance without being pushy and allowing for a lot of freedom of choice."
> "My parents instilled independence. Firm parenting with ample freedom and trust." (Riesch et al., 1996, p. 17)

In contrast, the men whose parents set *chaotic* boundaries, "exemplified by low parental control and involvement," felt that they were deprived of attention and guidance that would have been beneficial, while the responses of those whose parents set *rigid* boundaries can be summed up in the statement "I often thought (as a teenager) that my parents were dictators!" (Riesch et al., 1996, pp. 18–19).

Quantitative research on the topic supports the idea that parents who occupy the midrange of the boundary-setting continuum do have an advantage. A meta-analysis of parenting practices that promote academic success identifies seven parenting practices that, in conjunction with one another, have the most positive impact on student achievement (Rosenzweig, 2001):

- *Educational aspirations and expectations:* This practice entails specifically conveying high expectations for children's academic success.
- *Engagement:* Engagement is demonstrated by spending time with children, showing interest in their activities and their friends, demonstrating that they are committed to their children's well-being.
- *Authoritative parenting style:* Authoritative parents set guidelines for responsible behavior while allowing their children to pursue their own interests, facilitating autonomy, and encouraging independent problem solving and decision making.

- *Autonomy support:* Encouraging independence and autonomy facilitates academic success, while encouraging conformity has a negative impact; autonomy support promotes self-confidence and self-efficacy.
- *Emotional warmth and support:* Like autonomy support, emotional warmth and support are linked with authoritative parenting; children learn to make choices and take risks within a supportive environment.
- *Providing resources and learning experiences:* This one is a no-brainer—parents who create a positive learning environment at home and provide children with enriching learning experiences convey the message that learning is valuable.
- *Specific types of participation in school:* Engaging in volunteer activities and participating in school governance were the two specific activities correlated with academic success; on a more general level, being involved in school activities reinforces the message that learning and school really count.

Consistent with the fathers' perceptions of their childhood experiences (Riesch et al., 1996), excessive control and surveillance, permissiveness, and disengagement are negatively linked with academic success (Rosenzweig, 2001). Some differences exist about the degree to which parents encourage autonomy in special education and regular education students, but the need for parental warmth, encouragement, and positive support is ubiquitous (Deslandes, Leclerc, & Dore-Cote, 2001). In fact, virtually all sources recommend parenting workshops to enhance positive parenting practices.

Numerous studies confirm that positive engagement is an essential parenting skill. With respect to discouraging violence and fostering prosocial behavior, Steinberg (2000) states categorically that "parental engagement in their children's lives is one of the most important—if not the single most important—contributor to children's healthy psychological development" (p. 8). Parental engagement that provides warmth and support while encouraging autonomy is also associated with children's involvement in planning and decision-making (Gauvain & Perez, 2001), essential skills for deciding when it is right to have children as well as how to parent them.

Conflict resolution is also an essential parenting skill. Violence prevention has recently become part of the school curriculum, but parents who instill in their children respect for others combined with a strong sense of self-efficacy are taking the first step in preventing their children from becoming bullies or victims at school (Schmalz & Jalloh, 2003). At home, parents can model prosocial behavior and, through positive parenting practices, help children to develop strong self-concepts that serve as a buffer against negative peer influences (Steinberg, 2000). Adolescents, in particular, tend to base their awareness of their rights on the rights of others and on their experiences within the family (Day, Peterson-Badali, & Shea, 2002). Helping siblings to resolve disputes peacefully is a prime example of conflict resolution at home (Patten & Robertson, 2001).

Conflict resolution skills also enable individuals to use conflict constructively (Cross & Brodt, 2001). Creative problem solving entails presenting conflicting ideas and exploring adversarial positions. Parents who are adept at weighing alternatives and exploring different perspectives can effectively defuse potentially negative situations while encouraging independent thinking. Based on their own experiences as well as imaginations, students can brainstorm ways in which, as parents, they would use conflict resolution skills.

As virtually all parents admit, stress management is an essential parenting skill. In the Avon Longitudinal Study of Parents and Children (ALSPAC), participating parents expressed a variety of stressors, including children's behavior (often the greatest area of stress), financial concerns, time pressures, achievement and academic pressures, juggling home and work, social pressures, and safety concerns (Sidebotham & the ALSPAC Study Team, 2001). Coping with each of these issues involves learning specific skills in each domain as well as learning to prioritize needs. In fact, knowing how to balance the needs of the child with the needs of the parents may be the single most essential parenting skill.

Respecting Diversity

While extolling the advantages of flexible parenting roles over the rigidly gender stereotypes of past generations, Curran (2002) also advises today's parents not to be overly critical of their parents' adherence to strict cultural norms. Some parents may have wanted to step out of—or even reverse—the prescribed gender roles but were afraid that defying social conventions would cause the family to be ostracized and the children to be rejected and ridiculed. Stated succinctly, "We can't judge yesterday's parents with today's lenses" (Curran, 2002, p. 20).

Interestingly, Curran (2002) points out that the proportion of two-parent families today parallels that of a century ago: 71 percent. The difference is that, in the past, single parents were generally widowed, whereas today they are more likely to be divorced, separated, or never married. In defense of today's single mothers, she stresses that greater independence and opportunities for education and economic support give them a major advantage over their counterparts of yesteryear.

Families today can take on a myriad of forms. Divorces create blended families. Hispanic and African American families often have extended family networks. Hispanic parents are also more likely to engage children in planning activities involving the family (Gauvain & Perez, 2001). Interracial families are more common, and two-parent families may consist of parents of the same gender. Although it may be important not to view yesterday's parents with today's lenses, it is even more important that today's parents are not judged by rigid assumptions about what a "real" family should be.

Even very young children are capable of brainstorming about the different types of families they see and the fact that each one has intrinsic strengths (Matiella, 1990). In fact, because of increasing peer pressure, adolescents may be less accepting of nontraditional families than younger children (Jackson, 1998). For adolescents, discussions that frame diversity within the context of rights and individual freedom may be a valuable adjunct to more concrete exercises in understanding family diversity.

Promoting Family Health

An essential part of an effective parenting program is helping students to understand infant and child development, with a particular emphasis on the way parent–child interactions influence physical and emotional health (Zoline & Jason, 1985). Very young parents, in particular, frequently have unrealistic expectations about infant development, expecting their babies to reach developmental milestones such as walking and talking at an improbable young age (Higgenson, 1998). These idealized expectations may cause them to exaggerate their infants' cognitive or physical development, which may have the opposite effect if they deny or minimize real developmental delays.

Worries about children's health are a prominent parental concern (Sidebotham & the ALSPAC Study Team, 2001). The more well informed parents are and the better equipped they are to deal with problems, the less stressful these concerns are.

Social support is a major stress reducer for virtually all parents and contributes to both physical and psychological health. In particular, adolescent and single parents need strong social networks (Higgenson, 1998; Mazza, 2002; Sidebotham & the ALSPAC Study Team, 2001). The social needs of teenage parents can differ dramatically from those of adults. Not only do social networks help young parents combat the social stigma that many experience, but formal and informal networks also provide them with essential information and skills training about effective parenting.

Ethnicity also has an impact on expectations for social support. Anglo parents are more likely to form social networks outside the family, whereas Hispanic and African American parents are more likely to seek support through strong family ties.

Although parents may seek social support through different channels and in different ways, the need for support is universal. In classroom exercises, students can explore the myriad of ways in which parents seek out support and the different impact of different sources. For example, what happens when family advice conflicts with expert advice? Is bigger better when it comes to developing social networks? How do parents cope with social pressures in areas such as providing children with material things or promoting academic success? What impact do social networks have on physical health? How do social networks support childcare needs or impact decisions made about childcare during times parents are at work? These are only some of the questions that can be explored from an ecological perspective on family health.

SUMMARY

Many parents today base their parenting practices on what their parents did *not* do, such as provide them with emotional support or encourage them to be independent. Implementing parenting classes in schools can help future generations to learn from positive family role models as well as encourage them to wisely plan their futures so that they will not find themselves facing parental responsibilities before they are ready to take them on.

It may be a cliché to say that parenting is an art and a science, but it is undoubtedly true. To be effective parents, students need to learn both the concrete, practical skills of parenting and the social, cognitive, and interpersonal skills that will allow them to be successful parents in a complex environment that demands flexibility, creativity, self-confidence, and, above all, the ability to juggle multiple roles.

WEBSITES

Parents, Families, and Friends of Gays and Lesbians: www.flag.org

The Henry J. Kaiser Family Foundation: www.kff.org

Parenting Resources: www.educationindex.com/parents

Parenting Education Resources: www.parent-education.com

Realityworks: www.realityworks.com

University of Minnesota Parenting Education Resources: www.parentingumin.com

Family Education Network: www.fen.com

The Parenting Project: www.parentingproject.org

New York States Parenting Education Requirements Q&A's: www.emsc.nysed.gov/sss/parentingqa.html

Parent Education Network: www.parentednet.org

Education World: The Educator's Best Friend: www.education-world.com

The Great Body Shop: www.thegreatbodyshop.net

Sexuality Information and Education Council of the United States: www.siecus.org

Don't Laugh at Me curriculum: www.operationrespect.org

New York State Skills Matrix, The State Education Department: www.nysed.gov

New York State Parenting Education Scope of Instruction, The State Education Department: www.nysed.gov

Encouraging Multiple Intelligences into the Curriculum and the Classroom: www.masterteacher.com

REFERENCES

Bignell, S. (Ed.). (1980). *Family life education curriculum guide* (rev. ed.). Santa Cruz, CA: Network Publications.

Cross, R. L., & Brodt, S. E. (2001). How assumptions of consensus undermine decision-making. *Sloan Management Review, 42,* 86–94.

Curran, D. (2002, July). The good old days are now: What families are doing right. *U.S. Catholic,* pp. 19–22.

Deslandes, R., Leclerc, D., & Dore-Cote, A. (2001). *Longitudinal studies of special education and regular students: Autonomy, parental involvement practices and degrees of reciprocity in parent–adolescent interactions* (Report No. PS 029-541). Paper presented at the Annual Meeting of the American Educational Research Associates. (ERIC Document Reproduction Service No. ED453-957)

Day, D. M., Peterson-Badali, M., & Shea, B. (2002). *Parenting style as a context for the development of adolescents' thinking about rights* (Report No. PS 031-369). Paper presented at the Biennial Meeting for Research on Adolescents. (ERIC Document Reproduction Service No. ED464-746)

Elsters, A. B., Lamb, M. E., & Kimmerly, N. (1989). Perceptions of parenthood among adolescent fathers. *Pediatrics, 83,* 758–765.

Friedan, B. (1963). *The second sex.* New York: Norton.

Gauvain, M., & Perez, S. M. (2001). *Parenting practices and children's participation in planning* (Report No. PS 029-965). Paper presented at the Annual Meeting of the American Psychological Association. (ERIC Document Reproduction Service No. ED458-996)

Halter, M., & Lang, B. F. (1994). *Making choices: Life skills for adolescents.* Santa Barbara, CA: Advocacy.

Higgenson, J. G. (1998). Competitive parenting: The culture of teen mothers. *Journal of Marriage & the Family, 60,* 135–149.

Jackson, D. W. (1998). Adolescents' conceptualizations of adult roles: Relationships with age, gender, work goal, and maternal employment. *Sex Roles, 38,* 231–250.

Knox, M. (1998). Adolescents' possible selves and their relationship to global self-esteem. *Sex Roles, 39,* 61–80.

LaRossa, R., Jaret, C., Gadgil, M., & Wynn, G. R. (2000). The changing culture of fatherhood in comic-strip families: A six-decade approach. *Journal of Marriage & the Family, 62,* 375–387.

Matiella, A. C. (1990). *We are a family: Children's activities in family living.* Santa Cruz, CA: Network Publications.

Mazza, C. (2002). Young dads: The effects of a parenting program on urban African-American fathers. *Adolescence, 37,* 681–693.

Morfei, M. Z., Hooker, K., Fiese, B. H., & Cordeiro, A. M. (2001). Continuity and change in parenting possible selves: A longitudinal follow-up. *Basic & Applied Social Psychology, 23,* 217–223.

Patten, P., & Robertson, A. S. (2001). *Violence prevention resource guide for parents.* Champaign, IL: ERIC Clearinghouse.

Riesch, S. K., Kuester, L., Brost, D., & McCarthy, J. G. (1996). Fathers' perceptions of how they were parented. *Journal of Community Health Nursing, 13,* 13–29.

Rosenzweig, C. (2001). *A meta-analysis of parenting and school success: The role of parents in promoting students' academic performance* (Report No. TM 032-518). Paper presented at the Annual Meeting of the American Educational Research Associates. (ERIC Document Reproduction Service No. ED452-232)

Schmalz, K., & Jalloh, M. G. (2003). Preventing school violence. In E. Weinstein & E. Rosen (Eds.), *Teaching children about health* (2nd ed., pp. 303–328). Belmont, CA: Thomson Wadsworth.

Sidebotham, P., & the ALSPAC Study Team. (2001). Culture, stress and the parent–child relationship: A qualitative study of parents' perceptions of parenting. *Child, 27,* 469–485.

Steinberg, L. (2000). *Youth violence: Do parents and families make a difference?* (Report No. CG 031-821). Washington, DC: U.S. Department of Justice. (ERIC Document Reproduction Service No. ED465-924)

Zoline, S. S., & Jason, L. A. (1985). Preventive parent education for high school students. *Journal of Clinical Child Psychology, 14,* 119–123.

LEARNING EXPERIENCES

The learning experiences included in the following section will allow students to

- Describe how families may be similar and different, and how those similarities and differences influence parenting.
- Demonstrate, through writing, discussion, and role playing, effective communication skills to foster positive relationships.
- Develop perspectives through writing and discourse on the roles, responsibilities, and realities of parenting.
- Practice decision-making skills with peers through role plays and peer tutoring on topics related to the responsibilities of parenting.

[When approaching the topic of parenting, the teacher should be well versed on the many responsibilities that come with being a parent and differences in perspectives about parenting. Factors that influence different perspectives include gender, race, ethnicity, income, geography, education, and personal experiences, as they pertain to both being parented and being a parent. Understanding how perspectives have changed over time will also help the teacher to give context to students about how they may see their potential future roles as parents. Above all, sensitivity to the different parent and family situations of the students in the classroom is critical for this to be a positive learning unit. The teacher may want to refer back to the reflective questions in the opening scenario as a means to set the stage for the learning experiences.]

LEARNING EXPERIENCE 1

TITLE: I Am Part of a Family

GRADE LEVELS: K–3

TIME REQUIREMENTS: Five 30-minute activities; one 30-minute activity for summative assessment

LEARNING CONTEXT

This learning experience is an introductory lesson to get children to understand basic behaviors that are necessary in a family to build relationships. The teacher will have already introduced the concept of family and what that means and also how families are different. This learning experience will reinforce those messages and take the students further in understanding that they have some responsibility related to family dynamics and relationship management. It also is based on the assumption that the teacher has introduced concepts such as pair/share, cooperative learning, and comparison.

The focus of this experience is to help children understand the dynamics of relationships within a family. The students will be exploring ways to build trust and respect within a family unit, whatever its makeup, and how their behavior enhances or disrupts their relationships within their family. The students will also understand how simple communication can help build relationships. This experience is based on the assumption that children have had previous discussions related to the definition of a family and that families are different. After this activity, students will

- Understand the definition of a family.
- Understand the similarities and differences that exist among families.
- Explain and demonstrate positive behaviors to foster good relationships.
- Describe and demonstrate how to communicate effectively to foster positive relationships.
- Understand and demonstrate how to access resources to foster positive relationships.

Concepts

- A family consists of two or more people who care for each other in many ways.
- There are different kinds of families.
- Every family member has a role and individual needs.
- Family members take care of each other.
- Family members show love for each other.
- Family members have responsibilities.

NATIONAL LEARNING STANDARDS

5:   Students will demonstrate the ability to use interpersonal communication skills to enhance health.

7:   Students will demonstrate the ability to advocate for personal, family, and community health.

PROCEDURE

Although this learning experience is geared toward K–2 students, simply changing some of the strategies for children to respond increases the rigor of the lesson. This experience offers the teacher flexibility in teaching strategies to help children to meet the objectives.

Activity 1

Prior to the beginning of this experience, have the students bring in a picture of their own family or a picture of a family. The teacher should have pictures of families on hand so that those who do not bring one will have something to work with.

As a diagnostic assessment, ask the class, "What do we know about families?" Record their answers. Then ask, "How are families different and how are families the same?" Record likenesses and differences, using a T chart graphic organizer.

Have the students get into groups of two; the students will do a pair/share with their pictures and talk about the similarities and the differences of their own families. (Older students could share and record the similarities and differences on a Venn diagram.) Have them share the differences and likenesses of their own families as a large group, again using a T chart to illustrate the differences and similarities of the families of the whole class.

Activity 2

In a large-group discussion, ask the students, "How should we treat people we love and care about?"

Read to the class the children's book *Stellaluna*. The students will show their understanding by drawing what the story was about and will share their interpretations of the story. Ask the following questions of the large group:

- What was different about Stellaluna's family?
- What did Stellaluna's family do that showed they loved and cared for her?

Activity 3

In a class discussion, ask, "Has anyone in your family ever been mad at you? Why? What do we do sometimes that make our families mad at us? What does our family do that sometimes makes us mad?"

Students will be given a "Feelings Journal." One half of the journal should have a smiling face; the other should have a frowning face. Students will write or draw how it feels when things are going well in their family on the smiling side and how it feels when things are not going well on the frowning side. (Teachers may have to help with the writing aspect.)

Have students direct their attention to the frowning side of the journal. In large groups, the students will discuss how they could change the things on the frowning side. Remind them of their answers from the discussion of "what families do to show they love and care for each other." In a large group, ask, "What are the consequences of behaving badly?"

Activity 4

Hold a minilecture: The way that we communicate with one another shows how much we love and care for one another. There is verbal and nonverbal communication; demonstrate both forms to the class. Also talk about "I statements" and how they can be used so that we do not hurt each other's feelings.

Ask the students, "What happens when we say mean things to one another?" Hold a paper cutout of a child. Explain that when we say mean things to someone else, it is hurtful. Demonstrate this point by saying something mean and ripping a small piece from the paper cutout.

"You aren't very smart"—rip a piece of the child; "Give me that!"—rip another piece; and so on. Explain that to make someone "whole," we must say nice things to them daily, and then have the students one by one say nice things. Tape back the pieces that were ripped to make the cutout whole again. Ask the students to remember this when they are talking to their families, friends, teachers, and other people.

Next, give the students scenarios, and have them act out how they could communicate more positively. "How do you respond? How should you respond? How can you use 'I' statements?" Demonstrate the difference between saying, "Give me the swing," and using an "I" statement by saying, "I feel bad when you won't share the swing." Students will demonstrate the change. Ask the students, "How does this show respect for one another?"

Activity 5

Have the students pair up, and call out a nonverbal feeling (using both positive and negative feelings). Students will show that emotion to their partner. Both will do it at the same time.

To the whole class, ask, "How did you feel when your partner showed you a mad face? A happy face?"

Show the video clip from the curriculum "Don't Laugh at Me," and, as part of a large-group discussion, ask, "In the video clip, what emotions did you see, either verbal or nonverbal?"

For group reflection, ask the class, "Can nonverbal communication show family members that you care and love them?" and "Sometimes our feelings get in the way of good communication. What feelings might get in the way of being nice to someone?"

INSTRUCTIONAL/ENVIRONMENTAL MODIFICATIONS

This learning experience lends itself to different learning styles and developmental stages of the children involved. It can easily be modified to include more or less rigor. For example, instead of having students draw, they can write. Instead of writing, they could draw or orally discuss the lessons. The activity may require more one on one time with certain students in some parts.

RESOURCES

For the students, crayons, paper, and pictures of their families. For the teacher: the children's book *Stellaluna* (Harcourt Trade Publishers: phone [212] 592-1000 or e-mail trade.sales@ harcourt.com); videotape from "Don't Laugh at Me" curriculum (Operation Respect: phone [212] 904-5243 or visit www.operationrespect.org); T chart graphic organizer; pictures of families; Feeling Journals; paper cutout of a child; and premade postcards (see the section later on summative assessment).

ASSESSMENT PLAN

Diagnostic

- What do we know about families?
- How should we treat people we know and love?

Formative

- Assess the children's understanding of *Stellaluna*. (Use a checklist of concepts and components of the story.)
- Assess the students' understanding of feelings in the Feelings Journal (observation).
- Assess the students' understanding of the use of "I" statements and saying positive things, via observation and a checklist.
- Assess the students' understanding of nonverbal communication.

Summative

Ask the students to reflect on the lessons they have learned, and have them look at the products they have created. Hand out a postcard for each child, and on the front the students will draw a picture of something that they do to show that they love and care for a family member. On the back, on the message side of the postcard, the student (with the teacher's help) will write a positive message that illustrates their understanding of good verbal communication. Let the students know that the postcards will be sent home. Students share their pictures with others in the class. Send the postcards home to the family of the child.

REFERENCE

Submitted by Colleen M. Hurd, Elmira, New York; and Elizabeth Mastro, Hudson Valley Student Support Services Center, New Paltz, New York.

LEARNING EXPERIENCE 2

TITLE: Yes or No, Not Maybe

GRADE LEVELS: 7–9

TIME REQUIREMENTS: Five 45-minute sessions, not necessarily consecutive

LEARNING CONTEXT

"Yes or No, Not Maybe" takes place during middle school health or consumer science classes. The student is guided in identifying a decision; reviewing values, goals, needs, and priorities; seeking out and interpreting information; recognizing and managing resources; determining and evaluating a course of action. Some of the benefits of this approach include a sense of personal control, ease in predicting consequences, and the hope of a healthy future. The combination of self-awareness, recognition of family and peer relationships, and an understanding of the decision process, management of stress, and communication skills can empower students to act responsibly within their own life situations, both in the present and in the future.

Students will demonstrate decision-making skills in selecting choices that promote personal health when faced with pressure to the contrary. Because pressures involving choices often create stress, the role play must also incorporate stress management sills. Using communication skills as the content for the script as well as the tool to convey the message of the role play is important. The student's response must clearly be a yes or no, not maybe. The task is the summative assessment for units on the process skills and teen stress issues.

After this activity, students will

- Know and do to succeed (taught to students during the course before the assessment is given).
- Separate needs from wants.
- Identify personal values, resources, goals, and priorities.
- Name and recognize feelings.
- Apply the decision-making process.
- Form favorable relationships.
- Recognize consequences that risk personal health.
- Manage stress.
- Communicate verbally and nonverbally.
- Resolve conflicts.
- Demonstrate responsibility.
- Use graphic organizers.
- Interact with others in a positive manner as a team member.

NATIONAL LEARNING STANDARDS

3: Students will demonstrate the ability to practice health-enhancing behaviors and reduce health risks.

5: Students will demonstrate the ability to use interpersonal communication skills to enhance health.

6: Students will demonstrate the ability to use goal-setting and decision-making skills to enhance health.

PROCEDURE

Students plan, script, and execute a decision-making role play. This role play clearly promotes health in a realistic life situation with a believable healthy solution, using all team members, and maintaining the audience's attention. Students use information from previous class activities on decision making, stress management, communication, and conflict resolution, as background learning in accomplishing the task. Sample scenarios such as parenting are provided, or students may invent their own situations.

Provide and explain the worksheets, rubric, and reflection questions (see the section on resources):

- "Yes, No, Not Maybe" describes the task.
- The "Checklist for Necessary Expectations" parallels the rubric to help students to assess themselves during the process of working on the script and performing.
- "Sample Scenario Format" shows the style of writing for the role-play script.
- "Plan Sheet for Role-Play," "Planning Calendar," "Story Pattern," "Deciding," "Sentence Map," and "Resources Used" are graphic organizers to assist students in organizing their thoughts and time. Students will have had previous instruction in the use of graphic organizers and cooperative learning before completing this activity.

All groups present on Performance Day. Students are asked to notify parents of this date, in advance, to avoid doctor appointments and the like. Upon completion of the task, students assess themselves using the rubric provided and submit graphic organizers, the script, their personal reflection, and the rubric.

Each team and the teacher collectively assess individual team members using the rubric during checkpoint conferences and at the final conference session. If a student is absent on Performance Day, eliminate the "Presentation" strip from that child's rubric and adjust the score.

INSTRUCTIONAL/ENVIRONMENTAL MODIFICATIONS

Provide small-group computer stations and writing tables during planning and scripting. A large area to accommodate performers and audience during role play should be designated.

Special needs students have group support and a place to participate without any reason for exclusion. Teacher conferencing allows for one-on-one attention without drawing attention to special needs.

RESOURCES

Props to be supplied by individual group members; *Graphic Organizers,* by Chris Flynn, 1995 (n.p.: Creative Teaching Press); *Five under Cover,* 1989, p. 123 (Boston: Houghton Mifflin)

ASSESSMENT PLAN

Ask students to review the teacher-developed task and rubric, which may be edited accordingly before being used. At the end of the project, ask students again for feedback for continuous editing purposes.

Evidence of meeting the learning standards' performance indicators is achieved through the use of graphic organizers, a checklist of criteria, observation, and conferencing to demonstrate progress awareness for the teacher and student. Reflective questions summarize and document the student's personal experiences. The rubric is the final tool used to document the student's work.

REFLECTION

When students practice applying the decision-making process in real-life stress situations, the process becomes more natural for them, particularly in times of pressure. Role playing and peer tutoring have been found to be effective ways to empower students to change behavior.

REFERENCE

Submitted by Pat Loncto, Lewiston Porter Middle School, Youngstown, New York.

LEARNING EXPERIENCE 3

TITLE: A Document-Based Question (DBQ) Essay: The Role, Responsibility, and Reality of Parenting

GRADE LEVELS: 10–12

TIME REQUIREMENTS: Three 40-minute sessions

LEARNING CONTEXT

In this learning experience, students are given the task of writing a letter to their future child. The student takes on the role of parent in this DBQ essay; the performance task is designed to facilitate the development of a realistic personal vision of self in the role of a high-quality parent or citizen positively influencing youth.

A DBQ is a time-efficient way to engage students in high-level thinking and infuse content quickly, freeing classroom time for skill development. Given the documents in a DBQ format, each student can articulate a thesis by using the information to come to his or her own conclusions as he or she develops and supports an argument using the documents and background knowledge. The scaffolding questions are formulated to allow the student to uncover many of the essential skills and responsibilities of a quality parent. The student task is to weave ideas from the documents to support a viewpoint and to develop a personal vision of self in the responsible parent role.

The DBQ task is a solid foundation that can easily lead into goal-setting skill development. The activity is designed to provide young people with an opportunity to look ahead, consider future, and use cognitive rehearsal before being in the actual situation. The completed essay can be used as a tool providing content for assessment of personal characteristics necessary for their vision of a parent.

After this activity, students will be able to

- Analyze and synthesize information from a variety of sources and media.
- Support a thesis through accurate use of the documents.
- Consider evidence in individual documents as well as establish connections among them and relationships to outside information and experience.
- Use logic and organization as they present their points to an audience, supporting English language arts.
- Use the DBQ process with greater skill, supporting the social studies curriculum.
- Take on a personal readiness expectation for parenthood, based on conscious, thoughtful consideration of self in future role as parent.

NATIONAL LEARNING STANDARDS

5: Students will demonstrate the ability to use interpersonal communication skills to enhance health.

6: Students will demonstrate the ability to use goal-setting and decision-making skills to enhance health.

PROCEDURE

Students analyze documents by constructing short-answer responses to scaffolding questions, individually or in cooperative groups. Individually, students use a graphic organizer to organize and record their thinking about the analysis of documents as well as related outside information and personal experience to support their thesis statement. Students use all documents and cite them. (See the Instructional Modifications section for directions on adapting the scaffolding questions segment to a cooperative task.)

Students write a letter to their future child. The letter is their vision of the role of a parent. The student must state a thesis as to what he or she thinks is the degree of influence of parents on the health, safety, and positive development of youth. The students create supporting paragraphs, referring to and citing all documents. They may also include personal outside information. The concluding paragraph requires students to reflect on their personal readiness for the responsibilities of parenting.

Ask students to use green to highlight words in their essay that describe traits that come naturally to them, yellow for words that relate to developing personal characteristics, and pink for traits that they need to acquire. Students can write achievable short-term goals that they predict will help them to become the parent they described in their essay. Ask the students to develop a plan for achieving their goal and identify possible supports and strategies to overcome barriers. Students can use agenda books to post notes to remind themselves to stay focused and document and reflect on their progress over time.

Prepare document packets with a corresponding rubric. Begin by briefly reviewing the documents and scaffolding questions, the rubric for that part of the task, and the due date.

On the due date for the scaffolding questions, explain how to plan for writing the essay. Review the remaining parts of the rubric. Read past student work to use as models to clearly articulate expectations. Provide individual mentoring as needed.

INSTRUCTIONAL/ENVIRONMENTAL MODIFICATIONS

The scaffolding questions can be done in cooperative groups in a strategy called "expert jigsaw." With this strategy, students are assigned to an "expert group" and given the task of analyzing one or more of the documents cooperatively. The group must make sure that each group member is prepared to share the information with their home base. Later, the teacher reviews material with the large group.

Another useful modification is chunking: Break the DBQ task into smaller parts with a due date for completion of each part.

The task has been easily modified to accommodate students with various challenges by decreasing the number of documents for some students. However, documents 1 and 2 are necessary foundational documents.

Technology can be used when the DBQ is online and students can access from home and print or e-mail to the teacher.

RESOURCES

DBQ student packet; a computer with Internet linkage

ASSESSMENT PLAN

A review of the task and rubric facilitated by the teacher is done to ensure that expectations are clear. Students are encouraged to ask questions. Later, when models of student work are shared with students, they are asked to rate the models using the rubric. Students will self-assess before submitting an essay.

Evidence of student progress toward meeting the performance indicators of the learning standards is shown in the essay itself as well as the responses to all scaffolding questions and the graphic organizer. The graphic organizer is a written record of the writer's organization of thoughts and serves as a checklist to make sure that all documents are skillfully grouped and cited. "Data Boxes" graphic organizer is an overall plan of strategy for the essay that frees the student to develop ideas rather than getting caught up in details.

REFLECTION

This DBQ provides a way to encourage the development of realistic personal expectations in the role of a quality parent. Students articulate their current readiness for the responsibility of parenthood. The lesson also supports academic achievement in social studies and English language arts.

The learning experience is relevant because today many young people may not have the opportunity to observe young children and focus on the role of parenthood. We live in a culture that seems to glorify sexuality but the reality is that our young people need to learn that they have control over their lives. They can postpone sexual involvement and complete their educational goals. We must direct young people to give thought to the responsibility of parenting before it is their reality.

The letter to the student's future child is a written demonstration of how to express needs, wants, and feelings in healthy ways and to consider the impact of present behavior on one's vision for the future.

REFERENCE

Submitted by Carol Nochajski, Alden Senior High School, Alden, New York.

PREGNANCY AND CHILDBIRTH

SHANNON WHALEN AND JENINE DEMARZO

OBJECTIVES

After reading this chapter, students will be able to

1.   Identify content that is appropriate for and understandable at the different grade levels.
2.   Begin a dialogue on reproduction, pregnancy, and childbirth that is inviting even to the youngest learner.
3.   Identify appropriate terminology and definitions for all reproductive structures and pregnancy events.
4.   Promote communication and decision-making skills and describe how they are necessary for a safe and healthy pregnancy, labor, and delivery (treatments, testing, medications, procedures, and alternatives).
5.   Encourage setting goals for life.
6.   Identify factors that influence fertility and infertility and how stress management skills can be applied.
7.   Identify birthing alternatives, and integrate dialogue concerning advocacy skills.
8.   Discuss the postpartum experience: the significant physiological and psychological changes and how they influence the family dynamics.
9.   Introduce how problem-solving and conflict resolution techniques can be utilized to facilitate mature parenting.

REFLECTIVE QUESTIONS

Elementary School Students

1.   Have you ever known someone who was pregnant—a person or pet? What did you notice about them? Did they behave in any special ways?
2.   Have you ever had a chance to ask your mother what her pregnancy with you was like? Were you a good baby? Did you kick a lot or give your mom heartburn?
3.   What kinds of things do you think your mom did or didn't do to keep you healthy when she was pregnant with you?
4.   Do you want to have children when you grow up?

Middle School Students

1.   When you were younger, did your parents ever talk to you about where babies come from? What did they tell you?

2.   Why do people tell children "stories" about where babies are from?
3.   How old were you when you first learned how babies are really conceived and born?
4.   What are some things that improve a woman's chance of getting pregnant?
5.   What are some things that decrease a woman's chance of getting pregnant?
6.   Have you ever known someone who had a hard time getting pregnant?
7.   If a couple cannot get pregnant, what are some of the options available to them?

High School Students

1.   Are most teen pregnancies planned?
2.   What are some complications that can be prevented if a person has accurate knowledge about the steps to a healthy pregnancy?

3. Why do people continue to smoke and drink during pregnancy if they know it is unhealthy for the baby?

4. Are there any behaviors that boys and men participate in that contribute to a healthy or unhealthy pregnancy? Or is it simply the behavior of the girl or woman that affects the pregnancy?

5. Have you ever thought about having children in the future? At what age do you think you might want to have a child?

6. People often learn about labor and delivery from the movies and television. Do you think this is an accurate portrayal of what really happens in the labor and delivery room?

7. What are some birthing options available to people giving birth, other than the hospital?

SCENARIO

Ashley is studying for her test in health class. For the past 2 weeks, the class has been studying about pregnancy, labor, and delivery. She doesn't understand why they have to know about this stuff anyway. As far as she is concerned, everyone her age should be trying not to get pregnant instead of worrying about how it works. She shares her complaints with her friend Beth, who had health last semester. Beth tells her that she learned a lot from the class and what she learned will help her in the future. Beth told Ashley about her aunt Susan who got married and tried to get pregnant for years. It turned out that she was doing everything wrong. Beth thought that if her aunt had learned about pregnancy when she was younger, she might have had an easier time getting pregnant—or at least her aunt would have known about some of the options available to her to improve fertility. As Ashley thought about it, she guessed Beth was right. It probably was better to be prepared with the right information ahead of time, instead of waiting until the last minute.

Before reading the scenario, whose opinion did you agree with more, Ashley's or Beth's?

Did your opinion change after reading the scenario? Why or why not?

How many opportunities do people have to learn about credible health information in their lifetime?

What other health issues does it help to be informed about ahead of time, instead of waiting until the last minute?

Why do boys and men need to know about pregnancy, labor, and delivery? After all, they don't get pregnant or give birth!

INTRODUCTION

Sexual reproduction is the story of the creation of a human life from the moment of conception through the development of the fetus and the birth of a newborn baby. Students of every age are interested in pregnancy and childbirth. Many school-age students have experienced the process of pregnancy within their own families or via their friend's families. Young elementary school children have varied understandings of this phenomenon. Many of them have been told that the "stork" brings the new baby or that the baby grows in the mother's stomach from a "seed." Others may believe that the newborn leaves the mother's body through the belly button. Older students may believe themselves to have a better understanding of this process. However, they, too, are often greatly misinformed.

Even the sexually "experienced" high school-age student may hold beliefs that are rooted in myth or fallacy. Thus, it is our job as health educators to educate in a way that utilizes simple, correct terminology about how babies are created, develop, and are born. We need to use developmentally appropriate techniques in an atmosphere that is comfortable and conducive to a shared learning experience.

This natural occurrence is a sound platform for many "teachable moments" in the classroom. The youngest learners can begin to appreciate their own sexuality and its place in the natural rhythm of the life cycle. Encouraging open communication between students in the classroom and within their own families is merely the tip of the iceberg. Teaching adolescent learners decision-making techniques as simple as a list of pros and cons will elucidate the fact that pregnancy can and should be a planned event between two committed individuals.

Introducing the concept of setting life goals at any age can aid in the appreciation of pursuing healthy behaviors and experiencing healthful, positive consequences. Discussions such as these will certainly contribute to their knowledge base as well as to their arsenal of life skill techniques, thus paving the way for responsible, accountable young adults.

CONCEPTION

Conception or fertilization occurs when an ovum is penetrated by and united with a sperm cell to form a viable zygote. Fertilization usually occurs in the upper third of the woman's Fallopian tube after the egg is released from the ovary during the fertile period of the woman's menstrual cycle. Following ejaculation into the vagina, approximately 400 to 600 million sperm are deposited into the woman's vagina. However, a total of about 400 will reach the region where union of egg and sperm occurs. Sperm cells are one of the smallest cells in the human body, measuring no more than 2/500th of an inch. The *ovum* or *egg*, measuring about 1/175th of an inch, is the largest. Most reproductive specialists believe that sperm can remain viable for up to 5 days after ejaculation. However, sperm have been detected in the female reproductive tract several days after sexual intercourse.

Both the egg and sperm are responsible for delivering the genetic material of each parent. Unlike other cells in the body, these sex cells contain only half of the genetic material required to form a human embryo. The sperm and egg contain a single copy of each chromosome, a total of 23, where other cells in the body have 23 pairs, or a total of 46. The process of uniting the two halves of genetic material is called *meiosis*. All other human cells are produced by *mitosis*, a process in which the genetic material in the nucleus of the cell doubles before cell division occurs.

Meiosis of the female sex cell or ovum occurs during the early phase of the menstrual cycle. The chromosome in the nucleus of an immature egg cell, called the *primary oocyte*, divides into the secondary oocyte and a polar body. Each of these cells contains only half of the genetic material of the original cell. The secondary oocyte divides into another polar body and a cell that will become a mature ovum. When released from the ovary, the ovum is ready for fertilization.

The sperm cell follows a similar procedure. An immature sperm cell, called a *primary spermatocyte*, divides into two new cells, each with only half of the genetic material of the original cell. These secondary spermatocytes contain either an X chromosome or a Y chromosome (not both, as in the primary cell). The two new secondary spermatocytes replicate the chromosomes and divide into two new cells called *spermatids*.

Each primary spermatocyte produces four spermatids, each containing half of the X and half of the Y chromosomes. The spermatids mature into sperm cells, which can pair with the 23 chromosomes of the mature ovum. The mature sperm cell, also called a *spermatozoa*, consists of a head, which contains the nucleus; a midpiece containing the energy source for motility; and the tail, which aids in locomotion.

When a woman ovulates or releases a mature egg, it is drawn into a Fallopian tube via the *fimbria* on which small hairlike projections called *cilia* push the egg toward the uterus. If fertilization does not occur, the ovum disintegrates within 24 hours.

Sperm must also make a journey through the male reproductive system in order to unite with a potential female egg (see Chapter 2). After ejaculation into the vagina, the sperm begin to move through the cervix into the uterus and Fallopian tubes. If the sperm unites with an egg, fertilization occurs.

How does the sperm know where to go? Scientists believe that the egg emits a substance that attracts the sperm to it. In addition, the female mucus produced by the cervix has channels to direct the sperm to the egg. Most often it is a single sperm that gets to the egg and undergoes a transformation called *capacitation*. This process enables the sperm to penetrate the egg. Once this occurs, the sperm secrete a gel-like substance called *hyaluronidase* that eats away at the top protective layer of the egg called the *zona pellucida*. Generally, several dozen capacitated sperm may be trying to penetrate the ovum and fertilize it. Eventually the combined enzymes of these sperm cells will break down the zona pellucida, and one "lucky" sperm cell successfully penetrates the egg. Once this occurs, the egg undergoes a chemical change in the gel covering so that no other sperm can penetrate the zona pellucida. The fertilized egg becomes a zygote, and cellular division and development commence.

FERTILITY

A healthy woman of child-bearing age, who is free from serious problems, well nourished, and receives regular health care, has a very good chance of conceiving and delivering a healthy baby. The effects of maternal age and fertility are well documented. Biologically, a woman's best time to have a baby is when she is in her 20s, although safe pregnancies and deliveries regularly occur outside this prime window of opportunity, and some women have delivered healthy babies as late as their 50s. Pregnancy for adolescent girls carries a higher risk of complicated pregnancy and delivery. These risks include low birthweights and premature delivery. After the age of 35, pregnancy is considered "high risk" due to the fact that the fetus and the mother have a greater risk for trauma. For example, women over the age of 35 have an increased risk for babies born with chromosomal abnormalities. One such condition is Down syndrome, which is associated with varying degrees of mental retardation. The chances of having a child with Down syndrome for a woman in her 20s is approximately 1 in 2,000 and for a woman in her 40s, 1 in 110 (Daniels & Weingarten, 1982; Westheimer & Lopater, 2004).

Prenatal Readiness

Relatively recent research has suggested that women can prepare their bodies for pregnancy. The American College of Obstetricians and Gynecologists recommend that women be in good overall health before and particularly throughout their pregnancies. Prenatal readiness may include exercise, proper diet, and stress management. Men make sperm up to 3 months before ejaculation. They should also choose a healthy approach toward pregnancy, avoiding tobacco, alcohol, or other drugs.

EXERCISE

Health professionals have learned much about the benefits of prenatal aerobic fitness. Any exercise regimen that increases cardiorespiratory fitness such as brisk walking, jogging, swimming, tennis, and cycling (stationary during pregnancy) can better prepare the women physically and mentally for the demands that pregnancy places on the human female. Healthy women who are physically active before they conceive can continue to exercise throughout their pregnancies. Women who are physically fit before and during their pregnancies may have an easier time adjusting to the bodily changes that accompany pregnancy (*PDR Family Guide to Women's Health and Prescription Drugs,* 1994). Maintaining coordination and endurance are vital for feeling well.

NUTRITION

A sound diet is also one of the basic elements for good health throughout the life span. A woman's dietary patterns and practices before pregnancy can have a great influence on the amount of weight she will gain during her pregnancy as well as a direct effect on the development of the embryo during the pregnancy. Unhealthy eating habits are difficult to break and often lead to women eating too much of the foods they should have in moderation or too little of the foods that would enhance their overall health. Changing eating habits at any stage of life is a daunting task, even more so during pregnancy. However, many women claim that pregnancy gives them the motivation to make positive changes.

The amount of weight gain for women during pregnancy depends on what they weigh before conception. If a woman is underweight, then a weight gain of 28 to 40 pounds is ideal. If the woman is overweight, a weight gain of 15 to 25 pounds is recommended. The weight gain occurs in the breasts, uterus, and the fatty tissue as the body stores protein and other nutrients in preparation for the baby. The fetus and the placenta account for a percentage of the weight gain, as well as an increase in blood volume and other fluids in the woman's body.

Most women have a diet that provides sufficient nutrients to support a developing fetus. However, pregnant women are often instructed to take a nutritional supplement (Mills & England, 2001). Many women take these "prenatal vitamins" a month or two before trying to conceive. The majority of these vitamins provide iron, folic acid, calcium, and zinc. Appropriate folic acid levels have been associated with the normal development of the fetal central nervous system and reducing the risk of neural tube defects (NTDs), which are birth defects of the baby's brain (anencephaly) or spine (spina bifida).

STRESS MANAGEMENT

Research has also shown that a proper diet and regular exercise can maintain or perhaps reduce stress levels for both men and women. By achieving healthy standards in both of these areas, many women will learn to live with their rapidly changing physique. Very often, the time set aside for exercise is a time to elevate not merely one's physical health but also mental health. This "me time" provides a well-needed respite from life's stressors. *Stressors* are events or actions experienced by an individual that cause a disruption in the daily flow of life. Daily stressors may be as benign as misplacing the car keys or as disruptive as a fender bender. Stressors cause the body to be knocked "off balance"; in other words, they disrupt the body's sense of homeostasis.

Regular exercise is just one way to manage stress. Others may include relaxation exercises, learned breathing techniques, meditation, and yoga. When women are proactive in their preconceptual care, as well as during their pregnancies, they feel that they are an integral part of their pregnancies, not merely a second to "mother nature" and their health care provider.

Fertility Awareness

The methods utilized to monitor a female's menstrual cycle in order to identify when intercourse is most likely to lead to conception are often called *natural birth control methods*. These involve the detailed observing, charting, and tracking of daily/monthly changes in the fertility cycle so that they may be interpreted to predict a woman's most fertile time. Some couples may only engage in coitus during certain times of the month to achieve pregnancy. Fertility awareness methods include cervical mucus monitoring, the calendar method, the basal body temperature method, and ovulation prediction kits (for more, see Chapter 9).

CERVICAL MUCUS MONITORING

Throughout a woman's menstrual cycle, the amount and texture of the cervical secretions change. These changes indicate when ovulation is approaching. Engaging in sexual intercourse when cervical mucus is present is a way of achieving pregnancy. This method is easy to monitor and costs nothing. However, it may be a less accurate way of predicting ovulation. The woman simply uses her own fingers and inserts them into her vagina removing a small amount of mucus and observes the look, touch, and feel of it. When documented, women, even those with irregular menses, will detect a mucus secretion pattern before and after ovulation. Throughout much of the menstrual cycle, the secretions are dense, white, and cloudy. This appearance is due to the level of estrogen, which impacts the follicle maturing in the ovum. As this follicle releases more estrogen, the composition of the mucus changes again. Just prior to ovulation the mucus can be clear, slippery, and stringy. The last day in which this clear, slippery, and stringy mucus is present is when conception is most likely to occur. This indicates that the woman is at her peak fertile time. However, a woman will not know it is the last day until it has passed!

The number of fertile days varies between 6 and 12 days. During menstrual bleeding, there is no or very little mucus secretion. Immediately after menstrual bleeding, the cervical secretions can be scant or completely absent.

The advantages to this method is that there is no cost or side effects, and it does not interfere with sexual spontaneity, unless you are not trying to get pregnant. The disadvantages are that this approach does not protect against sexually transmitted infections, requires vigilant monitoring of the woman's cycle, and offers no protection on the peak fertile days.

THE CALENDAR METHOD

Also called the *rhythm method,* this approach is the oldest and most widely used fertility awareness method. Fertile times are calculated based on three assumptions: (1) ovulation occurs 12 to 16 days before the onset of the menstrual flow, (2) sperm may remain viable for up to 5 days, and (3) the ovum survives for about 1 day. Generally, a set number of days, usually a number between 18 and 21, are subtracted from the shortest cycle length in the past 6 to 12 recorded cycles. This method is used to identify the woman's most fertile time. Recorded data on the past cycles provide an estimate of the peak fertile period.

To use this method a woman must record her menstrual cycle length for 6 months. A cycle begins on the first day of menstrual flow and continues until the day before the next menstrual flow begins. Days to avoid sexual intercourse and prevent conception will be determined by subtracting 18 from the number of days of the shortest recorded cycle. For example, if the woman's shortest cycle was 27 days, she would subtract 18, and day 9 would be the beginning of the fertile time. To estimate when this time was over, a woman would subtract 10 from the number of days of the longest recorded cycle. This number gives an indication of when unprotected sexual intercourse can resume.

This method is moderately effective; effectiveness rates will be enhanced if the woman is ardent about recording her cycle. However, miscalculations and changes in the menstrual cycle, such as stress, illness, and travel, can inhibit the effectiveness of this method.

There is no cost to the woman to use this method, and it poses no adverse side effects. In addition, it does not interfere with spontaneity of sexual intercourse unless a woman is trying to avoid pregnancy. The disadvantages are similar to those of other natural methods.

BASAL BODY TEMPERATURE (BBT)

The basal body temperature method also requires the daily monitoring of the woman's oral or vaginal temperature and recording the data. This method is accomplished by taking the woman's resting body temperature each morning and keeping track of this information for several months. The basal body temperature is lower in the first segment of the menstrual cycle and then rises after ovulation. The temperature remains elevated until the next menstrual flow begins. The woman's temperature is taken at the same time each morning before getting out of bed. The temperature will rise anywhere between 0.4 degree and 0.8 degree around the time of ovulation. If the woman notices 3 days of a continuous rise in temperature following 6 days of lower temperatures, the woman has ovulated and the infertile time has begun. Some woman may notice a temperature drop 12 to 24 hours before the rise caused by ovulation; others may detect none at all. The advantages and disadvantages are similar to the ones mentioned previously.

OVULATION PREDICTION KITS

These kits are available at drug stores and do not require a prescription from the doctor. This method is used to detect the increase in the luteinizing hormone that signals ovulation. The woman urinates on a test strip or into a collection cup. Generally, several tests are done over the course of a few days. Results may take several minutes or up to 1 hour. These kits cost several dollars but do contain several tests.

The advantages of this method are that women have less work to do, with no data recording and no temperature taking. The disadvantages are cost and the fact that some of the tests are less sensitive and may not be able to read a woman's urine sample.

INFERTILITY

The American Society for Reproductive Medicine considers infertility a condition in which conception is not achieved after a year of twice-weekly unprotected sexual intercourse. Approximately 6 million people in the United States are affected by infertility, representing about 10 percent of the reproductive age population. There has been a noticeable increase in the number of people affected by this condition due to the greater number of men and women in their 30s and 40s attempting first pregnancy. As mentioned earlier, it is a fact that fertility decreases with age.

Female infertility is experienced by 1 in 12 women aged 15 to 44 years of age (National Center for Health Statistics, 2000). Infertility may occur for a number of different reasons. Failure to ovulate is the most common problem for women, as a result of hormonal imbalances, poor overall health, genetics, or stress. Problems with the reproductive tract can also influence the fertility of women. Tubal disorders caused by *pelvic inflammatory disease* (PID) are often associated with infertility. Several types of bacteria and several viral strains can cause PID. Often associated with a sexual infection, PID can result from repeated infection and, on occasion, after a single exposure. *Endometriosis,* another common cause of infertility, occurs when the endometrial lining of the uterus overgrows, sometimes in other areas of the body, often on the Fallopian tubes and ovaries, causing scarring of the tissue and inhibiting passage of the mature ova. Many women may also be affected by cervical mucus that contains antibodies that attack sperm. Excessive exercise, obesity, and being underweight can also increase the risk of infertility.

Male Infertility

A man may be infertile due to low sperm production or poor sperm motility. Very often problems with sperm density can be linked to several correctable causes: frequent ejaculation, constricting underwear or clothing, regular usage of hot tubs or baths, or prolonged strenuous physical activity (Leary, 1990). Problems with the sperm's ability to move (sperm motility) through the woman's reproductive tract can be affected by prostate or hormonal difficulties.

Recent studies have indicated that both female and male infertility may be negatively influenced by exposure to environmental toxins such as pollution and or possibly radiation. In addition, exposure to alcohol, drugs, and tobacco can adversely influence fertility.

Coping with Infertility

Health care providers consider a couple infertile after 1 year of attempting pregnancy. However, in most cases, couples wait at least 2 years before seeking help for their condition. Very often couples who were once unable to conceive are successful with the help of fertility treatments that generally speed up the process. To date, several methods may be considered. The choice of method depends on the cause of infertility and on the couple's preference. Pursuing treatment for infertility is a serious endeavor, requiring a strong relationship and a shared level of commitment.

Infertility can have a disastrous impact on the most stable couple. The financial burden alone can place couples at odds. Even though most states have "mandate to access" legislation, visits to health care providers, attempts at artificial insemination, in vitro fertilization, and other costs associated with pregnancy attempts can be staggering. Each individual within the couple may deal with this problem differently. Some may seek social support; others may use avoidance. Both the coping strategies and the effects of infertility on each partner must be considered when choosing a method (Jordan & Revenson, 1999).

STIMULATION OF OVULATION

This method utilizes a particular class of drugs that overstimulates the release of ova. It increases the possibility of multiple births because more than one egg may be released at the time of ovulation. This method increases ovulation in about 80 percent of the women who use it, with approximately 45 percent of them becoming pregnant. It may also be used to stimulate release of ova for in vitro fertilization (IVF).

IN VITRO FERTILIZATION

In vitro is when eggs are removed from the woman and fertilized with the partner's sperm in the lab, and then they are planted in the uterus. When a woman's reproductive tract is blocked by scar tissue, this method may be employed.

ARTIFICIAL INSEMINATION

This treatment is used when a man's sperm count is low or when sperm motility through the cervix is challenged. The sperm is introduced directly into the cervix. Semen is placed in a plastic device, which remains in the woman's vagina for a few hours and can be removed by pulling a string attached to it. Most women will have to repeat this procedure four or five times before they are successful. Success rates vary. This method is the least invasive and least expensive.

GAMETE INTRAFALLOPIAN TRANSFER (GIFT)

A woman's eggs are removed from her ovary and the sperm are collected. The unfertilized egg and sperm are then implanted directly into the Fallopian tubes through a small incision in the abdomen. If successful, the egg and sperm will unite on their own.

ZYGOTE INTRAFALLOPIAN TRANSFER (ZIFT)

This procedure is similar to GIFT, but the transfer of the cells takes place only after fertilization has occurred in the laboratory. After fertilization occurs, the zygote is placed inside the woman's Fallopian tubes in a manner similar to the GIFT procedure.

DONOR OPTIONS

Egg donors or sperm donors can be obtained by the couple attempting a pregnancy. The GIFT or ZIFT procedures can be utilized using donor cells.

SURROGATE MOTHERHOOD

When a woman can ovulate but cannot maintain a pregnancy, surrogate motherhood is often used. A surrogate woman is implanted with an embryo from the host woman's ovum. Sometimes this approach is used for a woman who cannot ovulate. A donor egg is used, fertilized by the husband's semen and then carried to term by the surrogate mother. Once the baby is born, it is turned over to the biological parents. The surrogate is paid a fee for carrying the pregnancy—sometimes before, during, and after the birth.

ADOPTION

Adoption is the only method available for couples in which both partners are infertile. This method has several advantages and several disadvantages. If adoption is the first choice, then one advantage is that there are no invasive procedures to endure for either partner. However, if adoption is used as a last resort, the couple has usually already experienced invasive procedures that are unsuccessful.

One disadvantage is that adoptions in the United States are very expensive. Adoption of a healthy child can cost upward of $25,000, and the wait for such a child may be very long. Costs associated with adoption are related to agency overhead and operating expenses, advertising in local or college newspapers, and possibly travel to foreign countries. Adoptions that occur through private parties are more expensive, but the couple generally does not wait as long for a child. Adopting a child through a state agency is the least expensive but most restrictive. Many of the children in the state system have been in foster care or government agencies before being adopted. Thus, the average child is past infancy, the period in which most adoptive parents want their adoptive children to be. In the United States, some couples will adopt a child from outside the country rather than from within. In many cases, it is easier for couples to obtain an infant from a developing country than from the United States.

PREGNANCY DETECTION

Couples may react to discovering the pregnancy in many ways. Some women and their partners may begin to assess their psychological readiness, others their financial security. Knowing one is about to become a parent is a rite of passage, one that is certain to be remembered, positively or negatively, forever.

Missing a menstrual period is an occurrence that affects many women at one time or another. Missing a period is not necessarily a certain sign of pregnancy. The detection of a fetal heartbeat is the only certain method of confirming a pregnancy. However, women can sometimes recognize early signs or symptoms of pregnancy well before they have heard their babies' heartbeat. Many women may presume they are pregnant if they notice the absence of their menstrual flow accompanied by any or all of the following symptoms: nausea and/or vomiting at any time of the day (morning sickness), increase in breast size and perhaps breast tenderness, and darkening of the areola, the tissue that surrounds the nipple. Other signs and symptoms of pregnancy that are often thought to be more probable indicators of pregnancy might include more frequent urination (due to the growth of the uterus and pressure on the bladder), increase in the size of the abdomen, and a positive result from an over-the-counter pregnancy test.

Pregnancy tests use the woman's urine to detect a substance called *human chorionic gonadotropin* (HCG) that is produced by the membranes that surround the embryo. Home pregnancy kits can detect HCG between 10 and 12 days after conception. Some of the tests work by holding a test stick in the stream of urine, others by collecting a sample of the urine and dipping a diagnostic test strip into the sample. Results show up in similar ways. The presence of HCG in the urine is shown by a change in the testing device such as a stripe or a "+" sign in the result window. Over-the-counter tests provide a fairly inexpensive method of pregnancy detection. However, the accuracy of these tests may vary widely. Much of the diagnostic efficiency is lost due to human error in following the directions (Wheeler, 1999). A skilled professional through a pelvic examination can detect more positive indicators of pregnancy. About 30 days after conception, a softening of tissue, called the *Hegar's sign,* can be found by touch between the uterus and cervix during this exam.

PRENATAL CARE

The health of the fetus and expectant mother can be protected and possibly enhanced by good prenatal care. *Prenatal care* is the health care available to almost any pregnant woman who wants it, whether or not she can financially afford it, although women with insurance through Medicaid may have difficulty finding a health care provider who accepts this insurance. Most often, pregnancies go smoothly with the end result being a healthy baby and mother.

Today's technological advances are used to detect, and sometimes correct, the most miniscule problems with the developing fetus. Many of the available diagnostic tests can reveal problems before they can harm the mother or fetus. It is the responsibility of the expectant mother and her partner to maintain their own wellness, and the responsibility of both parents to be informed and proactive in the health status of the fetus. Obstetricians do their best in ascertaining all pertinent health and genetic information that may affect the development and delivery of the baby. Physicians will also utilize the latest technology to ensure the best possible pregnancy for all women. Several prenatal tests are performed on the pregnant woman with her consent.

Risks to Pregnancy

Problems with pregnancy can arise at any time and may be influenced by maternal risks. Women who engage in unhealthy lifestyle behaviors are at greater risk for delivering a child with irreversible birth defects, abnormalities, or babies that will be stillborn or die within the first few weeks of life.

Anything that can harm an embryo or developing fetus is called a *teratogen*. Prescriptive, over-the-counter, and recreational drugs can harm and/or cause a miscarriage of the fetus. Much of the irreversible damage occurs within the first 2 months of pregnancy. It is during this time that the major organs and body systems are being formed. Compromising these important developmental stages can alter the functioning of the brain, heart, and lungs and may also affect the baby's appearance. For example, alcohol consumption during pregnancy may cause fetal alcohol syndrome (FAS). Children born with FAS often experience developmental delays, hyperactivity, delayed motor development, visual defects, and behavioral difficulties (Mills & England, 2001). FAS also influences the physical appearance of the child. These children are often smaller in stature, with slowed growth patterns, and have wide-set eyes.

Cocaine use and abuse can damage the embryo in many devastating ways. Cocaine in the bloodstream causes fluctuations in blood flow for both the mother and fetus. These fluctuations can cause a stroke in the mother and child. Children of cocaine-addicted mothers may also be born with an addiction. These children often face a life of irreversible learning disabilities and behavioral problems.

The effects of heroin can also be life-threatening. The drug used by the mother crosses the placenta and enters the fetal circulatory system. This can cause problems with the development of internal organs and the infant's regulatory systems. Heroin-addicted babies can also die from heroin withdrawal.

Tobacco users are at risk of premature delivery, low-birth-weight babies, and spontaneous abortions. Smokers are often drinkers. Thus the two substances in tandem cause a mounting risk for unsuccessful fertility and fetal adversity.

Prenatal Testing

Birth defects, abnormalities in physical or mental form or function of the baby at birth, can be mild to life-threatening. Major birth defects affect a small portion of live births, approximately 4 percent. These defects can be caused by genetic factors, teratogenic or lifestyle influences, environmental exposures, or maternal illness. Even the smallest external influences can bring disastrous results to the fetus.

Birth defects can be detected early in the pregnancy in several ways. *Ultrasound imaging* is often one of the first prenatal testing procedures for many women. Ultrasound examination uses high-frequency sound waves to locate body tissue that is then used to form a picture of the fetus in the uterus. This technique not only can detect the physical manifestations of birth defects but is also used to monitor the growth of the fetus, identify twins, and sometimes aid in the diagnosis of other problems. This method is not invasive and offers little risk to the fetus.

Chorionic villus sampling (CVS) is a test of the *villi,* or little finger-like projections that stabilize the embryo to the uterine lining. These villi contain the embryo's genetic material and can disclose genetic abnormalities if they are present. This test can be performed in the 8th week of pregnancy. Like amniocentesis, CVS does place the fetus at higher risk for miscarriage.

Amniocentesis is a test performed around the 16th week of pregnancy. It involves the drawing of a sample of amniotic fluid (fluid that surrounds the fetus in the uterus and contains some of its cells). This fluid is analyzed for the presence of genetic disorders and sometimes to identify the sex of the baby. Amniocentesis does incur an increased risk for fetal damage, injury, or miscarriage. *Miscarriage* is the spontaneous expulsion of the fetus before it is able to survive outside the uterus.

Alpha-fetaprotein, a protein molecule produced by the fetus, can be detected in the mother's bloodstream at the 16th week of pregnancy. Elevated presence of this protein can indicate neural tube disorders that cause a spinal deformity such as spina bifida. This test cannot offer definitive proof of this disorder but does warrant further testing to rule out the possibility of its presence (Crandall & Chua, 1997).

Routine blood and urine tests are also performed throughout the pregnancy to monitor the overall health of the mother and developing fetus.

Blood tests look for anemia and the presence of hepatitis and sexual infections such as HIV. Urine samples are tested for diabetes and possible kidney problems. Weight gain and weight loss are also monitored each month at the prenatal "well baby" visits. Extreme weight loss or gain can have harmful effects on fetal development.

STAGES OF PREGNANCY

Pregnancy is the condition of a woman after conception until the birth of the baby. A normal, full-term pregnancy lasts between 37 and 42 weeks. Pregnancy is divided into three trimesters, and, within each segment of time, significant changes in the woman can occur. The beginning and end of each trimester is also marked by changes in the developing fetus. The first trimester is the first 3 months of pregnancy directly after fertilization. The second trimester is the 4th, 5th, and 6th months of pregnancy. The third trimester is the last 3 months of pregnancy and ends in delivery. Many women feel that their pregnancies last forever, but the majority of pregnancies end in the 38th week after fertilization, or 40 weeks after the last menstrual period. Few babies are actually born on their due date, with most deliveries occurring between 10 days before or after their due dates.

The First Trimester

Directly after conception has occurred, a developing mass of cells start to proliferate in a sequence that is genetically scripted. The early cells are grouped together according to how they will function in the future. Basically the cells are either outside cells or inside cells. The outside cells become the protective and nourishing membranes that help bring fetal development and ultimately, delivery of a baby, to fruition. The inside cells eventually form into the baby. These cells form the placenta during the embryonic stage of development (first 8 weeks after fertilization). The placenta is found in the lining of the uterus and is composed of a union of embryonic tissue and the uterine mucous membrane. This membrane provides for the nourishment of the fetus and the elimination of waste materials that it produces. The placenta allows only select material to pass through: oxygen is passed from the mother to the embryo, and carbon dioxide and other waste products from the fetus are passed to the mother's lungs and kidneys.

The fetus is ensconced in a protective environment within the uterus called the *amniotic sac*. This sac contains fluid that protects the sac from temperature fluctuations and cushions the embryo from the jolting and bouncing around that the mother may experience. Embryos are the same anatomically until 6 to 8 weeks of gestation when sex differentiation occurs. By the end of the 8th week, the embryo not only can be identified as male or female, but it has developed primitive circulatory, digestive, and central nervous systems. Facial features and limbs are formed as well as major blood vessels. The umbilical cord, which carries two arteries and a vein to the placenta, is now present. At about this time, the testicular tissue that differentiates male and female embryos is present. Ovarian tissue for females occurs at about the 3rd month of development. The 3rd month also offers more distinctively human features. The nails and hair follicles are present, and the appendages are more proportionate to overall body size. During this time of rapid growth and development, the pregnant woman may experience many of the signs and symptoms discussed earlier.

The Second Trimester

It is during this time that the greatest amount of fetal development occurs; all systems are formed and functioning. The mother may now detect fetal movement called *quickening* that is likely to feel like a little tickle or flutter. The fetal heartbeat is distinguishable with a stethoscope or fetal heart monitor. The fetus can open and close its eyes and can be sensitive to light and sounds. Although the fetus looks like a small human, it is still unable to survive outside the uterus. The mother at this time may be experiencing fewer bouts of nausea and more gastrointestinal disturbances, indigestion, or constipation. The expectant mother will also have an abdomen that has increased in size considerably, resembling something like a cantaloupe or a volleyball.

The Third Trimester

By the 7th month, the fetus experiences a rapid increase in brain development. Nerve cells and pathways that connect nerve cells to the sense organs also grow markedly. Pathways from motor areas of the brain have been developed and are present between the fetal muscles. At this point the fetus resembles a bony, wrinkled human. During the last trimester fat cells will be deposited beneath the skin, which will increase the size and weight of the fetus and increase its chances of survival at birth. By the end of the 7th month, a fetus has some chance of survival if born prematurely. Aggressive technology has been employed to save many fetuses delivered preterm, or before 38 weeks of gestation. At about the 8th month, the fetus usually turns so that its head is pointed down toward the cervix and vagina.

The expectant mother will often feel many symptoms as a result of her increasing weight and change in the center of gravity. Women may experience difficulty getting comfortable in any position, pressure when walking, and frequent urination and backaches. As the body prepares for delivery, some women may experience *Braxton-Hicks contractions,* also called *false labor pains.* Many women believe that these are true labor pains when indeed they are not. As the final weeks pass, the combination of strong fetal movements, Braxton-Hicks contractions, frequent urination, and increasing discomfort are true indicators that delivery time is near.

Childbirth

Most babies will be born between 37 and 42 weeks of a normal pregnancy. Some women may feel excited and some may feel anxious about the labor and delivery. The progression of the labor experience is predictable, yet each labor experience is unique.

STAGES OF LABOR

Although each woman has a different childbirth experience, labor and delivery can be divided into three distinct stages. These stages begin with the first true contraction and end with the delivery of the baby and the passing of the placenta and membranes through the vagina. Most women who are experiencing their first vaginal delivery go through these stages between 12 and 24 hours. Subsequent births are often shorter in duration.

First Stage of Labor.   Most health care providers will advise the expectant couple to report to the hospital when contractions are 5 minutes apart. After an internal examination, the professional will confirm that the contractions are either true labor pains or Braxton-Hicks contractions. Real labor, in the first stage, is marked by strong contractions of the uterine muscles at regular intervals. The contractions cause the cervix of the uterus to dilate (open) and efface (thin out). The progression of the dilation and effacement distinguishes the differences between early, active, and transition phases of the first stage of labor.

During the early phase, the cervix will dilate up to 4 centimeters; dilation between 4 and 8 centimeters demarks the active phase, and dilation of 8 to 10 centimeters occurs in the transition phase. There is wide variation in the length of labor from woman to woman and from pregnancy to pregnancy. Early labor is characterized by contractions of short duration, 10 to 20 seconds, and they may be as far apart as 10 to 20 minutes. As active labor progresses, the contractions become more uncomfortable, last longer, and may come as frequently as 3 minutes apart. During transition, the cervix dilates fully to allow the passage of the baby through the uterus and into the birth canal. This stage is the most demanding. The contractions come as quickly as 2 minutes and last for 60 to 90 seconds.

Few women who have had children would say that childbirth is without pain. Much of the pain derives from the contractions of the uterus and the pushing of the baby through the tight birth canal. Remedies for the pain associated with labor and delivery have been used for thousands of years. Contemporary medical professionals often use epidural anesthesia, which is administered in the hospital, via the spinal cord. This medication numbs the woman from the waist down. It allows her to feel the sensations of the contractions but not the pain associated with them. Some hospitals and birthing centers utilize hydrotherapy to alleviate pain; women will be placed in a warm whirlpool bath or hot shower with pulsating shower heads that massage the back and neck.

Second Stage of Labor. This stage begins when the cervix is completely dilated and the baby is pushed through the vagina. At this time, the baby's head is fully lodged in the cervix. Contractions tend to slow down to every 4 to 5 minutes. Women will now be encouraged to push with each contraction. Each contraction pushes the baby further down the birth canal until it appears from behind the pubic bone and into the perineal area. The perineal area may be stretched to the point at which it may tear. At this time the health care professional may perform an *episiotomy,* although they are no longer routine. This procedure entails a small incision between the vagina and rectum, called the *perineum.* This allows the baby to pass through the vagina more easily and prevents tearing of this tissue.

Once the baby's head is delivered, blood, mucus, and secretions are suctioned from the baby's nose, mouth, and throat. All of the vital signs are monitored and recorded. Silver nitrate is dispensed in the infants' eyes as a precaution against gonorrhea, and the umbilical cord is clipped and cut.

Third Stage of Labor. This stage is often referred to as the *afterbirth.* The placenta and fetal membranes are now expelled from the uterine wall. They are examined by the physician to ensure that no tearing has occurred.

Cesarean delivery, or C-section, is the removal of the fetus through an incision in the woman's abdomen and uterus. This procedure is done when vaginal delivery of the baby may compromise the well-being of the baby and or the mother. Two of the most common causes of Cesarean delivery are (1) the baby is not in a headfirst position and cannot be turned around, and (2) the pelvis is too small to allow the baby to enter the birth canal. This procedure can save the woman's life and the baby's life and reduces the risk of complications during delivery. It does have risks of its own, however: infection, blood clots, and excessive bleeding. Recuperation from this method of delivery takes longer than vaginal delivery. Vaginal childbirth is an experience that many women look forward to experiencing. Thus, most women would prefer to deliver their child vaginally if it is medically safe to do so.

CHILDBIRTH ALTERNATIVES

Although much of the process of childbirth may vary from culture to culture, this common experience for women has gone more or less unchanged for centuries. Most women in the United States proceed with the usual custom of hospital delivery. However, many alternative methods for labor and delivery are also possible. And women now have the option as to how and where their child will be delivered.

A hospital delivery provides the customary treatment, enhanced by the fact that the institution is well staffed and equipped in the case of an emergency. Birthing centers offer a more relaxed family-friendly environment, one that allows for support people to be present at every stage of labor and delivery. Some women may opt for home birth assisted by midwives and private nurses. Alternative birthing options offer the woman more autonomy and control over this life event than does the customary hospital delivery. More recently, hospitals have tried to make adjustments to the "traditional" environment to improve the labor and delivery experience.

BIRTHING OPTIONS

The expectation of pain, duration of labor, anxiety, and level of childbirth education are all factors that can work in concert or independently to influence the amount of pain experienced during this time. Many women will seek out birthing education techniques in hopes that increased knowledge will provide the tools that may reduce anxiety and possibly the likelihood of using pain medications during delivery.

The most well-known method is the *Lamaze method,* based on learning to relax the abdominal and perineal muscles, and controlling breathing to help with pain management. An important component of the Lamaze method is the use of a birthing "coach," who is generally the woman's partner. Basically it is the coach's job to offer support, encouragement, and advocacy.

The *Bradley method* emphasizes relaxation exercises coupled with a sound education. Participants and their coaches are taught 12 different relaxation exercises, any of which can be performed during labor, with the support and guidance of the coach. This method encourages women to change position often and not to lie on their backs.

The *LeBoyer method* is based on the premise that newborns should be delivered in a way that minimizes stress. The originator of the method, Frederick LeBoyer, refers to his method as "birth without violence." He believes that traditional hospital delivery is an unpleasant way to leave the womb and enter the world. After delivery, the baby is placed on the mother's abdomen and caressed, then placed into a warm bath. The bright lights are lowered, and the noise level is contained considerably.

SUMMARY

Although it may seem like pregnancy, labor, and delivery are issues that are in the distant future of young people, it is important to teach these topics to students. Teen pregnancy is occurring more frequently in today's society. Almost every school district has had to address at least one situation of teen pregnancy. In some school districts, teen pregnancy has become uneventful because so many young women become pregnant and give birth during their school-age years. If educators want to assist young people with healthy pregnancies and want to prevent occurrences of birth defects, it is essential that young people learn accurate information about pregnancy, labor, and delivery.

Misinformation about pregnancy can have dire consequences. Many unplanned pregnancies have occurred because young people did not understand the true nature of conception. Teaching accurate information about pregnancy in the context of decision making and goal setting can help prevent unintended pregnancy by dispelling myths about pregnancy and empowering students to make appropriate choices for themselves.

Even if students do not plan on becoming pregnant themselves for many years, they are still exposed to others who either recently had a baby or are trying to become pregnant. Teaching about pregnancy, labor, and delivery to young people will serve to provide a foundation of knowledge for what your students are already exposed to in a real-life context. The educator can capitalize on "teachable moments" when students ask questions about something they have heard, or overheard, related to pregnancy, labor, and delivery.

All adults, no matter what their personal and political interests, have a vested interest in assisting young people in delaying pregnancy until the appropriate time for themselves and their families.

WEBSITES

Reproductive Health:
    www.cdcgov/ nccdphp/drh /art
International Council on Infertility
    Information: www.inclid.org
American Infertility Association:
    www.americaninfertility.org
Courageous Choice:
    www.courageouschoice.com
Pregnancy Information:
    www.pregnancy-info.net
National Campaign to Prevent Teen Pregnancy: www.teenpregnancy.org
Pregnancy Today: www.pregnancytoday.com

MedlinePlus—Pregnancy and Reproduction
    Topics: www.nlm.nih.gov/medlineplus/
    pregnancyandreproduction.html
CDC Health Topic Pregnancy:
    www.cdc.gov/health /pregnancy.htm
Childbirth: www.childbirth.org
Planned Parenthood:
    www.plannedparenthood.org
Pregnancy and Childbirth Information:
    www.childbirth.org
Natural Childbirth:
    www.naturalchildbirth.org
LaMaze International:
    www.lamaze-childbirth.com

REFERENCES

Annie E. Casey Foundation. (1998). *When teens have sex: Issues and trends*. Baltimore, MD: Author.

Crandall, B. F., & Chua, C. (1997). Risks for fetal abnormalities after very moderately elevated AF-AFPs. *Prenatal Diagnosis, 17*, 837–841.

Daniels, P., & Weingarten, K. (1982). *Sooner or later: The timing of parenthood in adult lives*. New York: Norton.

Hatcher, R. A., et al. *Contraceptive technology* (16th rev. ed.). New York: Irvington.

Jordan, C., & Revenson, T. A. (1999). Gender differences in coping with infertility: A meta-analysis. *Journal of Behavior Medicine, 22*, 341–358.

Leary, W. (1990, September 13). New focus on sperm brings fertility success. *New York Times*, p. B11.

Marsiglio, W. (1987). Adolescent fathers in the United States: Their initial living arrangements, marital experience, and education outcomes. *Family Planning Perspectives, 19*(6), 240–251.

Mills, J. L., & England, L. (2001). Food fortification to prevent neural tube defects. *Journal of the American Medical Association, 285*, 3002.

National Center for Health Statistics. (2000). *Fertility/infertility.* Vital Health Statistics, Series 23, No. 19. Washington, DC: Author.

The PDR family guide to women's health and prescription drugs. (1994). Montvale, NJ: Medical Economics.

Westheimer, R., & Lopater, S. (2004). *Human sexuality: A psychosocial perspective* (2nd ed.). Baltimore, MD: Lippincott, Williams & Wilkins.

Wheeler, M. (1999). Home and laboratory pregnancy-testing kits. *Professional Nurse, 14,* 571–576.

LEARNING EXPERIENCES

Several learning experiences are offered here that teachers can use when teaching about pregnancy, labor, and delivery. The prospective teacher should modify the activities so that they are applicable to the district regulations and student population. Particular attention should be given to age-appropriate information whenever any information related to sexuality is taught in the classroom.

The learning experiences presented here will provide opportunities for students to develop the following skills and knowledge:

- Understand how an ova and sperm meet to create a pregnancy.
- Identify the factors to be considered before becoming pregnant.
- Describe the stages of pregnancy.
- Describe the process of labor and childbirth.
- Identify the meaning of their own birth to their family.
- Identify similarities and differences in pregnancy and childbirth among different species.
- Explain the impact of an unintended pregnancy on an individual's future goals and plans.
- Apply a decision-making process to sexual behavior to prevent or produce a pregnancy.
- Recognize the health maintenance activities associated with a healthy outcome of childbirth.
- Discuss options available in the selection of a practitioner and a place to give birth.
- Identify different components of a birth plan.

LEARNING EXPERIENCE 1

TITLE: Tell Me about the Day I Was Born

GRADE LEVELS: K–3

TIME REQUIREMENTS: One class period to share results of the interviews

LEARNING CONTEXT
Students will discuss their own birth with a parent/guardian. They will also write a reflection or draw a picture depicting what they learned in their interview.

NATIONAL LEARNING STANDARDS
    1: Students will comprehend concepts related to health promotion and disease prevention.
    2: Students will demonstrate the ability to access valid health information and health-promoting products and services.
    5: Students will demonstrate the ability to use interpersonal communication skills to enhance health.

PROCEDURE
1. Prior to the lesson, hand out the "Tell Me about the Day I Was Born" worksheet (included later). Allow students 3 to 5 days to complete this assignment.
2. Explain to students that to complete this activity, they must interview a parent/guardian in order to learn about their birth.
3. Older students with language arts skills should complete a written reflection of the interview. Younger students should draw a picture depicting what they learned about their birth. (Note: Participants have two options. One section includes questions for birth parents, and the second section includes questions for a guardian, adoptive parent, and so forth).
4. On the day the homework assignment is due, allow students to share some of the things they learned about the day they were born.
5. Conclude the lesson with the following questions:
   - How easy/difficult was this activity?
   - How did you feel about doing this activity?
   - What did you learn?

RESOURCE
"Tell Me about the Day I Was Born" worksheet

ASSESSMENT PLAN
Students will be assessed through the completion of their worksheet.

REFLECTION
Parent–child communication is an important part of preventing risk behavior among youth. This activity affords parents the opportunity to have a discussion with their child about the day they were born, but it also sets the stage for future communication about other health issues. Students enjoy the chance to share what they learned with classmates.

"Tell Me About The Day I Was Born"

Name: _____

Directions

Students: Interview a parent or guardian about the day you were born. Use the questions below to help you with your interview, but please be creative and think of questions on your own as well. If you were adopted, find out everything your adoptive parents know about your birth, and then answer the questions based on the day you were adopted. Use the space below to either write a reflection or draw a picture of what you learned.

Parents/Guardians: This assignment is part of a lesson on pregnancy and childbirth. Please use it as an opportunity to discuss issues that are not talked about in normal everyday conversation. If your child does not have the reading skills necessary to read the questions, please read the interview questions to your child and help with their reflection or picture.

1. What was my place of birth—city and hospital?

2. What time was I born? Was there any strange weather or historical events at this time?

3. Where were you when labor began? How long was the labor?

4. Who was present at my birth—family, medical, or others?

5. What was my weight and height at birth?

6. Were there any unusual happenings?

7. How was my name selected?

8. What sources of information about me do we have (such as baby books, family records, albums, photos, and traditional stories)?

9. Ask any other questions you would like to know about your birth and early childhood, such as diseases, first steps, and first words.

10. Use the space below to write a reflection or draw a picture about what you learned from your interview:

LEARNING EXPERIENCE 2

TITLE: Animal Life Cycles

GRADE LEVELS: 4–6

TIME REQUIREMENTS: 2–4 weeks

LEARNING CONTEXT

After this activity, students will

- Compare and contrast the life cycles of different species.
- Recognize a similarity in the basic needs of all living organisms and how they affect their own environment.

NATIONAL LEARNING STANDARD

1:   Students will comprehend concepts related to health promotion and disease prevention.

PROCEDURE

Almost every elementary school child has had the opportunity to directly observe the stages in the life of a plant or an animal. The study of the life cycles of different species helps put into perspective many aspects of human development, a topic that is often the subject of youthful curiosity. The connections are made between various real-life experiences, and, more often than not, the result is enthusiastic understanding.

Many hands-on experiences can assist students in learning about the life cycle. Here are some suggestions:

- Set up an aquarium for raising brine shrimp (sea monkeys). Brine shrimp are related to crabs and lobsters in a group commonly known as crustaceans.
- For each student or study group, place two or three mealworms in a capped jar. Provide the mealworms with bran and a slice of raw potato or apple. The mealworm is the larva stage of a beetle. Before reaching this final step in the metamorphosis, the mealworm goes through a pupa stage that resembles neither the "worm" or "beetle" developmental periods.
- Fertilized frog eggs are usually easy to find or purchase. Place them in an aquarium and observe each day. Tadpoles hatch from frog eggs in a week to 10 days, and the process from tadpole to frog is fascinating to observe.
- Incubate fertilized chicken eggs. The period of incubation for chicks is 21 days. Hold the eggs to your ears periodically. Days before hatching, you will be able to hear the chicks peeping inside. Some teachers will open an egg every day or so, to show the developing embryo in various stages of growth. The age of the students and the guidelines set by local animal rights organizations must be a consideration. The baby chicks should also be given a proper home shortly after birth.

Explain to the class that all living things are born, grow, and change; consume water and food, and die. This process is commonly known as the *life cycle*. Tell them that they are going to participate in a learning experience where they will have the opportunity to observe the life cycle of a [whatever species is selected]. Ask students to maintain a journal in which they will record the life cycle charts, descriptions of observations, and measurements where appropriate.

Following are some additional activities that can be assigned to enhance the life cycle experience:

- Have the students pretend that they are one of the creatures observed or researched. Tell students to write their life story, making certain they mention their life cycle somewhere in their tale.
- Ask the students, "If you had to be an organism that was studied, which one would you choose to be?" Instruct students to support their choice with scientific facts they learned, combined with personal reasons.
- Tell students to write a letter to an organization devoted to the care of animals or the preservation of animals in danger of extinction. Instruct them to ask for information about the animal, its life cycle, or suggestions on how they can help. Some possible places to start include the U.S. Fish and Wildlife Service, World Wildlife Fund, and National Audubon Society.
- Ask students, "In your opinion, what is the most successful organism in terms of the life cycle it goes through?" Tell them to summarize their choice in a reflective paragraph.

Once the students have fully observed, researched, and documented the life cycle of the animal the teacher has selected, lead a discussion using the following discussion questions:

- What did you learn from observing the life cycle of [whatever animal the teacher selected]?
- What do you know about the life cycle of human beings?
- How is the life cycle of human beings similar to that of [whatever animal the teacher selected]? How is it different?

INSTRUCTIONAL/ENVIRONMENTAL MODIFICATION

The teacher should place the animal(s) being studied in a place in the classroom that is easily accessible. Students should be able to observe the animal(s) readily.

RESOURCES

Most living specimens may be either purchased locally at pet shops, school biological supply companies, or captured outdoors.

ASSESSMENT PLAN

Students will be assessed through their journal entries and through their participation in class discussion. If additional learning activities are assigned, students will be assessed through the completion of those activities as well.

REFLECTION

Oftentimes parents and administrators believe that children in younger elementary grades are too young to learn about health issues such as pregnancy and childbirth. What they forget, however, is that students observe this behavior in household animals, creatures that live in the outdoors, and even in their family members. They see moms nursing babies. They may see animals on farms or ranches mate, give birth, and nurse as well. Younger children have an innate curiosity that allows for many teachable moments to take place. This learning activity approaches the topic of pregnancy and childbirth in an age-appropriate manner and provides the foundation for more complex learning in older grades.

LEARNING EXPERIENCE 3

TITLE: What Do You Want to Do When You Grow Up?

GRADE LEVELS: 7–9

TIME REQUIREMENTS: One session

LEARNING CONTEXT
Completing this activity, students will
- Draw images representing their goals and dreams for the future.
- Identify how their goals for the future will change if they get pregnant or get someone else pregnant.
- Discuss the impact of the activity on their health-related attitudes and behaviors.

NATIONAL LEARNING STANDARD
6: Students will demonstrate the ability to use goal-setting and decision-making skills to enhance health.

PROCEDURE
1. Hand out a worksheet with the shape of a tie outlined on it.
2. Explain that students are to draw pictures on their tie that represent what their goals and dreams are for the future.
3. If possible, show an example of his or her own tie, so students see what is expected of them.
4. Pass out markers and scissors, and allow students approximately 10 minutes to work on their tie. When students are done drawing, they should cut out their tie. Meanwhile, hand out tape to each student.
5. When the time is up, ask students to tape their tie to their chest and get up and make a circle in the middle of the room.
6. Students should then share what they drew on their tie and what it represents.
7. When all students have completed the sharing activity, apologize to the class and say, "I'm very sorry, but you and your partner were engaging in sexual intercourse, and either you or your partner got pregnant."
8. Instruct the class to turn their tie over and draw how their future has changed now that they or their partner is pregnant.
9. Use the following process questions to lead a class discussion:
   - How did it feel to think about your goals and dreams? How often do you do that? When was the last time you thought about what you wanted out of life?
   - How did it feel when I told you that you or your partner was pregnant?
   - What was the point of this activity?
   - How can you make changes in your life so your tie does not have to change?
10. Conclude with the following: "Oftentimes we don't think about the impact of our behaviors on our goals and dreams for the future until it is too late. Sometimes we make choices that are irreversible—we wish we could turn back the clock, but we can't. This lesson will be meaningful if you start to force yourself to think toward the future when you make decisions. Ask yourself, 'What will the consequence of this decision be? Will it help or hurt my chances for my goals?'"

INSTRUCTIONAL/ENVIRONMENTAL MODIFICATION
The teacher might want to arrange the desks in a circle on the perimeter of the room. This will allow students to observe each other's ties and face each other when they are sharing their goals.

RESOURCES
Markers, scissors, tape, and copies of the tie worksheet—one per student

ASSESSMENT PLAN
Students will be assessed through the completion of their tie and through participation in class discussion.

REFLECTION
One of the psychosocial characteristics of adolescence is present orientation. Young people do not often consider the impact of decisions on goals they have for the future—in fact, they do not often consider goals for the future at all. This activity allows students the opportunity to reflect on their goals for the future and how those goals would be affected if they got pregnant or got their partner pregnant.

REFERENCE
Health Quickies: Over 100 Exciting Interactive Activities to Use with Adolescents and Adults, by S. Whalen, D. Splendorio, and S. Chiariello (forthcoming).

LEARNING EXPERIENCE 4

TITLE: Want Ad for a Parent versus a Babysitter

GRADE LEVELS: 7–9

TIME REQUIREMENTS: One session

LEARNING CONTEXT
In this activity, students will

- Brainstorm about the responsibilities of a babysitter and a parent.
- Create want ads for babysitters and parents.
- Discuss the difficulty of being a parent.

NATIONAL LEARNING STANDARDS

1: Students will comprehend concepts related to health promotion and disease prevention.
6: Students will demonstrate the ability to use goal-setting and decision-making skills to enhance health.
7: Students will demonstrate the ability to advocate for personal, family, and community health.

PROCEDURE

1. Introduce the activity by opening the newspaper to the want ad section. Read a few want ads to the class and ask them to guess what job is being advertised. (Or prepare 6 to 10 packets of want ads, one for each small group, before class.)
2. Ask students whether they have ever babysat or looked after a younger sibling or other child. Ask those who have to share their experiences. The students will probably want to tell their own horror stories, but make sure they also include some of the basics of child care. Questions the educator might ask include:
   - What time of day do you usually babysit?
   - How many children do you look after? How old are they?
   - Are the children already fed? If not, what do you make them to eat?
   - How long do you babysit? Do you have to put the children to bed? Bathe them?
   - What kind of things do you do with them for fun?
   - What are the responsibilities of a babysitter?
3. Now ask the class how a parent differs from a babysitter.
4. Ask students to imagine what it would be like to take care of a newborn baby for one day. Go through a typical day of raising an infant. Ask students to name daily activities of raising a child. Write the responses on the chalkboard. Start from the time a child wakes up until the child goes to sleep at night. Some suggestions for daily tasks might include these:
   - Morning—get up when baby wakes up (maybe 5:00 A.M.), change diaper, change clothes, feed, and clean spit-up
   - Midmorning—another feeding, play; the baby may cry for long periods of time for unknown reasons; the parent needs to care for the child during this time

- Afternoon—nap, change diaper, and do laundry
- Midafternoon—feed baby, change diaper, play, and so forth, throughout the day
- Night—give the baby a bath, feed, and put to bed—but babies often do not sleep through the entire night when they are very young; they can often wake up crying several times throughout the night

5. Make sure students understand that some of the daily activities are not just playing and dressing a newborn; babies need special attention that are not always fun. For example, breast-feeding is a wonderful way to be close to your child, but it's not always easy or convenient to do so in public or when trying to do other things. Also, when babies are only a couple of days old, the remainder of their umbilical cord is still attached to their bodies and needs delicate, frequent care until it falls off.

6. Also make sure students understand that there may be different responsibilities of raising a baby that occur throughout the week, such as washing or doing dirty laundry and changing the sheets in the crib. Don't forget to include immunization shots or regular checkups the baby will need into this discussion.

7. Some students may think that parenting stops, or at least becomes easier, as the child gets older. However, each stage of the child's life includes a different set of responsibilities that typically continue until the child is 18 years of age.

8. Break the class up into small groups.

9. Tell half the groups that they must now write a want ad for a babysitter. Tell the other half of the class that they must write a want ad for a parent. Instruct the class that they will have 10 minutes to complete this assignment.

10. When the small groups have completed their assignments, ask them to share their want ads.

11. Ask the class to compare and contrast the want ads for the babysitters and the want ads for the parents. Some questions might include:
    - How are the ads alike, and how are they different?
    - Which is harder, to be a parent or a babysitter? Why?
    - On a scale from 1 to 10 (with 1 being "nothing" and 10 being "a lot"), how much do you know about child care?
    - Do you feel ready to take care of a child, possibly by yourself?
    - Is there time in your day to take care of a child?
    - What would you have to give up in order to take care of a child?

12. Point out that taking care of a baby is hard for anyone, regardless of their age, but teen parents may have a more difficult time with finances, parenting skills, and future job and educational plans. Hopefully this activity increased students' understanding and awareness of the difficulties in raising a child. Babysitting is temporary, but parents are legally responsible for their child until their child is 18 years of age.

13. Point out that if students are not ready to become parents, then they are not ready to put themselves at risk for pregnancy; therefore, they should not be engaging in sexual intercourse until they are ready for the possibility of becoming a parent.

INSTRUCTIONAL/ENVIRONMENTAL MODIFICATION

The teacher may want to set the desks up in small groups ahead of time to save time. Pair slower learners with faster learners in the small groups.

RESOURCES

Newspaper want ads for class discussion or 6 to 10 preprepared packets of want ad examples—one for each small group

ASSESSMENT PLAN

Students will be assessed through their creation of the want ads and their class discussion.

REFLECTION

Young people do not often think about the consequences of their actions. They make poor choices and then regret their actions after it is too late. This lesson increases student awareness of the difficulty of parenthood. The hope is that students will recognize that parenthood is a very hard job that they are unable to cope with at their age. Thus, perhaps students will be less likely to engage in sexual intercourse and put themselves at risk for parenthood. The teacher should make sure that the positive aspects of parenting are discussed as well.

REFERENCE

Adapted from Campaign for Our Children (www.cfoc.org).

LEARNING EXPERIENCE 5

TITLE: You Can't Beat the Odds

GRADE LEVELS: 10–12

TIME REQUIREMENTS: One session

LEARNING CONTEXT
In this activity, students will
- Define the following terms: *odds* and *probability*.
- Participate in an activity that illustrates the odds of teen pregnancy.
- Discuss ways to prevent teen pregnancy.

NATIONAL LEARNING STANDARD
1: Students will comprehend concepts related to health promotion and disease prevention.

PROCEDURE
1. Before students arrive, set an empty trashcan on its side on the floor about 8 to 10 feet away from the door. A golf club and ball will also be needed for this activity.
2. Greet students at the door before they take their seats. One at a time, have students try to putt the golf ball into the trashcan as they enter the room. On a sheet of paper record the number of people who get the ball in the trashcan. Students should take their seats after they take their putt.
3. When students take their seats, tally the total number of putts the class made. Write that number on the chalkboard. Next to that number write the total number of students in the class. Now express it in terms of odds. For example: Fifteen students made the putt, and there are 30 students in the class.
4. Write 15 to 30. This is a ratio. If you can reduce the number by the lowest common denominator, do so. For example, tell the class, "Divide by 15; therefore, the ratio is 1 to 2, and the odds are that 1 out of 2 people made the putt."
5. Point out that not everyone made a putt, but you all had no way of knowing what the outcome would be when you shot the putt. There was uncertainty about the outcome.
6. Write the following definitions on the board, and have the students copy them into their notebooks:
   - *Odds:* The probability that one thing will happen rather than another.
   - *Probability:* The chance that a given event will happen
7. Point out that some students in the class may play golf, so the odds that they will make the putt is higher. A golfer player may make 7 out of 10 puts.
8. Ask students, "What are some daily occurrences in your life that you can express in terms of odds?" Example: The school serves pizza once every month. What are the odds that it's today?
9. Next, take out the prepared bags of candy. Ask girls to pick one piece of candy from the 4:10 bag and take it to their seats without eating it or trading it with anyone. Have boys do the same for the 1:9 bag.

10. Find out the total number of students that picked each of the two candies. Write these numbers on the board next to the candy type and by gender. Inform everyone who received the purple lollipop (or whatever the lesser candy is) that they just became pregnant or got someone pregnant (hypothetically).

11. Calculate the ratio or odds of students in your classroom who selected a candy that indicated that they represented a teen pregnancy. Now compare that to the real national rates. The statistic is that 1 out of 9 males get someone pregnant as an adolescent and 4 out of 10 females become pregnant under age 20. Make sure students understand the odds are either getting pregnant or becoming a father.

12. Hold a class discussion about the activity. Following are some discussion questions:
    - How could someone protect him- or herself from these odds?
    - How do contraceptive methods change the odds?
    - What is the best way to avoid pregnancy and sexually transmitted diseases and infections (STDs/STIs)? (Abstinence is the correct answer.)

13. Discuss the following facts with students:
    - Normally, 3 milliliters (each milliliter contains 120 million sperm) of semen or sperm are secreted during ejaculation. That's less than a teaspoon. It only takes one drop of semen to get a female pregnant.
    - One in every 15 men fathers a child while he is a teenager (Hatcher et al., 1994, p. 572; Marsiglio, 1987).
    - Half of all initial teen pregnancies occur within the first 6 months after a person has sexual intercourse for the first time, and 20 percent happen within the first month (Hatcher et al., 1994, p. 580).
    - Four out of every 10 girls under the age of 20 becomes pregnant each year (Annie E. Casey Foundation, 1998).

RESOURCES
Obtain a golf club and ball. Before students enter the classroom, place two different kinds of candy in two bags in a 1 to 9 ratio and a 4 to 10 ratio. Students should not be able to see into the bags. Choose candies that are similar in shape and size. For example, one purple lollipop for every nine red lollipops. Make sure there are at least 50 or more candies in each bag in the appropriate ration, or make sure that every time a student selects a particular candy that the teacher replaces the same candy in the bag; otherwise, the odds will change from the first student who selects a candy to the last.

ASSESSMENT PLAN
Students will be assessed through their participation in the class discussion.

REFLECTION
The lesson allows students to learn about the odds of teen pregnancy through concrete activities. Putting the golf ball makes the concept of odds and ratio come alive. Selecting the candy as an analogy to teen pregnancy forces students to acknowledge their risk for pregnancy as real instead of abstract. Teachers may want to collaborate with math specialists to teach this lesson at the same time students are learning the concepts in math.

REFERENCE
Adapted from Campaign for Our Children (www.cfoc.org).

LEARNING EXPERIENCE 6

TITLE: Decisions, Decisions

GRADE LEVELS: 10–12

TIME REQUIREMENTS: One session

LEARNING CONTEXT
Students will review the GREAT decision-making model and apply it to a real-life scenario.

NATIONAL LEARNING STANDARDS
3:   Students will demonstrate the ability to practice health-enhancing behaviors and reduce health risks.

6:   Students will demonstrate the ability to use goal-setting and decision-making skills to enhance health.

PROCEDURE
1. As a "do now" activity, have the students count the number of squares that you have diagrammed on the board.
2. After the students have finished counting, call on each one for their answers. The guesses will probably vary from 16 to 30. Now show them the correct number of squares, which are 30.
3. Discuss with the students how it is important to look at all the possible consequences when making a decision. By looking at all of the possible consequences, hopefully they will consider the impact on their lives of certain choices before engaging in behavior that may bring negative consequences.
4. The following are some discussion ideas:
   - How many squares did you see immediately?
   - How many squares did you see after you had studied the diagram for a while?
   - Why did you keep discovering more squares?
   - Is it important to explore fully the consequences of our actions?
   - Who is responsible for the decisions you make?
5. Now review the purpose and objectives for the lesson. Ask the class how many of them have ever had trouble making a difficult decision. Ask them to share what the decisions were and why they were difficult to make.
6. Explain that today, students are going to be learning about and using the GREAT decision-making model to make decisions. Explain that a decision-making model is simply steps to making a decision listed out in an acronym format so the steps are easy to remember.

7. Put the GREAT decision-making model up on the overhead projector or write it on the board. Break down each letter and its meaning for the students, and have the students copy the information into their notebooks:

Great Decision-Making Model

Give thought to the decision/problem.

Review all your options.

Evaluate outcomes of each option.

Assess and choose the best option.

Think it over afterward—would you make the same decision next time?

8. Explain that the class is going to break up into small groups to practice using the GREAT decision-making model through a decision-making scenario.

9. Break the class up into small groups, and hand each group a worksheet with one of the two scenarios (cited later). Make sure that Scenarios 1 and 2 are evenly distributed around the room.

10. Allow the students 5 to 10 minutes to review their scenario and apply the decision-making model.

11. When all groups have completed the decision-making worksheets, bring the small groups back into the large group, and give groups an opportunity to share their scenario and answers.

12. Conduct a class discussion using the following process questions:

- How does the GREAT decision-making model help when making important decisions?
- What would you do if someone you were dating was pressuring you to have sex?
- What are the possible negative consequences of engaging in sexual intercourse at a young age?
- What are other ways couples can be intimate without having sexual intercourse?

13. Conclude the lesson by reminding the students that there are many different ways to make a decision; however, more difficult decisions require time and consideration. The GREAT decision-making model can help young people make the best choices.

RESOURCES

"GREAT Decision-Making Model: Scenario" worksheets

INSTRUCTIONAL/ENVIRONMENTAL MODIFICATIONS

The teacher may need to know which students may or may not be able to work as partners. The teacher may wish to make sure that those students aren't put in the same small group.

Make sure that the room is arranged so that the students will easily be able to move around the room when forming their small groups.

ASSESSMENT PLAN
Students will be assessed through the completion of their decision making worksheet, their participation in the group process, and their participation in the class discussion.

REFLECTION
Young people often make snap decisions without thinking about the consequences of their actions. If students are taught a decision-making model, perhaps the next time they are forced to make an important choice they will use the model and run through the steps in making a good decision before making a decision they might regret later.

Great Decision-Making Model: Scenario 1

Scott and Mary

Scott and his girlfriend Mary have been dating each other for 2 months. Scott has never had sex before. He has heard from his friends that his girlfriend, Mary, has had several boyfriends. He assumes that she will start wanting to have sex soon. All his friends have been bugging him and asking him whether they are having sex.

One day Scott and Mary get out of school early, and Mary invites Scott over to her house to watch TV. Scott wants his friend, Larry, to come with them, but Mary says that Larry gets on her nerves and she wants it to be just them. Scott is a little worried about going because he knows that Mary's mother is never home during the day and they will be all alone. Worried he may not be ready for sex, Scott tries to decide what to do.

Give thought to the decision/problem. What is the problem?

Review all your options. List them below.

Evaluate outcomes of each option. What are the consequences of each option?

Assess and choose the best option. What is it and why?

Think it over afterward—would you make the same decision next time?

Great Decision-Making Model: Scenario 2

Charlie and Anne

Charlie and Anne have been dating for almost 2 years. They are both seniors in high school and are getting ready to go to the prom. Charlie and Anne have discussed waiting to have sex until they are older. However, Charlie decides that he wants to make their prom night unforgettable and have sex for the first time. Anne says she loves Charlie but still wants to wait to have sex.

Give thought to the decision/problem. What is the problem?

Review all your options. List them below.

Evaluate outcomes of each option. What are the consequences of each option?

Assess and choose the best option. What is it and why?

Think it over afterward—would you make the same decision next time?

LEARNING EXPERIENCE 7

TITLE: Pregnancy, Labor, and Delivery: From Start to Finish

GRADE LEVELS: 10–12

TIME REQUIREMENTS: 25–30 minutes

LEARNING CONTEXT
Students will put the steps of pregnancy, labor, and delivery in sequential order and discuss each step.

NATIONAL LEARNING STANDARD
1: Students will comprehend concepts related to health promotion and disease prevention.

PROCEDURE
1. Explain to the class that they are going to be playing a game today. Tell them that each student is going to get a card. On each card is one step in pregnancy and birth. Following are the list of cards:
   a. Decision to have a child
   b. Male's erect penis put into female's vagina
   c. Ejaculation
   d. Sperm enter vagina
   e. Sperm swim up vagina
   f. Some sperm meet ovum in Fallopian tubes (if ovulation occurred)
   g. One sperm enters ovum's outer membrane
   h. Fertilization
   i. Fertilized egg (zygote) travels to uterus
   j. Zygote implants on wall of uterus
   k. Confirm pregnancy
   l. Good prenatal care
   m. 40 weeks pass
   n. Signs of labor (water breaks, back pains, contractions)
   o. Travel to hospital or birthing clinic
   p. Contractions of uterus opens cervix
   q. Baby enters birth canal
   r. Abdominal muscles propel baby into the vagina
   s. Head of the baby "crowns"
   t. Baby's shoulders pass out of the vagina
   u. The rest of the baby's body passes out of the vagina
   v. Umbilical cord cut
   w. Delivery of placenta
   x. Apgar and other tests performed on the baby
   y. Baby is swaddled and placed under warming lights
   z. Recovery time for the mother in the hospital
   aa. Mother and baby are released from the hospital

2. Students should move around the room reading each other's cards and trying to determine where their step is in the sequence of cards.

3. Students should line themselves up in the order they believe is correct.

4. Randomly distribute the cards to the class—one student per card. If there are not enough cards for the number of students in the class, give one card per pair of students. It is important that every student participates in this activity.

5. Once the class believes they are in the appropriate order, distribute a piece of tape to each student/pair. Instruct the class to tape their cards on the wall in the order in which they think they belong.

6. In the large group, discuss the sequence of the cards. Correct any mistakes students have made and make sure the cards are rearranged in the order in which they belong. Use the attached answer sheet to provide background information to students.

7. As each step in the sequence of pregnancy and birth is reviewed, make sure to prompt students to take notes. By the time the activity is finished, students should have all the steps recorded in their notebooks.

INSTRUCTIONAL/ENVIRONMENTAL MODIFICATION

The teacher might consider moving the desks into a large outer circle so there is room for students to circulate in the center of the room.

RESOURCES

"Pregnancy and Birth" cards (on 8.5 × 11-inch paper) with one stage of pregnancy/birth on each card; tape

ASSESSMENT PLAN

Students will be assessed through their class participation in the activity and the discussion as well as through their note taking.

REFLECTION

The steps of pregnancy, labor, and delivery activity allow students to be actively involved in learning. Instead of listening to a lecture, students have the opportunity to use critical thinking skills and participate in group process to put the cards in sequential order.

TEACHER'S NOTES

1. Decision to have a child—The first step toward pregnancy should be making the decision to have a child. This decision is based upon weighing parenting skills, understanding the day-to-day responsibilities of caring for a child, assessing finances and support of family and friends, and the age and health of the parents. The expense of raising a child from birth to age 21 is considerable.

2. Male's erect penis put into female's vagina—When a man and woman have vaginal intercourse, the man's erect penis is put into the woman's vagina. (For more mature groups, you may want to add that if a woman does not have a male partner or if her male partner is infertile, she can undergo artificial insemination where sperm is placed in her vagina.)

3. Ejaculation—During ejaculation, millions of sperm spurt out of the penis and enter the vagina.

4. Sperm enters vagina.

5. Sperm swim up vagina—The sperm swim up the vagina, using their tails to propel themselves forward. Some of the stronger sperm swim through the cervix to reach the uterus, or womb.

6. Some sperm meet ovum in Fallopian tubes—Some of these sperm move through the uterus into the Fallopian tubes. Fertilization occurs when the sperm must meet the ovum in the Fallopian tube. (If ovulation occurred, whereby the ovary releases one egg per month, and if the egg is not fertilized, a woman has a menstrual period. Ovulation occurs about 14 days prior to a woman's menstrual period which makes this a woman's most fertile time of month.) Once the sperm get up into the uterus and Fallopian tubes, they can live for 3 to 5 days. Sperm usually reach the Fallopian tubes within 90 minutes of ejaculation.

7. One sperm enters ovum's outer membrane—Despite the fact that millions of sperm are released during ejaculation, only one sperm penetrates the egg to fertilize it.

8. Fertilization—If an egg has been released by an ovary (approximately 2 weeks before a woman's menstrual period, a woman's most fertile time of month) and is present in the Fallopian tube, only one sperm is allowed into the ovum's outer membrane. The process of the sperm entering the ovum is called *fertilization* or *conception*.

9. Fertilized egg (zygote) travels to uterus—The newly fertilized egg travels through the Fallopian tube toward the uterus. The fertilized egg is now called a *zygote*.

10. Zygote implants on wall of uterus—In the uterus, the zygote will develop into a baby during 9 months of pregnancy.

11. Confirm pregnancy—Tests of urine and blood samples can be done in laboratories to confirm pregnancy on the 15th day after fertilization.

12. Good prenatal care—Diet during pregnancy is very important. If a woman's diet is healthful, she has a better chance of remaining healthy during pregnancy and bearing a healthy child. Women should not smoke, drink alcohol, or take drugs during pregnancy, as these actions harm the developing baby. Excessive and chronic alcohol use increases the risk of fetal alcohol syndrome. Most healthy women can continue regular physical activity during pregnancy. Vigorous and strenuous exercise should not start in pregnancy.

13. Forty weeks pass—The baby is ready to be born after 40 weeks. Most people say that pregnancy lasts 9 months, but it is really more like 10 months! Birth happens in three stages: labor, delivery of the baby, and delivery of the placenta.
14. Signs of labor (water breaks, back pains, contractions)—The woman will experience certain signs that alert her that labor is about to begin. One major sign is the "water" breaking, which is really the amniotic sac breaking and the amniotic fluid leaking out. Other signs are strong back pains and abdominal pains that may be contractions.
15. Travel to hospital or birthing clinic—The mother gets a ride to her hospital or birthing clinic—wherever she has chosen to give birth. Some women choose to give birth at home! Hopefully she remembers to bring her bag that she has prepacked!
16. Contractions of uterus opens cervix—Contractions of the uterus gradually increase in intensity and occur more frequently as labor progresses. The contractions of the uterus thin, soften, and open the cervix wide enough for the baby to exit.
17. Baby enters vagina—When the cervix has completely opened, the baby enters the vagina, which results in the delivery of the baby out of the mother's body.
18. Abdominal muscles propel baby through vagina—As the uterus contracts, the woman pushes with her abdominal muscles to propel the baby through the vagina.
19. Head of the baby "crowns"—The baby's head is the first thing to come out in a "regular" birth.
20. Baby's shoulders pass out of the vagina—The shoulders are the next body part to come out; they are the widest part of the baby's body and can be the most difficult part of labor.
21. The rest of the baby's body passes out of the vagina—once the shoulders have passed through, the rest of the body slides out.
22. Umbilical cord cut—After the baby is born, it is still attached to the mother by the umbilical cord. As soon as the baby begins breathing on its own or the cord no longer pulsates, the umbilical cord is clamped and cut.
23. Delivery of placenta—The delivery of the placenta, or "afterbirth," usually occurs 30 minutes after the baby is born. The placenta grows on the inner wall of the uterus and nourishes the baby during pregnancy. It is the size of a large dinner plate. After the birth of the baby, it separates from the uterus, which then contracts to push it out.
24. Apgar and other tests performed on the baby—Tests are performed on the baby to make sure all reflexes and other systems are in working order.
25. Baby is cleaned off—When babies are born, they are covered with amniotic fluid and other body fluids. The baby needs to be cleaned off.
26. Baby is swaddled and placed under warming lights—The baby loses body heat very quickly after it is born. The baby is swaddled with blankets and is placed under warming lights to help maintain body temperature.
27. Recovery time for the mother in the hospital—Mothers usually stay in the hospital for 48 hours for a vaginal birth and 3 to 5 days for a C-section or surgical delivery.
28. Mother and baby are released from the hospital.

LEARNING EXPERIENCE 8

TITLE: Taking Control of Labor and Delivery

GRADE LEVELS: 10–12

TIME REQUIREMENTS: One session

LEARNING CONTEXT
In this activity, students will
- Discuss options available to them in the selection of a practitioner and place to give birth.
- Review different components of a birth plan.
- Create their own birth plan.

NATIONAL LEARNING STANDARDS
1: Students will comprehend concepts related to health promotion and disease prevention.
7: Students will demonstrate the ability to advocate for personal, family, and community health.

PROCEDURE
1. Explain to the class that having a baby is one of the most rewarding and stressful times in a man and a woman's life. However, with planning and preparation ahead of time, a family can prevent and alleviate a lot of the stress that can occur.
2. Ask the class whether they know what types of practitioners help deliver babies. Most of the students will know that obstetrician/gynecologists, or ob/gyns, are the types of physicians who specialize in labor and delivery.
3. Ask the class whether they know of any other practitioners that are qualified to help a woman give birth—if students don't already know, explain the difference between using an ob/gyn and a nurse practitioner or a midwife.
4. Point out that if families choose an obstetrician, their labor and delivery are likely to be managed in a more medical manner, with more interventions. If they have an alternative health care provider, such as a midwife, they will have more freedom to make their own choices.
5. Next ask the class to identify where and how women can give birth. For example, a woman can deliver at a hospital—where else can she choose to deliver? Students may know that a woman can choose a birthing center or home birth. If students are not familiar with these options, explain.
6. Finally, point out that some women choose water birth (delivery in a tub). Discuss the reasons a person might choose this option.

7. Now ask the class what a woman brings with her to the hospital when she goes. Solicit student responses and write them on the board. Point out that a favorite nightgown, slipper, throw, or pillow will give the scent of home. Having pictures and music that you enjoy at your birthplace can help you relax. Point out that a woman may need something to do to fill the time. Some women give birth in 2 hours, whereas others may take 6 to 12 hours. It helps to have a book or a crossword puzzle to work on. What will the woman wear when visitors come? Remember to bring a change of clothes and clothes for the baby when you leave the hospital. Point out that it is mandatory to have a car seat installed to bring the baby home.

8. Tell the class that labor can be long and painful, but a family can take steps to ensure they have some control over their delivery by developing a birth plan ahead of time. Explain that a birth plan is a list of directions for what you wish to take place during labor, birth, and the delivery of your child. It is important that you let everyone know who is around you how you want to deliver your child. Explain the components of a birth plan:

   - *Your environment:* As you look at the rooms in the place where you'll give birth, think about how you can create an environment that will help you feel comfortable and confident. You'll need space to move around in freely as you try various birthing positions. The temperature of your room, lighting, pillows, and kinds of furniture will affect how you feel.

   - *Emotional support:* Whom do you want in the delivery room? Do you want your partner to be with you or a parent or a coach? Do you want to be alone? Think carefully about whom you'll invite to share in your labor. Women with continuous, nurturing care and support give birth more easily, so the people you choose must be supportive of your beliefs and plans for labor and must be able to convey to you a calm, competent, reassuring presence. You may decide to have a professional support person, or *doula,* join you and your partner during labor and birth.

   - *Pain:* How do you want to deal with the pain? Do you want to be able to walk around during labor? Do you want to use an anesthetic? Do you plan to have a completely natural childbirth? Do you want to have an episiotomy or not? Do you want heat packs or ice packs to help with back pain? Do you want to be able to take a bath or shower to help alleviate discomfort?

   - *Photos:* Do you want the birth videotaped? Do you want pictures taken immediately?

   - *After delivery:* After you deliver, do you want to hold your child? Who will cut the cord? Will you breastfeed or bottle feed or both?

   - *Emergency:* In case of an emergency Cesarean section, what do you want to do? Do you want someone with you in the room? What kind of anesthetic do you want? Do you want your family with you in the recovery room?

9. Hand out the "My Birth Plan" worksheet (included later). Break the class up into partners and tell them that they will be thinking about the future when they may have a child. Ask students to think about what options they want for labor and delivery. Tell the male students that they are to pretend that they will be giving birth or projecting what a partner might like during the birthing experience. Each student will be completing their own birth plan but can use their partner to discuss ideas.

10. Give the class 7 to 10 minutes to complete their worksheets; then bring the class back to the large group, and allow students to share the choices they made.
11. Lead a class discussion using the following questions:
    - How many of you knew about all the choices and options available to expecting parents during pregnancy, labor, and delivery?
    - Where do you think most people learn about what is "supposed" to happen during labor? (TV is the most likely source of information for students.)
    - Why do you think we had this lesson today? Why is it important for high school students to learn about options for labor and delivery? (Answer: So that they can make informed choices in the future.)
    - Why should male students have to learn about this? (Perhaps their partners will not have had such a class and the men can share what they learned; pregnancy, labor, and delivery should be a shared experience—men no longer wait in the waiting room.)
12. The teacher can choose to implement follow-up activities after this lesson:
    - Ask students to interview a parent about what went on and the choices their parent was afforded during the student's delivery.
    - Assign students a project to interview an ob/gyn, family practice physician, nurse practitioner, or midwife about choices during labor and delivery.
    - Arrange for a tour and take the class on a field trip to a birthing center.

RESOURCES

"My Birth Plan" worksheet (one per student). The teacher may want to visit www.ivillage.com for more information about any of the material covered in the lesson plan. This website provides comprehensive information about all aspects of pregnancy, labor, and delivery.

ASSESSMENT PLAN

Students will be assessed through their participation in class discussion and the completion of their birth plan.

REFLECTION

This lesson opens up a world to students that they never knew existed. Most young people think labor and delivery occur as they see on television. They are not aware that there are so many options available to them, from choosing a practitioner, to a birthing site.

My Birth Plan

Name: _____

Directions: You may or may not choose to have children when you get older; however, think about what you might want for your birthing plan if you do have children.
Use the space provided below to write your choices for each category.

Your environment:

Emotional support:

Pain management:

Photos:

After delivery:

Emergency:

CONTRACEPTION AND ABORTION

NANCY O'KEEFE

OBJECTIVES

After reading this chapter, students will be able to

1. Discuss contraceptive methods available in the United States, the advantages and disadvantages of each method, the effectiveness of each method, and indications and contraindications for their use.
2. Discuss abortion, the methods used, and the differences between surgical and medical abortion.
3. Gain insight into the some of the deep feelings and beliefs regarding contraception and abortion in the United States and how these impact how we educate our youth.
4. Understand how personal life skills affect the decisions young people make about their sexuality, sexual activity, contraception, and abortion decisions.

REFLECTIVE QUESTIONS

Elementary School Students
1. How many people are in your family?
2. How many adults and how many children?
3. Is your family the right size for you? Why?
4. Who decides family size?

Middle School Students
1. How many people are in your family?
2. Who are the members of your family?
3. Who decided your family size?
4. What can affect family size?
5. What can families do to determine the size of their family?

Senior High School Students
1. How many people are in your family?
2. Who decided your family size?
3. What can families do to determine their size?
4. Do contraception and abortion affect family size? If yes, how?
5. What are some of the pros and cons about contraception and abortion?
6. Can you list some of the contraceptive methods? Would abstinence be included?
7. Do young people (teenagers) determine family size? How about in their own family?

Casey comes home from school all excited; one of the girls in her first grade class has a new baby sister! Casey asks her mother when her sister is coming. Her mother is stymied. Casey has a 10-year-old brother, and both parents are happy with their family size. There are no plans for another child. She explains this, but Casey persists. She asks her mother how she knows that another baby won't come. Casey is a bright and inquisitive child and has often asked questions about babies. Until this point the answers have been relatively simple, but she now wants an answer to why a sister won't join their family. Casey's mother shares this conversation with Casey's teacher the next day. The teacher replies that she was asked some difficult questions by students the prior day also.

How would you respond to children's demands for a sister or brother if you were the mother? If you were the teacher?

How would you explain that families come in all sizes?

How would you answer Casey's question "How do you know another baby won't come?"

How do you explain contraception to a 6-year-old?

INTRODUCTION

Contraception and abortion are integral components of sexual behavior, and most women and men in their lifetimes will be touched by one or both. To fully understand contraception and abortion, the reader must have knowledge of the male and female reproductive systems (Chapter 2), sexual behavior (Chapter 3), and relationships (Chapter 6) because understanding contraception and abortion are involved in each of these.

Teaching children about human sexuality, and in particular about contraception and abortion, include many of the skills discussed in Chapter 1. For example, an adolescent who wishes to be abstinent will need communication/refusal skills if he or she is being pressured by a girl- or boyfriend. Along the same lines, if a young person is sexually active and wishes to prevent pregnancy, then he or she will need decision-making/problem-solving skills when looking for a place to go for contraception and then deciding which method of contraception to use. Each skill in Chapter 1 will be illustrated throughout this chapter.

Also, throughout this chapter the reader will find guidelines regarding the age appropriateness of the information being discussed. These guidelines are the author's suggestions and are not meant to be carved in stone. Throughout this book, the reader will read about the wonderful and mystifying individual differences in the physical and emotional development of young people. These differences need to be considered when discussing contraception and abortion.

CONTRACEPTION

Contraception is not a new phenomenon; there is knowledge of contraceptive techniques from ancient Egypt, Greece, and Rome (Family Education Network, 2000). The following sections look at contraception through the years, including issues that have affected its use and the various methods employed as contraceptives.

A Historical Perspective

In the past, women used the natural method—they nursed their children for 2 to 3 years and in doing so suppressed ovulation. Men withheld their ejaculate or withdrew before ejaculation. Women relied on potions and rituals as well. Barrier methods were also used: sea sponges, half of a lemon, and oiled paper were all used to prevent sperm from reaching the egg; condoms were invented in the 17th century.

The modern birth control movement began in Britain and found its way to the United States in the early 1900s. Margaret Sanger opened the first U.S. birth control clinic in 1916 in Brooklyn, New York. In 1936, the federal law prohibiting dissemination of contraceptive information through the mails was modified; the 1940s and 50s saw advocates fighting laws prohibiting contraception. In the 1960s, 30 states had statutes that prohibited the sale or advertisement of birth control. These laws had historical roots in the Comstock Act that was passed in 1873 defining contraceptives as "obscene and illicit and making it a federal offense to disseminate birth control through the mail or across state lines." The first successful challenge to this act was when Margaret Sanger was arrested in 1916. The resulting case loosened some restrictions on birth control (see www.pbs.org/wgbh/amex/pill/peopleevents/e_comstock.html). In 1965, the U.S. Supreme Court, in *Griswold v. Connecticut,* struck down state laws that had made the use of birth control by married couples illegal. This decision paved the way for the nearly unanimous acceptance of contraception that now exists in this country (Planned Parenthood Federation of America [PPFA], 2003).

Religious and Cultural Issues

Among religious bodies, the Roman Catholic Church has provided the main opposition to the birth control movement. The Church maintains that deliberate acts of artificial birth control are always gravely sinful if done with full knowledge and deliberate consent (Catholic Answers, 2001). Protestant denominations accept the use of contraception, as do many Jewish groups. The Conference of Leading Scholars of Saudi Arabia issued a verdict that concluded that women are not allowed to take birth control pills. "It is a must to avoid such things (as birth control) and not to use them except in the cases of dire necessity." Muslims are encouraged to "increase their numbers" (Muhammad bin Abdul-Aziz Al-Musnad, 2001, p. 1).

Although some religions frown on the use of contraception, the use of contraception in the United States is widespread. The proportion of U.S. women using a contraceptive method was 64 percent in 1995, including female sterilization, the pill, and the male condom being the most widely used methods (Modern Contraception, 1998).

It is important to be aware of potential religious or cultural barriers to contraceptive use when working with young people. It is also helpful to point out the contradictions of many young people's actions and statements. A young woman may say her religion forbids contraception, and that is why she resists using a birth control method even though she is sexually active. The same religion probably also forbids premarital sex.

In 2003, with much attention and money going to abstinence-only messages and programs, it is difficult for a young person to admit to being sexually active. Often, the use of contraception is an acknowledgment of sexual activity, and young people are not comfortable with any planning that involves sex. Young people are in a difficult place; they are sexual people with sexual feelings, bombarded with sexual images in the media, and they are being told to postpone sexual activity until marriage. With the median age of marriage at 26.8 years for men and 25.1 years for women (Center for Family and Demographic Research, 2002), this can be a long wait for adolescents who are falling in love and wanting to express that love in physical ways, especially since studies show that most young people begin having sex in their mid- to late teens, about 8 years before they marry (Alan Guttmacher Institute, 1994, 1999).

On the other hand, adolescents face peer pressure to have sex and may feel abstinence is not an acceptable choice. Our culture, religions, family and friends give conflicting messages to our youth about sex.

TEACHING CHILDREN

It is crucial for children of all ages to receive factual information so that they can understand all the consequences, both positive and negative, of being a sexually active person. The goal of teaching our children and youth about sexual issues is to give them the tools to make healthy informed decisions as they approach their middle to late teens.

Children between the ages of 5 and 8 often see their families change, or their friends' families change, by the arrival of a baby through childbirth or adoption. Often at this age there is also a desire for a baby sister or a baby brother. It is appropriate to discuss these changes in families and the desire children have for a baby by explaining that children are special and that they should be wanted and loved. Children this age can also understand that families can decide their size; some families may have many children, and others may have one or two. They also should be taught that some families include children, whereas others do not (some may have personal experience with aunts and uncles who do not have children) (Haffner & Yarber, 1996).

As children get to Grades 4 through 6, more information can be added to the discussion about family size and families having babies. At this age some children will be ready to learn that men and women can prevent pregnancy by using contraception. They can also learn some of the religious and cultural issues involved with an explanation that some religions find contraception acceptable and others do not. Children this age can also understand that families make decisions about family size based on many factors, including personal wishes, cultural traditions, and finances (Haffner & Yarber, 1996).

In seventh through ninth grades, educators will begin to teach young people about the different methods of contraception. At this time, young people between the ages of 12 and 15 should know the advantages and disadvantages of the various methods and the indications and contraindications. Effectiveness of the methods and availability should also be part of the learning. Interspersed throughout the discussions should be information about pregnancy, sexually transmitted infections, and HIV (Haffner & Yarber, 1996). Paramount should be the notion and skills of decision making.

As young people enter Grades 10 through 12, the information they received in earlier grades should be reinforced. A onetime discussion about the various methods of contraception may not have had relevance at an earlier time, and now, when there may be real need, an adolescent needs to have current factual information. (Hence, a one-time-only discussion as the only tool for teaching about contraception and abortion is insufficient.) This is an age when sexually active adolescents need to weigh their and their families' feelings and beliefs, and their religious feelings and beliefs, against their need to prevent pregnancy and disease (Haffner & Yarber, 1996). At this age it is helpful to ask the participants for their and their families' feelings and beliefs and their religions. Religious leaders may state the stance of their religion on contraception, but many followers of the religion do not follow or accept this stance. Also, the variations among people of the same faith make it difficult to make blanket statements about religion and contraception. Parents are encouraged to make it clear how they feel about their child having sexual intercourse, recognizing that the young person may feel and act differently.

Some adolescents, during these years, will begin exploring and taking risks. This is a time when young people may experiment with alcohol or drugs and may begin to explore their sexuality. Adolescents armed with factual information often postpone or abstain from risks and exploration. Studies have shown that adolescents want information from their parents, but when unable to speak about sexual issues with them, they look to books, the Internet, and their peers.

Methods of Contraception

The effectiveness of contraceptive methods is divided into two categories: "perfect use" and "typical use." *Perfect use* measures the effectiveness of a method when it is used "perfectly," or exactly how the clinical guidelines state it should be used. *Typical use* measures the effectiveness of a method when it is used by the average person who may not use the method correctly or consistently at all times (Daillard, 2003). When choosing a contraceptive method, the user must understand this distinction. For example, if a young woman chooses birth control pills as her contraceptive method and often misses taking pills, she needs to know that her risk of pregnancy is greater than if she took the pills on time every day.

ABSTINENCE

There are many definitions for abstinence when referring to sexual activity. *Abstinence* can be defined as refraining from all sexuality activity and behavior, including masturbation. Some definitions allow genital contact and oral sex. For this chapter, *abstinence* is refraining from any sexual behavior that can lead to pregnancy because this is a discussion about contraception. This means no genital-to-genital contact—the penis cannot be in close proximity to the vagina.

In preejaculate or "pre-cum," the fluid that is present at the tip of the penis prior to ejaculation contains sperm. Enough sperm exists in preejaculate to cause pregnancy. Penetration of the vagina or ejaculation near the vagina is not permitted when using abstinence as contraception. Anal intercourse is also included in this discussion since semen containing sperm can leak and drip into the vagina and cause pregnancy.

Abstinence can be continuous or variant. Virgins are abstinent. Young people who have engaged in sexual intercourse can become abstinent and then engage in sexual intercourse again in the future. There are numerous reasons for abstinence: virginity, a breakup with a boy-/girlfriend, health reasons, a fright about pregnancy, a sexually transmitted disease, and so forth. No matter what the reason, each is acceptable and subject to change.

Abstinence as a contraceptive method does not have a "typical use" effectiveness measurement because it has never been measured. When presenting abstinence as a method, the educator needs to make it clear that the possibility of failure does exist. When college students were questioned about the status of their virginity vows (Modi, 2000) to remain abstinent until marriage, more than 60 percent had broken their vow.

Advantages.   Abstinence is 100 percent effective when measuring "perfect use" in preventing pregnancy as long as the prohibitions listed earlier are followed. There is no worry about pregnancy and no stress with a delayed menses. Abstinence does not include the taking (ingestion) of hormones, so women will not experience any side effects related to hormones. Abstinence is free of cost and available to all. It not only prevents pregnancy but can also prevent disease. Abstinence for young women allows the cervix time to mature, which, in turn, means that there is less chance of future serious health complications such as infection with human papillomavirus (HPV or genital warts) and cervical cancer. Abstinence may also allow young men and women time to focus on other aspects of their relationships and their lives.

Disadvantages.   Abstinence can be difficult when one person in a relationship wants to be abstinent and the other does not. It can be difficult to withstand the pressure from a partner. This in no way means the person who wishes to be abstinent should give in to this pressure. Abstinence also has different meanings for people, which, in turn, can make it difficult to use as a contraceptive method. The skills that young people will learn through this book will help them deal with this potentially difficult situation.

Indications/Contraindications.   When a young person does not want to engage in sexual intercourse, abstinence is a healthy choice. When there are medical reasons to avoid intercourse, such as a sexually transmitted disease or painful intercourse, then abstinence is the obvious choice. As stated earlier, whatever the reason for choosing abstinence, as long as it is chosen willfully and freely, it is a good choice. There are no medical contraindications or medical reasons (or risks) why someone shouldn't use abstinence as a contraceptive method.

An important discussion to have with young people when talking about abstinence is alternatives to sexual intercourse such as touching, kissing, and masturbation. As discussed in prior chapters, we are all sexual beings, and expressing and exploring feelings is okay and appropriate. Just because someone chooses to be abstinent doesn't mean that he or she can't love someone and express that love.

Lastly, abstinence, as defined here, does not prevent the transmission of sexually transmitted diseases. Young people who abstain from vaginal/penile or anal/penile sex may engage in oral sex. But if, for example, one of the participants has oral herpes, then that partner can spread it to the genitals of the other.

Personal Life Skills.   Choosing abstinence as a contraceptive method can utilize all of one's personal life skills. A young man and young woman in a relationship will need to communicate his or her choice to abstain from intercourse. This communication may include refusal skills if there is opposition from the other person in the relationship. Being able to explain in clear and concise words why one has chosen abstinence may help to avoid conflict. Being able to say no may also be an important part of the contraceptive choice.

Choosing abstinence will often utilize decision-making/problem-solving skills. When young people are fully aware of the responsibility of being a sexually active person and of the advantages and disadvantages, then they are often more able to make good informed decisions about their lives and, in particular, about contraception. When one is able to weigh the advantages and disadvantages of being sexually active and is weighing the option of choosing abstinence versus other contraceptive methods, then one is problem solving. A typical thought process involves a statement such as

"I am in a relationship that is becoming intimate, and I don't know if I am ready to go the next step and engage in sexual intercourse."

Conflict management skills may come into play when one partner in a relationship chooses abstinence and the other does not. For example, a young woman who is reluctant to engage in sexual intercourse, but her partner wants to have sex, needs the skills to discuss the conflict and find a mutually agreeable solution with her partner. Just because she wants to be abstinent does not mean that she is not willing to touch and kiss and participate in other pleasurable and intimate behaviors.

Finally, stress management skills may also be a part of the decision of choosing abstinence. If a relationship is in conflict because of this choice, then there will be stress on the relationship and the individuals involved. It is important for young people to understand that stress exists in many relationships (and many will have experienced this in their families and among their friends). Managing stress and finding ways to alleviate some of the pressures will help in having healthier relationships. Encouraging a young person to talk to a family member or a close friend who will understand the conflict and support the decision without judgment may lessen the stress.

Although children in Grades K through 6 may not need to understand sexual abstinence, they are learning about saying no and abstaining from other behaviors. We teach children early that it is all right to say no when someone tries to touch them. We teach them to say no to drugs and no when strangers offer candy. The skill and comfort of saying no may be useful as they enter into relationships.

FERTILITY AWARENESS METHODS

Fertility awareness methods work by identifying the days of the menstrual cycle when pregnancy is most likely to occur. This can be done in a variety of ways. To avoid pregnancy, young people can "either abstain, use a barrier method, or practice withdrawal during the fertile time" (Hatcher et al., 1998, p. 309). Abstaining from intercourse is considered *natural family planning,* while using a barrier method, or withdrawing, is called *fertility awareness combined methods.*

Physical changes occur during a woman's fertile time in her menstrual cycle; when using fertility awareness methods, women look for these changes. When a woman is fertile, her cervical secretions increase and become clear, stretchy, and slippery. Her cervix also becomes softer and wider and pulls up higher in the vagina. When a woman's basal body temperature (while she is at rest) rises for three consecutive days, then she is ovulating (Hatcher et al., 1998, p. 310). Young women using fertility awareness methods would avoid intercourse while experiencing the increased and changed cervical secretions and when their basal body temperature is first increasing (it will remain elevated for the rest of the cycle).

Another fertility awareness method is the calendar method. This method is based on three assumptions: ovulation occurs on Day 14 (plus or minus 2 days) before the onset of the next menses; sperm remain viable for about 5 days; the ovum survives for about 1 day (Hatcher et al., 1998).

Young women have to keep a careful record of their menstrual cycles so they are able to calculate their fertile time. This is especially difficult for young women who are not yet having regular menses.

Another way to detect ovulation is ovulation tests that can be purchased over the counter at pharmacies and drug stores. Many of these kits were developed to assist couples who were experiencing fertility problems but they were not developed to avoid pregnancy.

Cycle beads are another way for a woman to determine when, during her cycle, pregnancy is likely to occur. Cycle beads are a color-coded string of beads that represents a woman's menstrual cycle and can be used by women with 26- to 32-day menstrual cycles. Each bead represents a day of the cycle, and the color of the bead determines the likelihood of pregnancy occurring (Cycle Technologies, 2003).

Advantages.   Fertility awareness methods can be highly effective in preventing pregnancy when used correctly. Among perfect users, the failure rate is between 1 and 9 percent (Hatcher et al., 1998). For women who wish to prevent pregnancy, but because of religious or other reasons cannot use a barrier or hormonal method of birth control, fertility awareness methods provide an acceptable alternative (when a barrier method is not used in conjunction with this method). Another benefit is that little cost is involved with these methods. Some couples may also like the control they have over their fertility. Fertility awareness methods do not use hormones, and there are no serious side effects. Fertility awareness methods can be used while breast-feeding.

Disadvantages.   Among typical users of fertility awareness methods, the pregnancy rate is close to 25 percent in the 1st year (Hatcher et al., 1998). In addition, many young women are uncomfortable with the normal changes that occur in their bodies during childhood and adolescence. Checking one's cervical secretions daily can be embarrassing and overwhelming. Checking one's temperature every day, at the same time while at rest, can present its own challenges. Young women's schedules often change daily. Privacy and quiet may not be available. Fertility awareness methods are also a cooperative endeavor between the man and woman, which can present additional challenges to the young woman. Fertility awareness methods provide no protection against sexually transmitted infections.

Indications/Contraindications.   As stated earlier, fertility awareness methods do not have serious side effects; almost anyone can use these methods. They are good for women who may be, because of health reasons, unable to use any hormonal method of contraception and for women whose partner is unwilling to use a condom. Some conditions, however, can make the use of these methods more difficult. Young women who do not have regular menstrual cycles, for example, may have difficulty calculating their fertile times. Women who have not had normal menses because of pregnancy or breast-feeding and women who have used a hormonal method of contraception need to establish regular cycles before using this method (Hatcher et al.).

Personal Life Skills. Fertility awareness methods include the need for communication and refusal skills. These methods include abstaining from intercourse during fertile times or using an alternate method and it is important that a young woman be able to communicate to her partner what is needed during her cycle. These methods will not work if a woman is unable to explain why she cannot engage in sexual intercourse or if a woman is unable to refuse to engage in sexual intercourse. They also require a lot of cooperation between partners.

Fertility awareness methods are probably most successful when goal-setting skills are used. Because these methods involve many steps and real communication between partners, it is important that both partners have agreed that using one of these methods of contraception is worth the work. The goals of this decision are often to contracept without using hormonal contraception, to utilize abstinence at times, and to have control over one's fertility.

Fertility awareness methods are quite involved and require a lot of dedication. They are best suited for mature women and couples with good communication and negotiation skills. It should be included in any discussion of contraceptive methods but is most appropriate for Grades 10 through 12.

WITHDRAWAL

Withdrawal, also known as *coitus interruptis,* is the practice of a man pulling his penis out of the vagina before ejaculation. This is done to prevent semen from getting into the vagina, reaching an egg, and causing pregnancy. Withdrawal has been used as a contraceptive method for centuries.

Advantages. Withdrawal has no cost and no serious side effects. There are no hormones involved, so there are no worries about side effects caused by hormones. It is available when a couple has no other method of contraception. Withdrawal can also help to reduce the risk of sexually transmitted diseases to some extent. Finally, there is no need to go to a health center for a prescription or exam.

Disadvantages. For the typical user, the failure rate with withdrawal is quite high—19 percent in the 1st year of use (Advocates for Youth, 2002). Withdrawal can fail because men have no control over their preejaculate, the fluid present at the tip of the penis that contains sperm. Another problem is that frequently men do not withdraw in time and ejaculate in the vagina. Some couples are so focused on the timing of withdrawal that they are unable to achieve any pleasure. Finally, another disadvantage is that there remains the chance of passing on a sexually transmitted disease.

Indications/Contraindications. If a couple has no other method of contraception, withdrawal is better than nothing. There are no medical reasons that a man cannot use withdrawal, although some men may have difficulty withdrawing on time.

Any discussion of withdrawal as a contraceptive method should also include information about emergency contraception. Emergency contraception is a method of pregnancy prevention that can be used after inter-course and will be discussed later in this chapter.

Personal Life Skills.   With withdrawal's high failure rate comes the need for decision-making/problem-solving skills. If a young man does not with-draw on time, the couple needs to decide what to do next. An immediate decision may be whether to use emergency contraception and then what to do the next time to avoid this occurrence. One decision may be to switch to a more effective method of contraception. Another may be for the young woman to use a spermicide as a backup to withdrawal.

When withdrawal fails, there may be conflict and the need for conflict management skills. Yelling, crying, or apologizing profusely will not solve the problem of a young man ejaculating in his partner's vagina. Deciding to use emergency contraception can be an agreeable solution; using sper-micide is another.

Withdrawal is often the first method of birth control a couple uses. This method should be discussed in Grades 7 through 9, and emphasis should be placed on its high unpredictability. It is true that withdrawal is better than nothing, but a more effective method is even better.

BARRIER METHODS

Barrier methods of contraception include: the male condom, diaphragm, cervical cap, spermicides, the sponge, and the female condom. Barrier methods create a barrier so that sperm cannot enter the cervix.

THE MALE CONDOM

The male condom, a thin sheath that is placed on the penis and rolled down toward the base of the penis, has been around for centuries and is the most widely available and popular male contraceptive in the United States (Hatcher et al.). Male condoms come in latex, lambskin, and polyurethane. They also come in different sizes, textures, colors, and flavors.

The male condom is used to prevent semen from entering the vagina. It must be put on an erect penis prior to any genital contact and must be used during the entire act of intercourse. Condoms are to be used only once. Upon ejaculation, the man must hold onto the condom before with-drawing from the vagina to avoid leaving the condom in the vagina.

Before intercourse, the expiration date of the condom should be checked (it can be found on the wrapper). A visual inspection of the wrap-per should also take place; if any holes are noted, the condom must be dis-carded. Care should be taken when opening the wrapper. Beware of teeth and sharp objects, rings, and fingernails that can damage the condom. Do not use oil-based lubricants such as Vaseline, baby oil, massage oil, and veg-etable oil—they can weaken the condom. Suppositories, contraceptive films, creams, and gels can be used along with a condom to increase effec-tiveness. Condoms should not be stored in warm places (a pants pocket, the glove compartment of a car, a spot in the warm sun, and the like) or in frigid temperatures because heat and cold can also damage the condom.

Spermicides (described more fully later) such as creams, jellies, and foams can increase the effectiveness of the condom by providing a backup contraceptive measure. If a male condom breaks, slips, leaks, or comes off, the spermicide can often kill the sperm before they reach the egg.

Advantages.   Condoms have a high effectiveness rate when used consistently and correctly. Approximately 3 percent of couples will have an unintended pregnancy during the 1st year of use (Hatcher et al., 1998). Condoms are inexpensive and accessible; they require no prescription. Condoms prevent many sexually transmitted diseases and HIV as well as pregnancy. Condoms do not contain hormones, so there is none of hormones' possible accompanying side effects. Condoms can help some men maintain an erection longer and share the responsibility for contraception. For women, condoms prevent semen from entering the vagina so there is no semen (or "mess") after intercourse.

Disadvantages.   Condoms are a barrier between the penis and the vagina, and some men and women complain about the decrease in sensitivity that they experience during sexual intercourse. For men, this can lead to a loss of erection (although stimulation can often bring the erection back). Some couples don't like having to stop during sexual activity to put on the condom. Condoms do break and can slip off. Leakage is also possible if the man does not withdraw quickly enough after ejaculation. Some condom users may experience allergic reactions to the latex of the condom or to the spermicidal lubricant (alternatives are available such as nonlubricated condoms and polyurethane condoms).

Indications/Contraindications.   Young men and women with sexually transmitted infections such as genital warts (HPV) or herpes should always use condoms to help prevent spreading the disease. Although condoms do not always prevent these infections, they do offer protection. Women who cannot use or do not want to use a hormonal contraceptive method can have their partner use a condom.

The main contraindication for the male condom is when a latex allergy exists. Fortunately, other condoms are available that are made of polyurethane and offer many of the same advantages.

Once again, any discussion of male condoms as a contraceptive method should include information about emergency contraception. If the condom, or the user, fails, then emergency contraception can be used to prevent pregnancy.

THE DIAPHRAGM, CERVICAL CAP, AND SPONGE

Diaphragms and cervical caps are soft latex barriers that are placed in the vagina and cover the cervix. They create a barrier between the vagina and the uterus. The diaphragm is a shallow, dome-shaped cup with a flexible rim. It fits into the vagina and covers the cervix. The cervical cap is thimble shaped and smaller than the diaphragm. It fits snuggly onto the cervix. Both must be used with a spermicidal cream, jelly, or foam (PPFA, 1998–2003a).

Diaphragms and cervical caps come in different sizes and must be fitted by a medical professional. The appropriate size for a woman can change after a pregnancy, whether the pregnancy went to term or ended in miscarriage or abortion. The size may also need to be changed if a woman gains or loses more than 10 pounds.

The diaphragm and cervical cap are approximately 80 percent effective in preventing pregnancy for the typical user. When used perfectly, the effectiveness rate increases to more than 90 percent effective in the 1st year. To be a "perfect user," young women need to fully understand how to use their barrier device. Information on the Planned Parenthood Federation of America website (www.plannedparenthood.org) provides a detailed description of how to use a diaphragm and cervical cap.

Advantages.   Diaphragms and cervical caps do not contain hormones, so they do not have the side effects that can sometimes occur with hormonal contraception. They offer some protection against certain sexually transmitted diseases by covering and protecting the cervix from infection. Diaphragms can be inserted up to 6 hours prior to intercourse, and cervical caps can be inserted for up to 48 hours to avoid any interruption in sexual activity (Hatcher et al., 1998). Numerous acts of intercourse can occur without having to remove the diaphragm or cap, although another application of spermicide is recommended.

Disadvantages.   Some young women find the thought of touching themselves "down there" distasteful, and the process of inserting a diaphragm or cervical cap may prove to be too great of an obstacle. Other women may be unable to insert the device even after many tries. If a woman does not insert one of the barrier devices ahead of time, then the sexual activity is interrupted. A diaphragm should be held up to a light source and searched for any tears or holes. A woman may need to make another trip to her health care provider to be fitted with a new size. Some sexual positions, penis sizes, and thrusting techniques and angles can push diaphragms out of place (PPFA, 1998–2003a). It is recommended that a condom also be used when a woman is first learning to use this method.

Indications/Contraindications.   Women who wish to use contraception, but want or need to avoid hormones, can use either the diaphragm or cervical cap. Women who do not engage in frequent sexual intercourse may find a barrier method that they control an attractive choice (Hatcher et al., 1998). Women who are breast-feeding can also use these and other barrier methods as well as natural family planning.

Women with a history of toxic shock syndrome (TSS) should not use a diaphragm or cervical cap because each can increase the risk for TSS. Women who have had recent cervical surgery (such as LEEP or a cone biopsy) or a recent second-trimester abortion should also avoid these methods. Cervical caps are not recommended for women who have had a recent abnormal pap smear or other reproductive tract problems (PPFA, 1998–2003a).

THE SPONGE

The contraceptive sponge is made of polyurethane and contains spermicide. It provides a barrier between the cervix and the uterus and kills sperm. It is available without a prescription and is currently available online in the United States.

The sponge is similar in shape to the diaphragm and is inserted the same way. The sponge should be inserted prior to any sexual contact and must remain in the vagina for at least 6 hours after intercourse. The sponge can be left in the vagina for 24 hours, during which time repeated intercourse may occur (Hatcher et al., 1998). Use of a condom with the sponge increases effectiveness.

Advantages. The sponge contains no hormones and the potential side effects that go with hormones. It does not require a prescription or a visit to a medical provider. It provides more effective contraception than spermicides alone and can be used for multiple acts of sexual intercourse.

Disadvantages. The sponge is not widely available in the United States, and because it is currently available online, extra shipping expenses can make it more expensive than other methods. Some women and men may experience irritation from the spermicide. Some users may experience difficulty inserting and removing. Since the sponge only comes in one size, it offers decreased effectiveness in women who have had a full-term pregnancy and vaginal birth.

Indications/Contraindications. The sponge is an effective method for women who are willing and able to insert the device into the vagina. Almost any woman can use it. The sponge is not an option for women unable or unwilling to insert it into the vagina. If a woman experiences irritation, then use should be discontinued. As with any item (a tampon, for example) left in the vagina for long periods of time, there is a low risk of TSS. Women with a prior history of TSS should not use the sponge.

THE FEMALE CONDOM

The female condom is a polyurethane device with two flexible rings, one at each end. It is inserted deep into the vagina like a diaphragm. The ring at the closed end holds the pouch in the vagina. The ring at the open end stays outside the vaginal opening (PPFA, 1998–2003b). The female condom works by collecting semen and preventing sperm from getting into the vagina. It looks like a very large condom for the vagina.

Advantages.   The female condom contains no hormones. It does not require a visit to a medical provider, so no prescription is needed. The female condom can prevent sexually transmitted infections. Female condoms can be used by women who are allergic to latex. It gives women more control over protection.

Disadvantages.   The user of the female condom must be willing and able to insert the condom into the vagina. The male must be careful when inserting the penis to ensure it is actually in the condom. This act can prove difficult if the condom is twisted at the outer ring. The condom does make some noise, which can be embarrassing for some people. The female condom is not as widely available as the male condom, nor is it as effective. The female condom and the male condom should not be used together.

Indications/Contraindications.   Most any woman can use the female condom as long as she is willing and able to insert the device.

Personal Life Skills.   Barrier methods of contraception are most often used in close proximity to the time of sexual intercourse. A male condom is put on moments before intercourse. A diaphragm is inserted in the moments leading up to intercourse, as are the sponge, cervical cap, and female condom. Ensuring that a barrier is in place at the proper time requires communication/refusal skills. Someone needs to call a halt to the activity and make sure the barrier is in place. Another may need to say, "Stop—we need a condom." This communication may be difficult without a prior discussion about contraception.

Decision-making/problem-solving skills are essential with the use of barrier methods. Because each method often requires both partners' participation, decisions must be made as to who will take responsibility for contraception and when. And when a method is not used, then problem solving needs to occur as to the next step—"Do we need emergency contraception?" "What do we do next time?"

Resource management skills will also be useful in helping sort through the various barriers and deciding on the best method. Numerous websites for young people provide information in a format that is understandable and informative. Searching the web and other media will allow young people to make informed, healthy decisions.

Teaching about barrier methods is appropriate for Grades 7 through 12. The male condom is easily obtained, requires no doctor's visit, and provides prevention of disease and pregnancy. Many couples use condoms and withdrawal until a visit to a doctor occurs.

SPERMICIDES

Spermicides are a combination of a base, such as a cream, gel, foam, film, or suppository, and a chemical that kills sperm (Hatcher et al., 1998). They are inserted into the vagina up to an hour prior to intercourse and form a barrier between the vagina and the uterus. They can be used alone or in combination with some of the aforementioned barrier methods. Their effectiveness is increased when used with barrier methods such as a condom. A man's ejaculate can contain millions of sperm, and spermicides may not be able to kill all of them.

Advantages.   Spermicides contain no hormones, so some of the side effects that hormonal methods can cause are not an issue. Spermicides are low-cost and do not require a prescription. They may help prevent bacterial infections (Hatcher et al., 1998). Spermicides are one of the few methods for women that do not require a visit to a medical provider.

Disadvantages.   Spermicides, when used alone, have a failure rate of 29 percent during the 1st year of use. They provide little protection against sexually transmitted diseases, and because they can cause irritation to some women, there may be an increased risk for diseases, including HIV.

Indications/Contraindications.   Any woman can use a spermicide. If irritation occurs, another type can be tried, but spermicides should be discontinued if irritation persists. Again, spermicides are most effective when used with a barrier method.

Emergency contraception should be part of the discussion of spermicides. It can provide a good backup when a spermicide is used alone.

EMERGENCY CONTRACEPTION

Emergency contraception (EC) refers to pills or devices (IUDs) that are used after intercourse to prevent a pregnancy. EC can be used after unprotected intercourse, when a condom breaks, and after a sexual assault. Emergency contraceptive pills (ECPs) are often referred to as the "morning after pill," but this term is misleading since ECPs can be taken up to 120 hours (5 days) after intercourse (not just the morning after) and involve more than one pill. Although ECPs can be taken up to 120 hours, they are most effective when taken soon after unprotected intercourse. ECPs work by inhibiting ovulation, preventing fertilization or implantation. The IUD, another EC approach, is inserted within 5 to 7 days and prevents fertilization and implantation.

Advantages.   Emergency contraception is a good backup to another method or user failure. If a condom breaks, EC can reduce the risk of pregnancy. If a condom isn't used, EC can reduce the risk of pregnancy. There is no physical exam required for ECPs, although they are currently by prescription only in all but a few states. Thus, a visit to a doctor or clinic is necessary at this time (some states provide ECPs online or by telephone), but there is discussion about making them available over the counter. Some pills are manufactured solely for EC use consisting of two or four pills that can be taken during a short period of time (for example,

12 hours). They have few side effects and risks, and just about anyone can take them. ECPs will not harm an existing pregnancy.

Disadvantages.   Emergency contraceptive pills are not as effective as a reversible method of contraception (birth control pills, patches, rings, and so forth). They are called "emergency" contraceptive pills because they are for an emergency, such as a condom failure. The IUD is more effective, but the cost can be prohibitive. Since ECPs still require an office visit in most states, the timing of initiation may be delayed. Women should be encouraged to ask their medical provider for ECPs during an office visit so they can have them available at home if they are needed. ECPs can cause nausea, breast tenderness, irregular bleeding, and dizziness. These side effects are usually short in duration, lasting not more than 24 hours.

Indications/Contraindications.   Any woman who believes she is at risk for pregnancy can use emergency contraceptive pills within 120 hours of unprotected intercourse. A woman already pregnant should not use EC since it will not work. Some people confuse ECPs with the "abortion pill" (RU-486), so it is important to clarify the woman's needs. A woman who has had a heart attack, blood clots, or a stroke may be prescribed progestin-only pills to reduce the risk of complications. A woman at risk for a sexually transmitted infection should not have an IUD inserted for emergency contraception (including women who have been raped) because the risk for serious infection can occur.

Personal Life Skills.   In states that require a prescription or doctor's visit, young women will need to use resource management skills in order to obtain emergency contraception. A doctor's office or clinic will need to be located, timing will need to be taken into account, and money will be needed to pay for the visit and EC. Decision making/problem solving will also be useful skills because couples need to decide whether they consider the risk of pregnancy great enough to seek out EC. The condom may have slipped off, but there didn't seem to be any leakage of semen into the vagina. Is there a risk of pregnancy?

HORMONAL METHODS

Hormonal contraception includes oral contraceptives, injections, implants (not currently available in the United States), patches, vaginal rings, and an intrauterine device called Mirena. Hormonal contraceptive methods affect a woman's hormones in one or more of the following ways: they inhibit ovulation, change the mucus (by thickening it) around the cervix to prevent sperm from entering the uterus, and alter the lining of the uterus in order to prevent implantation.

Hormonal contraception is widely used throughout the United States, and some children may know that "Mommy is on the pill," and now, with the patch, some children may have seen Mom wearing her patch. Hormonal contraception should be included in the discussion of contraception that occurs in Grades 7 through 12. Some information should be shared earlier if younger children ask questions.

ORAL CONTRACEPTIVES

Oral contraceptives (OCs), or birth control pills, are one of the most popular birth control methods in the United States, second only to female sterilization. Many women, when asked about birth control, assume the interviewer is referring to birth control pills. It is important to make this distinction when speaking with young people.

OCs were first approved by the Food and Drug Administration (FDA) in 1960. Since then, many changes and advances in formulations have occurred. Today's birth control pill is highly effective and safe for most users. Unfortunately, some common myths about the pill continue to linger and cause fear among young people. In reality, OCs have been associated with health benefits: they may lend some protection against ovarian cancer, endometrial cancer, salpingitis, and ectopic pregnancy. OCs also may reduce the incidence of benign breast disease, dysmenorrhea, and iron deficiency anemia (Grimes & Wallach, 1997). For young women who believe that using birth control pills will "make them fat," it is useful to inform them that as many young women lose weight as gain weight while taking OCs. Tackling the myth about needing to "take a break" from the pill is also important. No medical evidence supports this claim, but there are negative consequences to taking a break (Grimes & Wallach, 1997). Young women who temporarily stop taking their OCs may be at increased risk for pregnancy and have difficulties with their menstrual cycle upon cessation—they may bleed heavier than normal, have irregular cycles, and even be without periods for a few to many months.

OCs' primary mechanism in preventing pregnancy is suppressing ovulation. If there is no egg, there can be no fertilization, no implantation, and no pregnancy. It is extremely important that women take pills consistently, one pill at the same time every day, so that they are protected against pregnancy.

Advantages.   In addition to their possible health benefits, oral contraceptives are very effective. When taken properly, they are between 92 and 99 percent effective (Hatcher et al., 1998). Women on the birth control pills have very predictable periods. Their periods are usually shorter in length, lighter in flow, and with less severe cramps. Some pills even improve acne. Pills do not interfere with the spontaneity of sexual intercourse.

Disadvantages.   Oral contraceptives contain hormones that can cause side effects such as nausea, breast tenderness, weight gain or loss, and breakthrough bleeding. They provide no protection against sexually transmitted diseases and may actually increase the risk for some infections. OCs may also cause some users to develop headaches, a loss in sexual desire, and depression. Fortunately, some side effects go away after the first few months of use, and with the numerous different oral contraceptives available for doctors to prescribe, many of these symptoms can be eliminated simply by switching pills.

Significant risks are possible with the pill. They include an increased risk for developing blood clots, risk of heart attack and stroke in smokers, benign liver tumors, and high blood pressure (Princeton University, 2000). Women should be educated about the warning signs of these problems. Additional information about side effects and risks can be found in the package insert of the birth control pills.

Some medications, including antibiotics, interfere with oral contraceptives. All women need to know that a medication prescribed to them, as well as some herbs, may decrease the efficacy of the pill. Women should ask the prescribing physician or pharmacist if a backup method is required during and immediately after the use of the medication. In addition, some over-the-counter medications, such as antacids, also interfere with the pill and put a woman at risk for pregnancy. All oral contraceptive counseling must include this information.

Indications/Contraindications.   Many women use the birth control pill because it is highly effective. Other women use it for menstrual complaints. Because the pill can shorten the length of time a woman bleeds, decrease cramping, and lighten the flow, it is a good method for women who bleed for more than 3 to 4 days, women who have severe cramping, and women who bleed heavily. It can also help to regulate a woman's menstrual cycle.

The pill is also a good method for women who want a method of contraception that they control. It is appropriate for women who can take pills and remember to take them at the same time every day. Birth control pills are a benefit to women with a family history of ovarian cancer or a personal history of ovarian cysts (Hatcher et al., 1998).

Women should not take the pill if they are 35 or older and smoke more than 20 cigarettes a day; have high blood pressure; have a history of blood clots or vein inflammation; have unexplained vaginal bleeding; have had an abnormal growth or cancer of the breast or uterus; have high cholesterol; have a severe liver disease or have had growths of the liver; have certain conditions associated with diabetes; can't remember to take them on schedule; think they may be pregnant.

Oral contraceptives are a prescription medication, and it is important for young women to discuss their medical history with their medical provider. Additional medical conditions need to be addressed before taking birth control pills, and a physician and a young woman can make the best decision about pills after reviewing all pertinent medical conditions.

As stated, oral contraceptives are highly effective when used correctly. Women will be told by their medical provider when to begin their pills. Once begun, consistency is the key—one pill a day, at about the same time every day (for example, after brushing your teeth before bedtime).

A backup method, such as abstinence or a condom, is recommended for the 1st month of use while the woman's body is adjusting to the hormones.

Personal Life Skills. Obtaining oral contraceptives for a young woman can be a frightening proposition. A visit to a health center or private doctor's office can feel overwhelming. First, one must find where to go and once she knows where to go she must then call and schedule an appointment. Concerns about confidentiality may be an issue as well as payment. Fears about having a pelvic examination may cause a woman to postpone the whole process. Good communication and decision-making skills may give confidence to a young woman and enable her to take the first steps.

INJECTIONS

Currently one injectable contraceptive method is available in the United States: Depo-Provera. Depo-Provera is a long-term method of birth control that contains progesterone. It is begun during the first 5 days of a woman's menses and then again every 12 to 13 weeks. The injection is given intramuscularly in the arm or buttocks and is effective within 24 hours. Depo-Provera works in similar ways to oral contraceptives in that it inhibits ovulation. Less often, it changes the lining of the uterus and thickens the mucus around the cervix. In contrast to most oral contraceptives, Depo-Provera does not contain estrogen and may be used by some women who cannot use oral contraceptives.

Advantages. Depo-Provera is more than 99 percent effective for women who receive their injections on time. There is no estrogen and therefore none of the serious, but rare, side effects that are attributable to estrogenic agents. Another benefit to Depo-Provera not containing estrogen is that women who are breast-feeding can use it. Menses are lighter or nonexistent, and cramping is diminished. It also seems to offer some protection against endometrial cancer, ovarian cancer, and pelvic inflammatory disease (Hatcher et al., 1998). Depo-Provera is considered a long-term contraceptive method and appropriate for women who wish to prevent pregnancy for long periods of time. Lastly, Depo-Provera does not require a daily reminder like having to take a pill every day, and it does not require any intervention during sexual intercourse like inserting a diaphragm.

Disadvantages. Women may experience changes in bleeding, including the absence of continuous bleeding during their first injection of Depo-Provera and, in rare instances, for an even longer period of time. Because it is hormonal, women may experience side effects associated with hormonal methods of birth control such as headache, nausea, breast tenderness, and weight gain. Some women may experience hair loss, depression, and some loss in bone density (Hatcher et al., 1998). There is no way to stop the effects of Depo-Provera once the injection is given; side effects may not subside until the injection wears off in 12 to 14 weeks, or longer. Depo-Provera does not provide protection against sexually transmitted diseases.

Indications/Contraindications. Depo-Provera is appropriate for women who are looking for a long-term method of contraception. Women who cannot use estrogen can use it, including those who are breast-feeding.

Depo-Provera is a good method for women who cannot take pills or for women who forget to take their pills. It is also appropriate for women who are uncomfortable using or relying on a barrier method.

As stated previously, women using Depo-Provera may experience heavy or irregular bleeding for their first injection or even longer; women using Depo-Provera must be able to tolerate this effect because there is no reversing an injection. The Depo-Provera injection is given intramuscularly, and deep, which can be painful (though brief). Women unable to tolerate this form of delivery will need to use an alternate method of contraception. Women wishing to get pregnant within 18 months should not use Depo-Provera because a return to fertility can take 9 to 10 months and at times even longer (PPFA, 1998–2003a).

Personal Life Skills.   A young woman will need to use decision-making/problem-solving skills when choosing Depo-Provera as her contraceptive method. Deciding on a contraceptive method should include a weighing of the pros and cons of each method. A woman will also need to decide whether she is willing to tolerate and accept irregular bleeding. Problem solving may be needed if there are issues relating to getting to a health center or doctor's office every 12 weeks.

IMPLANTS

Implants (not currently available in the United States, where they were once known as Norplant) are small rods inserted under the skin of the upper arm that constantly release a hormone similar to progesterone. Progestin is the same hormone found in Depo-Provera, and its mechanism is the same. It thickens the cervical mucus and, less often, inhibits ovulation and changes the lining of the uterus. Implants are highly effective and considered long-term contraception.

Advantages.   Similar to Depo-Provera, implants do not contain estrogen. They can be used by breast-feeding women and are good for women who want a long-term, effective, reversible method of contraception. Once inserted, implants require little work—no remembering to take a pill or putting on a condom.

Disadvantages.   Menstrual irregularities are frequent with implants; women may experience heavy and frequent bleeding. Implants require a small incision in the arm, and some discomfort may occur during insertion (numbing medication is used to minimize pain). Implants are cost-effective over time, but the initial cost can be prohibitive. Removal can be difficult because scar tissue grows around the capsules. Implants are hormonal so can cause possible side effects that are common with hormonal contraceptives.

Indications/Contraindications.   Implants are appropriate for women who are looking for a long-term, reversible method of contraception. Implants are good for women who do not want to bother taking a pill every day or getting an injection every few months, and for women who want something more effective than barrier methods. Implants are also good for women who can tolerate the irregular bleeding.

Women who cannot tolerate irregular bleeding should not use implants. Other contraindications include women who have unexplained bleeding from the vagina, have had breast cancer, have had growths of the liver, are breast-feeding in the first 6 weeks after delivery, and have a sensitivity to the ingredients in Norplant, as well as other medical conditions about which a physician should inquire (Grimes, 2000).

Personal Life Skills. Decision-making/problem-solving skills are important for all contraceptive methods including implants. Deciding on a long-term contraceptive method is a serious decision and one that should be made after weighing all options. Coming up with the money for implants may take some problem-solving skills as well as resource management skills because programs (such as the Norplant Foundation) do exist that may provide financial assistance.

THE PATCH

Ortho Evra is a contraceptive patch, about 2 inches square, that works very similarly to the pill; the patch contains progestin and estrogen, the two hormones found in oral contraceptives. The patch inhibits ovulation and thickens the mucus around the cervix that, in turn, makes it extremely difficult to get pregnant. It is 99 percent effective and appropriate for women who are able to use hormonal contraception. The patch is changed weekly for 3 weeks and is worn on the buttocks, abdomen, upper torso (front and back, excluding the breasts), or upper outer arm; it stays in place during bathing, swimming, and typical activities. During the 4th week, the woman does not wear a patch and should get her period (Ortho-McNeil Pharmaceuticals, 2003). As with birth control pills, the patch comes with instructions that include information on how to apply, when to change, and what to do in the event the patch comes off or is not changed on time.

Advantages. The patch only requires changing once a week. It is good for women who can use hormonal contraception but may have difficulty taking a pill or remembering to take a pill at the same time every day. Women who use the patch will often have lighter periods and shorter ones. A woman's return to fertility upon termination of use is almost immediate. Other advantages of the patch are still being learned because it is a relatively new method of contraception. At this time many of the benefits of the birth control pill are believed to exist for the patch also.

Disadvantages. As with any hormonal method of birth control, women using the patch may experience bleeding between periods, weight gain or loss, breast tenderness, nausea rarely, vomiting, and changes in mood. The patch may also cause skin irritation at the site of application.

Indications/Contraindications.   Women who are medically cleared to use a hormonal method of contraception can choose the patch as their birth control method (see indications/contraindications under "Oral Contraception"). Women who have blood clots, certain cancers, a history of heart attack or stroke, as well as those who are or may be pregnant should not use the patch. Women who experience irritation from the patch and its adhesive may want to switch to another method. The patch is not recommended for women weighing more than 198 pounds. Finally, as with all hormonal methods, the contraceptive patch does not protect against HIV or other sexually transmitted diseases (Ortho-McNeil Pharmaceuticals, 2003).

Personal Life Skills.   In choosing the patch as a contraceptive method, a young woman will need to use decision-making/problem-solving skills. Some decisions that will need to be made are, "Is hormonal contraception the best option?" "Is the patch the best option of the hormonal methods?" "How do I stay on schedule and remember to change the patch?" "Where should I place the patch on my body?" and "Should I use a barrier method for disease prevention?" Some problem-solving skills may address what to do if the patch causes irritation, what to do if the patch comes off, and what to do if the woman forgets to change her patch.

NUVARING

NuvaRing is a hormonal method of contraception similar to oral contraceptives and the patch. It is a flexible ring that is inserted in a woman's vagina for 3 weeks and releases progestin and estrogen, which inhibit ovulation and thicken the mucus of the cervix. At the end of the 3rd week, the ring is removed and a new one is inserted 1 week later; menses will occur during the 4th week.

Advantages.   The ring protects against pregnancy for 1 month. It does not involve taking a daily pill, require the use of spermicide, or require a fitting by a clinician. The ring has menstrual benefits as well. Periods are lighter and shorter. As with the patch, NuvaRing is relatively new, and all benefits are not known at this time. However, it is assumed that the benefits are similar to those of oral contraceptives and the patch (see advantages listed under "Oral Contraceptives").

Disadvantages.   The NuvaRing is a hormonal contraceptive and carries the same side effects as the others; women may experience irregular bleeding, weight changes, breast tenderness, and nausea.

The ring may also cause an increase in vaginal discharge and vaginal irritation. It is not appropriate for women uncomfortable with touching their genitals and women unable to insert the ring into the vagina.

Indications/Contraindications.   Women who are medically approved to use hormonal contraception can use the ring. The ring is a good alternative for women who can't take pills or forget to take them daily and for women who don't want to wear or can't wear the patch. The contraindications to the ring are the same as those for oral contraceptives.

Personal Life Skills. Decision-making and problem-solving skills are some of the skills needed when deciding to use NuvaRing. A young woman needs to weigh the advantages and disadvantages of all the methods of birth control and then, more specifically, weigh the pros and cons of the various hormonal methods.

Problem-solving skills may come into play if the ring falls out of the vagina (very rare) or is left in too long. A young woman may also need to use communication skills if her partner feels the NuvaRing while it is inserted in the vagina and conflict skills if he is bothered by the idea that something is in the vagina during intercourse.

INTRAUTERINE DEVICES

The intrauterine device (IUD) is a small T-shaped flexible device inserted into the uterine cavity. There are two types of IUDs; one is copper-releasing and the other, progestin releasing. Copper-releasing IUDs interfere with the ability of sperm to pass through the uterine cavity and with the reproductive process before ova reach the uterine cavity. Progestin-releasing IUDs also thicken the cervical mucus and change the endometrial lining (Tapestry Health, 2003). Both types of IUDs have strings that hang from them into the vagina. This string allows women and their medical providers to check that the IUD is still in the correct place, and the string also helps in removal.

Advantages. The IUD is highly effective, and the copper IUD can stay in the uterus for 10 years and Mirena for up to 5 years. The copper IUD is hormone-free, so it has none of the side effects associated with hormones. The progestin IUD (Mirena) releases small amounts of a synthetic progesterone hormone. This hormone works to decrease the excessive bleeding and cramping that some women have with the IUD. Because it entails little user involvement, effectiveness of typical and perfect use are very similar. Only one woman using the IUD will get pregnant in the 1st year of use. Women breast-feeding can use the copper IUD.

Disadvantages. Women using the copper IUD may experience spotting between periods. If the bleeding is heavy, it may lead to anemia. There can also be an increase in menstrual cramping. Some women expel their IUD, sometimes without the woman's knowledge. If expulsion occurs, pregnancy is possible. If a pregnancy occurs while the IUD is in place, then there is risk for ectopic pregnancy. The IUD provides no protection against sexually transmitted infections.

Indications/Contraindications. Women who are looking for a long-term and highly effective contraceptive method, have children, and are in a mutually monogamous relationship are good candidates for an IUD. Women with an active pelvic infection including gonorrhea and chlamydia, known or suspected pregnancy, or an unresolved cervical abnormality and women in nonmonogamous relationships should not use the IUD (Tapestry Health, 2003).

Personal Life Skills.   Decision-making/problem-solving skills are important when choosing an IUD as a contraceptive method. IUDs are considered long-term, and a woman needs to decide whether she truly wishes to postpone future pregnancies for many years or stop having children altogether. Because sexually transmitted infections can result with serious consequences (pelvic inflammatory disease, infertility, and so forth), it is important that a woman using an IUD limit the number of sexual partners. IUDs are cost-effective, but the initial payment can be quite large and require some problem solving.

STERILIZATION

Sterilization is considered a permanent method of birth control. Sterilization for women can be done by tubal ligation or essure (the insertion of microinserts into the Fallopian tubes to cause scarring and blockage) and for men by performing a vasectomy. Sterilization is one of the most popular methods of birth control in the United States and is highly effective. It is generally not performed on young men and women, especially if the man or woman seeking it has no children. Facts on sterilization can be found at the Planned Parenthood website (see also Alan Guttmacher Institute, 1998).

ABORTION

Historical, Cultural, and Legal Perspectives

Abortion has occurred throughout the ages. In ancient Egypt, Greece, and Rome, herbs or manipulation were used as forms of birth control. In the Middle Ages in Western Europe, abortion was generally accepted in the early months of pregnancy. However, in the United States in the 19th century, opinion about abortion changed, and in 1869, the Roman Catholic Church prohibited abortion under any circumstances (Lagassé, 2003).

Until the last third of the 19th century, when it was criminalized state by state, abortion was legal before "quickening" (approximately the 4th month of pregnancy). Many abortions occurred using herbal tonics and medicinal remedies, some of which proved fatal. The campaign to criminalize abortion was waged by physicians. The American Medical Association's crusade against abortion was partly a professional move, to establish the supremacy of "regular" physicians over midwives and homeopaths (*Atlantic Monthly,* 1997).

By 1900, 49 states had antiabortion laws on the books. Although abortion became illegal in the 1900s, abortions did not stop. Estimates of the number of illegal abortions in the 1950s and 1960s ranged from 200,000 to 1.2 million per year (Gold, 2003).

The number of deaths attributed to these illegal abortions alarmed many people, and a movement began to again legalize abortion. Beginning in 1970, four states—Alaska, Hawaii, New York, and Washington—repealed their antiabortion statutes and generally allowed licensed physicians to perform abortions on request before fetal viability. In 1973, the U.S. Supreme Court legalized abortion in the United States in the case of *Roe v. Wade.* Since *Roe v. Wade,* many laws have been passed that affect access to abortion. For example, some states require parental consent or parental notification before a minor can obtain an abortion, some states require a 24-hour waiting period, and most states do not provide Medicaid coverage for abortion. Although the majority of United States citizens believe abortion should be legal (ABC News/*Washington Post,* 2003), some favor restrictions.

Teaching about Abortion

Children in kindergarten, first, second, and third grades should learn that some women become pregnant when they do not want to or when they are unable to have a child. They also need to know that sometimes babies don't grow or develop right and that women may not bring that baby home (Sex Information and Education Council of the United States [SIECUS], 1996).

Some children may have experience with a late-term abortion due to severe fetal abnormalities and speak about their brother or sister dying. In Grades 4 through 6, children should be taught that some women have babies, some women place a baby for adoption, and some women have abortions. It should be explained that abortions are safe and legal in the United States, and they are performed by licensed professionals. As children go through Grades 7 through 9, more information about abortion should be given: that abortions are provided in some clinics, hospitals, and doctors' offices; that early abortion has few risks or complications; and that no one can force a woman to have an abortion. Teachers may also want to include information on religious beliefs. Some religions forbid abortion; others support a woman's right to choose. Young people need to be aware that abortion is legal but that there are restrictions that could affect their ability to access an abortion (SIECUS, 1996).

Young people in high school should understand that abortion is not a method of contraception. Young people need to learn that men and women share responsibility for contraception and when that fails, both should share the responsibility and the decision making about a pregnancy. They also need to understand that it is ultimately the young woman's decision (except where there is parental consent or notification) whether to continue the pregnancy or not. Lastly, young people should learn that abortion is a legal right and one that could be taken away.

Methods of Abortion

In the first 9 weeks of pregnancy, women who have decided to have an abortion have the option of having a surgical or medical one. A surgical abortion, up to 12 weeks of pregnancy, is most often performed by vacuum aspiration. *Vacuum aspiration* includes dilation of the cervix (stretching of the opening of the uterus) and suctioning (vacuuming) of the uterus. The procedure takes approximately 3 to 5 minutes. *Medical abortion* is an abortion that occurs after ingesting and inserting medications and takes approximately 3 days. The first pill that is swallowed causes the pregnancy to detach from the uterus. The four pills that are inserted 2 days later into the vagina cause the uterus to contract and expel the pregnancy.

Prior to having an abortion, women should receive counseling. Most abortion providers offer counseling that includes information about a woman's options to ensure that she is aware of her choices and that she is making the best decision for herself and her family. The counseling also includes detailed information about available abortion methods (surgical and medical), with a discussion of benefits and risks of the different procedures and possible complications. The purpose of the counseling is to provide women with information that allows them to make informed decisions and consent prior to an abortion. A discussion of follow-up care and contraception also occurs.

EARLY SURGICAL ABORTION
(UP TO 14 WEEKS OF PREGNANCY)

A woman having a surgical abortion will have lab tests performed prior to her procedure. An abortion provider will want to know her Rh status (part of her blood type), hemoglobin, and often weight and height. A Pap smear (culture that checks for ovarian cancer) and tests for sexually transmitted infections may also be performed. Most providers will also want an ultrasound to size the pregnancy accurately. The provider may perform a bimanual pelvic exam to feel the pregnancy in the uterus. Upon completion of these tasks, the provider or anesthetist will begin giving some anesthesia.

A surgical abortion can be performed under local anesthesia, conscious sedation, or general anesthesia. Local anesthesia is given into the cervix so that some of the discomfort during the dilation is decreased; most women will experience cramping and pain during the stretching of the cervix and the evacuation. Conscious sedation is administered through an intravenous tube. It relaxes women and sometimes puts them into a light "sleep." Women may experience cramping and pain with the sedation, although many have no memory of this since conscious sedation can cause an amnesia-type affect. General anesthesia may be given intravenously; with it, women will not feel the procedure or have memory of the procedure. After the procedure, the woman may have some discomfort, most commonly cramping.

As with all surgery, physical complications are possible. However, major complications such as hemorrhage, serious pelvic infection, or a tear in the uterus are very rare, occurring in less than 1 percent of abortions, according to Choice, USA (2002).

Over 88 percent of all abortions performed in the United States are performed in the first 12 weeks of pregnancy. Abortions are the safest when performed early. The mortality rate for abortion is very low: less than one death for every 100,000 abortions. This figure is even lower than the mortality rate for pregnancy in the United States: 7.5 maternal deaths for every 100,000 live births (Choice, USA, 2002).

SECOND-TRIMESTER ABORTION (15–24 WEEKS)

A second-trimester abortion is usually performed over a period of days. Unlike a first-trimester abortion, when the dilation of the cervix takes minutes, a second-trimester abortion requires greater stretching of the cervix, which, in turn, takes more time. On Day 1 of the process, a dilator will be inserted into the cervix. This dilator expands overnight and slowly dilates the cervix. On Day 2, the dilator is removed and the contents of the uterus are removed. This procedure is done with anesthesia. Although complications are still rare, the further into the pregnancy an abortion is performed, the greater the chances for a problem.

THIRD-TRIMESTER ABORTION (BEYOND 24 WEEKS)

Third-trimester abortions are very rare and are most often performed when serious fetal abnormalities or genetic defects are present or when the life of the woman is at risk.

MEDICAL ABORTION

The most common type of medical abortion provided in the United States uses the drug mifepristone, or Mifeprex. Mifeprex can be used up to 63 days from the last menstrual period and is given by a provider who has done all of the preliminary steps listed under surgical abortion (lab tests, ultrasound, and so on). Mifeprex (also known as RU486, or the "abortion pill," and sometimes used to treat several medical conditions, including endometriosis) blocks the hormone progesterone. Without progesterone, the lining of the uterus breaks down, ending the pregnancy. Another drug, misoprostol, is used to cause the uterus to contract and expel the pregnancy.

Methotrexate is another drug that can be used in place of Mifeprex. Methotrexate works a little differently than Mifeprex in that it stops rapidly growing cells (such as pregnancy) from further development. Misoprostol is used with methotrexate and will cause the uterus to contract and expel the pregnancy.

Personal Life Skills. When a woman is faced with an unplanned pregnancy, she will need to use many personal life skills. Her first step in her decision-making process is communication. She will need to communicate with a medical provider, and she will hopefully have supportive relationships. She will need to communicate her feelings about the pregnancy. She may need to put forth a strong argument as to why she has made this decision if she is facing opposition from others.

Decision-making skills have already come into play if a woman is seeking an abortion. Since a woman has the options to parent, place a baby for adoption, and seek an abortion, she will have gone through the decision-making process prior to seeking the abortion. The decisions she now needs to make are the type of procedure to have (medical or surgical) and the type of anesthesia to select (although some of these may be out of her hands if she has progressed too far for a medical abortion, and the provider does not offer all types of anesthesia). Because most providers provide counseling before the abortion, she will receive information that will make the decision-making process easier. Some problem-solving skills may be needed if there are financial, confidentiality, and consent issues. In states that require parental notification, a young woman will need to negotiate the process, especially if she feels she cannot notify a parent.

Other skills that may be used are conflict management skills and stress management skills. A woman having an abortion may be conflicted, especially since most young women never expect to have an abortion. It may be helpful for women to know that 43 percent of women will have had an abortion by the time they are 45 (Modern Contraception, 1998). The stress of the decision-making process, negotiating the health care system, and possibly dealing with keeping the abortion a secret can seem overwhelming. Young women and men should prioritize the various steps and include the support of others. Many young people are afraid to tell a parent about a pregnancy. This fear should be explored to assess how real the consequences of sharing may be. It can be very helpful to have a parent or an adult help with the abortion process, from making the decision, to finding a provider, to paying for the procedure, to accompanying the woman for the abortion.

SUMMARY

Families come in many different sizes. They also consist of numerous variations. It is important for children to understand that their family may look different from their friend's, but they provide the same love and support (for most). As children get older, they may voice a desire for a sibling or start asking questions about babies. Parents and teachers can start the dialogue with simple nonjudgmental lessons about families and decisions.

As children develop, they will ask more questions and demand more detail. Young children will accept that babies come from their mother's stomach, but older children will not. This chapter on contraception and abortion provides age-appropriate guidance about when and how to discuss challenging issues regarding family size, decision making, contraception, and abortion.

Many adolescents will require information about sexuality, sexual activity, and contraception and abortion for themselves. Studies show that many high school students are sexually active and that comprehensive sexuality education can help students postpone sexual activity and assist them in making informed decisions and choices when they do become sexually active.

WEBSITES

Alan Guttmacher Institute (AGI):
    www.guttmacher.org
AGI Review of Contraception by State:
    www.guttmacher.org/pubs/state_data/
    index.html
AGI Report on Contraception and Abortion:
    www.agi-usa.org/pubs/ib19.html
Planned Parenthood Federation of America:
    www.ppfa.org
Planned Parenthood Federation of America,
    Emergency Contraception:
    www.plannedparenthood.org/ec
LifeNews.com Pro Life Community:
    www.prolifeinfo.org
National Right to Life: www.nrlc.org
NARAL Pro-Choice America: www.naral.org

Advocates for Youth:
    www.advocatesforyouth.org
Pro-Choice America:
    www.prochoice america.org
Sexuality Information and Education Council
    of the United States: www.siecus.org
Contraception: An International Journal:
    www.arhp.org
Office of Population Research, Princeton
    University: www.ec.princeton.edu
Office of Population Affairs:
    www.opa.osophs. dhhs.gov
Go Ask Alice:
    www.goaskalice.columbia.edu/
    2349.htm

REFERENCES

ABC News/*Washington Post.* (2003). *Conditional support poll: Thirty years after Roe vs. Wade, American support is conditional.* Horsham, PA: TNS Intersearch. Available online: http://abcnews.go.com/ sections/ us/DailyNews/abortion_poll030122.html.

Alan Guttmacher Institute. (1994). *Sex and America's teenagers.* New York: Author.

Alan Guttmacher Institute. (1998). Trends in contraceptive use in the U.S. *Family Planning Perspectives, 30*(1). New York: Author.

Alan Guttmacher Institute. (1999). *Facts in brief: Teen sex and pregnancy.* New York: Author. Available online: www.guttmacher .org/pubs/fb_teen_sex.html.

Atlantic Monthly. (1997, May). Abortion in America's history. *279*(5), 111–115. Available online: www.theatlantic.com/ issues/97may/abortion.htm.

Catholic Answers. (2001). *The divinity of Christ.* Available online: www.catholic .com/library/Birth_Control.asp.

Center for Family and Demographic Research. (2002). *Ohio population news: Marriage in U.S. and Ohio.* Bowling Green, OH: Bowling Green State University. Available online: www.bgsu.edu/ organizations/ cfdr/ohiopop/ opn8.pdf.

Choice, USA. (2002). *Surgical abortion.* Available online: www.choiceusa.org/facts/ surgical.php.htm.

Cycle Technologies. (2003). *Plan or prevent pregnancy naturally.* Washington, DC: Institute of Reproductive Health of Georgetown University. Available online: www. cyclebeads.com.

Daillard, C. (2003). Understanding abstinence: Implications for individuals, programs and policies. *Guttmacher Report, 6*(5). Available online: www.guttmacher.org/pubs/ journals/gr060504.html.

Family Education Network. (2002). Birth control: History of the birth control movement. *Columbia Electronic Encyclopedia.* Available online: www.factmonster.com/ ce6/sci/A0856928.html.

Gold, R. B. (2003). *The Guttmacher report on public policy.* Available online: www.agi-usa.org/pubs/ib_5-03.html.

Grimes, D. (2000). History and future of contraception: Development over time. *Contraception Report, 10*(6), 15–25.

Grimes, D., & Wallach, M. (1997). *Modern contraception.* Warren, NJ: Emron.

Haffner, D. W., & Yarber, W. L. (1996). *National Guidelines Task Force guidelines for comprehensive sexuality education* (2nd ed.). New York: Sex Information and Education Council of the United States.

Hatcher, R., Trussell, J., Stewart, F., Cates, W., Stewart, G., Guest, F., & Kowal, D. (1998). *Contraceptive technology* (17th ed.). New York: Ardent Media.

Lagassé, P. (Ed.). (2003). History of abortion. In *The Columbia encyclopedia* (6th ed.). New York: Columbia University Press. Available online: www.encyclopedia.com/ html/section/abortion_HistoryofAbortion .asp.

Modern contraception. (1998, January/ February). *Family Planning Perspectives, 30*(1), 1–20.

Modi, M. 2000. National Longitudinal Study of Adolescent Health, Surveys measuring well-being. Available online: www.prince ton.edu/Nkling/surveys/Addhealth.html.

Muhammad bin Abdul-Aziz Al-Musnad. (2003). *Information from Islamic fatawa regarding women*. Available online: www.themuslimwoman.com/offspring/ birthcontrol.htm.

Ortho-McNeil Pharmaceuticals. (2003). *Frequently asked questions: Ortho Evra.*

Available online:www.orthoevra.com/ faqs/faqs.htm.

Planned Parenthood Federation of America. (1998–2003a). *Diaphragms*. Available online: www.plannedparenthood.org/bc/ Diaphragms.htm.

Planned Parenthood Federation of America. (1998–2003b). *Female condom*. Available online: www.plannedparenthood. org/bc/ bc facts16.html#FEMALECONDOM.

Planned Parenthood Federation of America. (2003). *Fact sheet*, Griswold v. Connecticut—*The impact of legal birth control and the challenges that remain*. Available online: www.plannedparenthood.org/ library/facts/griswoldone.html.

Princeton University. (2000). *Contraception*. Available online: www.princeton.edu/ puhs/SECH/contraception.html.

Sex Information and Education Council of the United States. (1996). *Guidelines for comprehensive sexuality education* (2nd ed.). New York: Author. Available online: www. advocatesforyouth.org/teens/health/ contraceptives/withdrawal.htm.

Tapestry Health. (2003). *Paragard IUD*. Available online: www.tapestryhealth.org/ services/paragard.html/#conditions.

LEARNING EXPERIENCES

This chapter contains detailed information about contraception and abortion. Educators (both teachers and parents) can use the information to tailor learning experiences that are appropriate and accurate for the young people with whom they work and live. These activities prepare students with knowledge and skills related to contraception and abortion. Specifically, students will

- Express that individuals need to decide to or not to have children.
- Be able to make personal decisions about birth control and abortion.
- Be able to communicate their decisions to a partner.
- Know that there are choices people make when they experience an unintended pregnancy.
- Explain the circumstances under which abortion is a legal choice.
- Know that some belief systems do not support abortion as a choice.
- Be able to identify and describe the various methods of birth control.
- Clarify their own attitudes and values regarding birth control and abortion.
- Identify family planning and abortion resources for information and services.

LEARNING EXPERIENCE 1

TITLE: "No!"

GRADE LEVELS: K–3

TIME REQUIREMENTS: Total time: 90 minutes; 30 minutes per session

LEARNING CONTEXT
Students will develop communication/refusal skills. Following this activity, students will
- Know that it is all right to say no.
- Have some skills and practice in saying no.
- Know that it is important to tell someone when someone is trying to engage them in an unwanted activity.

NATIONAL LEARNING STANDARD
5: Students will demonstrate the ability to use interpersonal communication skills to enhance health.

PROCEDURE
Ask the children to share all the things they do to prepare for school. The list will include activities such as getting dressed, brushing teeth, and eating breakfast. The teacher can add others (making the bed, washing one's face, and so forth). Make sure the children include activities that also got them to school by asking, "Did you walk to the bus stop? Did you take the bus? Did someone drive you to school?"

Once the list is completed, add some variables and ask additional questions:
- If you got up late this morning, could you have skipped getting dressed? Your mom told you not to forget to brush your teeth. Is it OK to skip brushing your teeth?
- You're waiting at the bus stop and a stranger stops in his car and asks if you want a ride in his car to school. What would you say? Who would you tell?
- Your dad is driving you to school, and you don't feel like buckling your seatbelt. Is it okay to drive in the car without it?
- Our friend on the bus keeps running in the aisle while the bus is moving. She says, "Come on!" What do you say?
- Your grandma wants a kiss, but you don't want to kiss her. What do you say?

Each time these (or similar) questions are asked, the students will respond with "No!" Continue asking about everyday occurrences interspersed with events that can endanger or harm children, and have them practice saying no.

The second and third sessions will follow the same pattern. The second session will focus on activities to which their parent(s), guardian, or other person say no. Ask, "Tell me some things you ask to do that your mom says no to. Why do you think you are told no?" The children will learn that people often say no so no harm is done.

The third session will focus on activities to which children should say no. Again, ask the students to share activities/events that could be harmful or dangerous. Begin with an example from the first session: "If someone stops his car and asks if you want a ride, what do you say (or do)?"

All sessions should include a discussion about children telling a parent or adult when something happens that frightens them.

INSTRUCTIONAL/ENVIRONMENTAL MODIFICATIONS
Teachers are aware of the differences among their students' families and should use appropriate language, such as "Uncle Mike" instead of "Dad."

RESOURCES
Movies and books teach children to say no that can be incorporated into this learning experience. In addition, organizations do programs for young children on how to say no (whether it is to drugs, strangers, and so on).

ASSESSMENT PLAN
Teachers will periodically ask students questions that contain harmful scenarios and have the children practice saying, "No!" Reinforcing this learning is important.

REFLECTION
Children age 5 to 8 learn refusal skills early with the hope that they will be able to say no to someone trying to touch them inappropriately or snatch them. We also teach children to say no to drugs (and candy from strangers). These refusal skills can be translated as they get older into refusal skills involving drugs, smoking, and sex. Saying no can help young people to be abstinent—the first contraceptive method discussed in this chapter.

LEARNING EXPERIENCE 2

TITLE: Families

GRADE LEVELS: K–3

TIME REQUIREMENTS: 1 hour

LEARNING CONTEXT

This learning experience develops communication/refusal skills and decision-making/problem-solving skills. Following the activity, students will

- Learn that families consist of different sizes and that some families have children, some do not.
- Understand that families can decide their size.
- Learn that children should be loved and wanted and they need families to take care of them.

NATIONAL LEARNING STANDARDS

5: Students will demonstrate the ability to use interpersonal communication skills to enhance health.

7: Students will demonstrate the ability to advocate for personal, family, and community health.

PROCEDURE

Ask students to describe their families and to bring in or draw an illustration or picture(s) of them as a homework assignment. Point out the similarities and differences among the students, focusing on family size and discussing the reasons families may be large or small. There will be no pictures of families without children, so ask whether children have aunts or uncles or friends who don't have children. Some families will have babies, and the discussion can consider how some families are still growing and some will remain the current size. This learning experience will contain information that was learned during both the contraception and abortion sections of the chapter.

During the learning experience, focus on differences found in families. Share that families come in all shapes and sizes but that their primary function is the same: to take care of and love one another. Ask students about ways that their families show their love of one another. This exercise can be done during a reading circle after reading a book about families. A reading circle is more intimate and supportive than sitting at individual desks or tables, and students may be more comfortable sharing family stories.

INSTRUCTIONAL/ENVIRONMENTAL MODIFICATIONS

Teachers need to be prepared for all variations of families, including ones headed by a grandparent and ones that consist of two mothers or two fathers. They also must recognize that some students may not be in a healthy family receiving the love and attention that is being discussed.

ASSESSMENT PLAN

As children learn about each other and about families, they will see how communities are created and how they care about each other. Children may ask how someone's new sister is or how a child's grandmother is. As they express interest in each other, the lesson of creating families and caring for children will be evident.

LEARNING EXPERIENCE 3

TITLE: My Family Is Growing

GRADE LEVELS: 4–6

TIME REQUIREMENTS: 1 hour

LEARNING CONTEXT
Communication/refusal and decision-making/problem-solving skills are developed in this lesson. Following this activity, students will
- Learn that families can decide how large they will be by choosing among the options of parenting, abortion, and adoption.
- Know that some religions believe abortion is wrong and others believe in a woman's right to choose.

NATIONAL LEARNING STANDARD
4:   Students will begin to learn the steps that will allow them to analyze the influence of culture, media, technology, and other factors on health.

PROCEDURE
Students in Grades 4 through 6 may have experience with a new baby joining their family or someone close to them. Ask students about their families and whether any students are going to have a baby sister or brother (if there are no siblings expected, ask whether any student would like a baby brother or sister). Invite students to share their feelings about having a new brother or sister. All students can share their thoughts about having a baby brother or sister, whether one is expected or not. Guide the students into a discussion about the changes that will occur in the family that is growing.

As the learning experience continues, ask for other ways in which families can grow, and begin a discussion about adoption. Ask students whether they know anyone who is adopted or of a family who has adopted a baby. Then pose additional questions about family size:
- Why do you think some families don't have children?
- Why do some have one child? Why do some have two? Or three?
- Why are some families very big, with more than 10 children?
- Can families decide their size? How?
- What makes some families decide to have few children and some many?
- What may influence a family's decision about family size?

Encourage students to answer the questions and explain their answers. They may need assistance in listing some of the factors that determine family size, such as income, religion, and culture. Some children may be ready to learn about abortion, and some children may already be aware of abortion. Inform the students that some families choose to have an abortion because they feel that it is best for their family and that a doctor helps them, just like one does when a family is having a baby.

INSTRUCTIONAL/ENVIRONMENTAL MODIFICATIONS

Any discussion about abortion can cause upset with students (as well as upset with parents), depending on what they have been taught about abortion, and can jeopardize a teacher's position. A teacher can state that some families decide not to have any more children without explaining how that may occur.

RESOURCES

Several books about adoption can be used during this lesson. One such book was written by Fred Rogers (of *Mr. Rogers' Neighborhood*) called *Let's Talk about It: Adoption* (New York: Putnam, 1994). Other books or videos can be used to facilitate this learning experience.

LEARNING EXPERIENCE 4

TITLE: I Want a Sister (but My Mom Said No)

GRADE LEVEL: 4–6

TIME REQUIREMENTS: Two 30-minute sessions

LEARNING CONTEXT

This learning experience develops communication/refusal skills as well as decision-making/problem-solving skills. Following this activity, students will

- Learn that many factors impact on a family's size.
- Know that some religions don't approve of the use of contraception, others do, and that some women and men use contraception.

NATIONAL LEARNING STANDARD

6:   Students will demonstrate the ability to use goal-setting and decision-making skills to enhance health.

PROCEDURE

Students will learn that moms and dads make many family decisions, including decisions about having babies. Some young people desire a baby and ask their mom or dad for one: "I want a baby sister!" Some children may know that their mother uses birth control, and others just know that there is no baby sister on the way.

List the factors that impact a family's decision to have children. The list may include financial reasons, the size of the current family (it may be just right), an illness in the family, careers that don't allow for more children at this time, inability to get pregnant, lack of a partner (a single mother may not have a sexual partner), or lack of desire to have children. Students should be encouraged to add to the list.

During the activity, ask the students whether they know how moms prevent having a baby, and build on the students' replies. Students will learn that some people use contraception so they can decide whether and when to get pregnant. Students will also learn that although many people use birth control, some don't because their religion doesn't approve.

Ask students to ask their mother or father (or grandparent, other relative, or guardian) about their family size. Is it going to stay the same? Will it get bigger? Has Mom decided how many children she wants? What made the family decide on its size?

ASSESSMENT PLAN

Once the students have questioned their family/guardian, the next class session will allow the teacher to evaluate whether children and families can have an open and honest discussion about having babies versus not having babies. All children know when their mother is having a baby, but we don't often hear about discussions that include why mom is not having a baby.

REFLECTION

This activity is designed to have students begin to communicate about issues that are not always discussed in a family. Parents want to participate in the education of their children on sexual issues, and this learning experience provides an easy place to start. Parents don't have to share information that they are uncomfortable with (such as their method of birth control), but they can discuss how they feel about their family and having babies. Students will share their families' response with the class, with the teacher leading the discussion.

LEARNING EXPERIENCE 5

TITLE: Consequences

GRADE LEVELS: 7–9

TIME REQUIREMENTS: Two 45-minute sessions

LEARNING CONTEXT

Following this activity, which develops communication/refusal skills, students will

- Understand that all actions have consequences and what looks fun and glamorous may also be harmful and dangerous.
- Practice saying no.
- Have skills to discuss difficult issues with a parent/adult.

NATIONAL LEARNING STANDARDS

4: Students will analyze the influence of culture, media, technology, and other factors on health.

6: Students will demonstrate the ability to use goal-setting and decision-making skills to enhance health.

PROCEDURE

Ask students to share their thoughts on images they see or things they hear in the media that look and sound funny and exciting, even glamorous, but have potentially serious consequences. For example, students may have seen an advertisement for beer on television that has a group of young people in their 20s laughing and having fun in a bar. The commercial shows only positive images of drinking beer; ask the students for some of the negatives to drinking.

Then encourage students to discuss experiences from their families' and friends' lives. For example, lying to one's parents about one's whereabouts may seem funny and exciting—until one is caught. Actions have consequences, and students need to understand this. The students should come up with a list of images that are glamorous and the resulting consequences that aren't shown or talked about by the media (television shows are a good source of examples).

In the next session, students will share a picture or describe an image selected from the media that illustrates something glamorous. They will then tell a story about the picture or image that includes an ending (such as what happened to the people when they left the bar after drinking?). Ask the other students whether they want to add to the story and share other possible consequences; they don't all have to be negative.

During both sessions, explore the consequences with the students and discuss ways to avoid the negative ones. Also speak about the pressures that students encounter to engage in risky behavior such as drinking and lying, and strategies that students can use to avoid them. Strategies that students can use are avoiding the situation, saying no, and talking with an adult about the pressures.

Students will keep a journal of images they see that, upon closer inspection, could have serious consequences. They will write their thoughts and feelings about these images. They will also write in their journals about pressure that they feel personally or experience through others. The teacher will ask students to share these experiences throughout the year and spend some time on problem solving so that students can develop their own strategies to avoid negative consequences.

ASSESSMENT PLAN

Journals will be reviewed and graded for content, clarity, grammar, spelling, and so forth.

LEARNING EXPERIENCE 6

TITLE: What Is Abortion?

GRADE LEVELS: 7–9

TIME REQUIREMENTS: 90 minutes

LEARNING CONTEXT

This learning experience develops communication/refusal skills, decision-making/problem-solving skills, resource management skills, and conflict management skills. Following this activity, students will

- Learn that abortion is safe and legal in the United States, but there are some restrictions depending on where one lives.
- Know some religions believe that abortion is wrong and others believe in a woman's right to choose.
- Know that no one can force a woman to have an abortion.

NATIONAL LEARNING STANDARD

4:   Students will analyze the influence of culture, media, technology, and other factors on health.

PROCEDURE

Prior to beginning this learning experience, explain to the students that there are many differing views on abortion, and this lesson will not focus on the moral aspect of abortion. This lesson is to give factual information about abortion. It will not touch on those aspects that have no clear-cut answer, such as when life begins. Ask the students what they know about abortion, clarify some information, and dispel myths and misinformation.

During the discussion, list the information that students state into two columns, one called "Facts" and one called "Myths." A third column labeled "Agree to Disagree" for the issues that have differing opinions will go there. Information that should be listed under "Facts" include that abortion is legal in the United States, there are restrictions to abortion—some states require parental consent or notification, abortion is performed by professionals, abortion is safe, no one can be forced to have an abortion, some religions forbid abortion except for specific circumstances, and some religions believe in a woman's right to choose.

Some myths are abortion is dangerous (having a baby carries more risk than having an abortion), abortion is not legal, abortions are performed in secret and dangerous places, all religions forbid abortion, and young people cannot have an abortion without their parent's permission (all states that require parental consent or notification have a judicial bypass).

Arrange the class in small groups, and ask students to develop a story about a woman who chooses to have an abortion. They will share her decision-making process with the class and explain her reason(s) for choosing to terminate her pregnancy. The story should contain factual information, but it can include some of the contentious issues in relation to her decision-making process. For instance, a Catholic woman who has always believed abortion to be wrong may make her decision to have an abortion with that belief foremost in her mind.

An important trait that students can learn during this exercise is empathy. One should not have to experience something to understand or feel the emotions that another may feel going through the actual experience.

Many women don't "believe in abortion" until they are pregnant with an unplanned, unexpected pregnancy. Developing scenarios of women who choose to have an abortion may provide insight into the process women go through to make this decision and the reasons women have abortions.

INSTRUCTIONAL/ENVIRONMENTAL MODIFICATIONS
Teachers will need to stay close to their lesson plan during this exercise; otherwise, it could become a debate on abortion.

RESOURCES
Useful resources about abortion can be found on the Internet at www.naral.org or www.plannedparenthood.org.

REFLECTION
Students in Grades 7–9 may have some knowledge of abortion from the experience of a friend or family member, through the teachings of their religion, from the teachings of their family, or through the media. Abortion is a difficult subject to teach because it is such a contentious issue throughout the United States. However, the fact that almost one in every two women will have an abortion in her lifetime speaks to the need for young people to have information about abortion. At the least, young people should have their questions answered.

LEARNING EXPERIENCE 7

TITLE: Decisions! Decisions!

GRADE LEVELS: 10–12

TIME REQUIREMENTS: 1 hour

LEARNING CONTEXT

This learning experience will include information from both the contraception and abortion sections of the chapter. Students will explore the various methods of birth control and the different abortion methods so that they can make the best decisions for themselves, their families, and other special people in their lives.

Decision-making/problem-solving skills and conflict management skills are developed in the following learning experience. Following this activity, students will

- Understand that making good informed decisions requires factual information.
- Understand that many factors influence decisions.
- Obtain insight into why people choose one option over another.

NATIONAL LEARNING STANDARDS

5: Students will demonstrate the ability to use interpersonal communication skills to enhance health.

6: Students will demonstrate the ability to use goal-setting and decision-making skills to enhance health.

PROCEDURE

Either develop scenarios or ask the students to develop scenarios (the number should be based on the number of students—the more students, the fewer the scenarios) prior to the session that include issues of sexual activity, contraception, pregnancy, and abortion. Each scenario requires a decision, and the teacher will ask students to choose a decision and to explain their reasoning. Depending on the time and size of the group, all students can give their reasons, or a select few per scenario will share their reasons. Here are some examples of scenarios:

> You are 16 years old and have been going out with your boyfriend for 2 years. You and he have begun having sex and want to use contraception. He says he'll use a condom, but you want to use the pill. What do you use?

> Your best friend is 6 weeks pregnant and has decided to have an abortion. She isn't sure whether to have a surgical abortion or a medical abortion. Which should she have? Why?

> You and your girlfriend have been using condoms and the condom broke. What do you do?

The students should make their decisions based on the information they learned about contraception and abortion. This activity has no right or wrong answers.

ASSESSMENT PLAN

The teacher will assess the students' acquisition of the content through their responses, decisions, and ability to identify the pros, cons, advantages, and disadvantages sought in the activity.

LEARNING EXPERIENCE 8

TITLE: Contraception

GRADE LEVELS: 10–12

TIME REQUIREMENTS: Two 45-minute sessions

LEARNING CONTEXT

This learning experience develops communication/refusal, decision-making/problem-solving, conflict management, stress management, and resource management skills. Following the activity, students will

- Have knowledge of the available birth control methods.
- Assess which method is best for different circumstances.

NATIONAL LEARNING STANDARDS

2: Students will demonstrate the ability to access valid health information and health-promoting products and services.

6: Students will demonstrate the ability to use goal-setting and decision-making skills to enhance health.

PROCEDURE

During the first session, educate the students about the various methods of birth control available in the United States. Share with the students resources that are available for additional information about the methods (such as books, websites, and medical journals). Students will be assigned a group and a method of birth control. During a specified period of time, each group will research their method and create a presentation to "sell their product." Each group will make a presentation to the class using various media (posters, PowerPoint presentations, handouts, and so forth) that will provide all the information necessary for students to make informed decisions about their birth control method.

INSTRUCTIONAL/ENVIRONMENTAL MODIFICATIONS

Presentations will use the available technology in the school and the community. The time frame for preparing the presentation may need to be longer if access to the Internet is limited. Students may not be able to use various media if the technology is not available, such as a laptop computer for a PowerPoint presentation.

RESOURCES

Any search engine on the Internet will provide numerous sites for contraception research. Students just need to type in "birth control" or "contraception." Planned Parenthood's website (www.plannedparenthood.org) is a great source for information, as is Advocates for Youth (www.advocatesforyouth.org).

ASSESSMENT PLAN

The teacher will grade the presentations on accuracy, thoroughness, clarity and understanding. Is the material accurate? Did it include all the elements? At the end of all the presentations, the teacher will create a test based on the information contained in the presentations and assess the students' learning by how well they perform on the test.

SEXUALLY TRANSMITTED INFECTIONS AND HIV/AIDS

RHONA FEIGENBAUM AND ANDRINA VEIT

OBJECTIVES

After reading this chapter, students will be able to

1. Describe how the human immune system fights disease.
2. Describe the various sexually transmitted infections and sexually related diseases, including HIV/AIDS.
3. Discuss modes of transmission, type of infection, symptoms, diagnosis, and treatment of specific STIs, including HIV/AIDS.
4. Describe methods of prevention, including life skills.
5. Examine social attitudes and fears that prevent open communication about STIs and thus contribute to continuing epidemics.
6. Identify resources in the community that provide information and health services.

REFLECTIVE QUESTIONS

Elementary School
1. If I share my friend's lunch, will I become infected?
2. My friend scraped his knee in soccer today, and the coach said, "Do not touch his blood." Why?
3. Do children become infected with HIV? How?
4. Can I get AIDS from kissing?
5. Can I get infected from having oral sex?
6. Does everyone who becomes infected with HIV die?

Middle School
1. How do I know if someone has AIDS?
2. Can I become infected from just one sexual encounter?

3. Is it true that most people with AIDS are homosexual?
4. Are condoms 100 percent effective in preventing the transmission of HIV?
5. Can I get infected by having oral sex?

High School
1. Do most people with HIV get AIDS?
2. How long from infection to AIDS?
3. Can an infected woman ever have a baby safely?
4. Do all infected people get AIDS?
5. Do all people with AIDS die from one of the opportunistic diseases?
6. If I am not homosexual, what is the likelihood of my getting infected with HIV?

——————— **SCENARIO 1** ———————

John and Mary are high school seniors. They have been dating for almost 2 years. Recently, they decided to begin having sex. Since this would be their first sexual experience, they decided that it would be a good idea for Mary to take birth control pills. They would not have to worry about an unplanned pregnancy. However, one night Mary goes to a party without John, drinks too much, and has sex with someone at the party. A month later John begins to feel a painful burning sensation when he urinates. He goes for a medical examination and discovers that he has chlamydia.

How did this happen?
What should John do now?
How should he tell Mary?

——————— **SCENARIO 2** ———————

Manuel is a ninth grade student. His mother has been very unhappy lately because her sister, Aunt Carmella, is dying of AIDS. The family is embarrassed, and they don't want anyone to know what is wrong with Carmella. It is the family secret. Manuel had heard his mother telling his aunt that she should have been more careful with her boyfriends, and she would not have gotten AIDS.

Manuel and Henrietta have been going out for more than 6 months, and their relationship is becoming closer and closer. There is lots of pressure to have sex—"all of their friends are doing it." Manuel is panicked about getting infected with AIDS because he sees how sick his aunt is. He doesn't want to tell Henrietta why he has been avoiding her.

What would you do if you were Manuel?
What can Manuel say to Henrietta?
Does Manuel really have anything to be afraid of? Can he become infected with AIDS? Can he infect Henrietta with AIDS?
What do both of them need to know about HIV so that they will not become infected?

INTRODUCTION

It is the goal of sexuality educators to reinforce the notion that sexual behavior among consenting adults is a healthy, natural, and pleasurable experience. It is also their responsibility to arm students with the skills and information with which to maintain their sexual health. The connection between sexual behavior, illness, and death especially associated with sexually transmitted infections (STIs) is an important component of sexuality education. All too often this becomes the focus of such programs. How does one provide students with the information and skills necessary to assure that they protect themselves, with a positive, empowering message without creating fears? In this chapter, we will attempt to provide the prospective teacher with the sociomedical information about STIs, allay the myths and misconceptions that interfere with prevention, and introduce the potentially protective life skills that they, in turn, can use in teaching young people, in the context of a health-maintaining model.

Adolescents are an especially vulnerable population. They cannot easily make the connection between illness, death, and sexual intercourse. Moreover, they "magically" believe that only "dirty" people get STIs (Powell, 1996) or people who are in "every way" different from themselves, particularly by race or culture. They also believe one can detect someone who has "it" (an STI). Furthermore, they believe that if they had "it," they would have symptoms, all of which constitute mythical thinking. Many cases of STIs are asymptomatic or have few symptoms and thus may go untested and untreated. Moreover, STIs can lead to serious long-term health problems for both women and men.

Adolescents are a risk-taking bunch, functioning on the notion that "it can't happen to me" in many aspects of their lives. This idea is probably among their best assets, when carefully harnessed. Taking chances on new and exciting things is what moves us ahead, motivating us to accept challenge, but knowing which chances are worth taking and minimizing the risks take some knowledge and maturity. And, when it comes to STIs, one can, with knowledge and skills, practically eliminate the risks entirely.

STIs fall into the category of communicable diseases. This means they are transmissible from one individual to another primarily through sexual activity. There are approximately 25 diseases that fall under this category (Sexuality Information and Education Council of the United States [SIECUS], 2003). STIs are caused by infectious agents such as viruses or bacteria. Some are curable but, upon exposure, can be contracted more than once. Some remain dormant, and infected people live with the illness for the rest of their lives. Still others cannot be treated and will die as a result. Besides being life-threatening, the more common complications from STIs range from pelvic inflammatory diseases (PID), sterility, and health complications in babies born from infected pregnant women. The immune system plays a determining role in the disease's etiology, prognosis, and treatment.

SOME IMPORTANT DATA

STIs are a significant health problem in the United States. An estimated 15 million people become infected each year with one or more STIs, and 65 million people live with one that is incurable (SIECUS, 2003). One in four sexually active adolescents will be at risk for giving and/or getting an STI, resulting in 3 million teens between the ages of 15 and 19 infected each year in the United States (Eng & Butler, 1997). Teens are becoming infected more frequently than young adults, and they represent more than one-fifth of all cases nationally (Hedgepeth & Helmich, 1996).

Several factors increase the risks for infection with STIs among sexually active young people, including the use of alcohol and other drugs, multiple partnering, and lack of condom use. During 2001, almost 43 percent of females and 49 percent of males, ages 15 to 19, had sexual intercourse. Of the students who ever had sexual intercourse, only slightly more than 50 percent of the females and 35 percent of the males used a condom at last intercourse. Although a considerable decrease in the number of students who ever had sexual intercourse (16 percent) and those who had multiple partners (24 percent) is being observed among upper-level high school students over a 10-year period, no decreases were found among younger high school students (9th and 10th graders). Moreover, the younger the age of initiation, the more likely for multiple partners—hence, the more likely for exposure to an STI. Furthermore, there is an increase in the number of teens who used alcohol or other drugs when participating in sexual activity—20 percent of females and 30 percent of males (Centers for Disease Control and Prevention [CDC], 2002)—rendering them less likely to make safer sexual decisions. But our educational efforts over the last decade seem to be having a positive impact on adolescent sexual behavior. Nevertheless, we still have a long way to go.

HOW THE IMMUNE SYSTEM WORKS

The body has an elaborate defense system against a wide variety of pathogens (agents) and chemicals that may damage or destroy it. Normally this system is effective in keeping out unwanted foreign matter and often keeps people from contracting the associated diseases. A brief description of the immune system is necessary to understand how the various sexually transmitted diseases occur.

FIRST LINE OF DEFENSE

In the first barrier, hair follicles in the nose trap dust and other particles, preventing them from getting into the respiratory system. Small cilia in the nasal passages and trachea direct debris outward and trap it in mucous secretions that are expelled by coughing, blowing the nose, or swallowing (in which case the foreign matter will be destroyed or eliminated by the digestive system). Thus, by keeping out most potential invaders, the skin (when unbroken) and mucous membranes constitute the first line of defense.

SECOND LINE OF DEFENSE

If foreign matter gets past the skin and mucous membranes, chemical barriers go to work. These consist of digestive enzymes and acids in the stomach that kill bacteria and break down unwanted chemicals. Tears, sweat, skin oils, saliva, and mucus also contain enzymes that can kill pathogens. In addition, the kidneys are continually washing out bacteria that are killed by the acidity of urine and eliminating metabolized chemicals.

THIRD LINE OF DEFENSE

When pathogens get past the first and second lines of defense, the immune system comes into play. It is on constant alert for foreign substances that might threaten the body and swings into action when needed. More than a dozen different types of white blood cells make up the immune system and are concentrated in the organs of the lymphatic system. By way of blood and lymph vessels, these white blood cells patrol the entire body.

The immune system has four stages:

1. *Recognition of the invading pathogen:* Specialized white blood cells called *phagocytes* and *macrophages* confront the foreign substances, called *antigens,* and attempt to engulf them. At the same time, they call upon helper *T cells* (a type of white blood cell that originates in the thymus gland) to identify the antigens.
2. *Rapid replication of T cells and B cells:* The *helper T cells* alert *B cells* (white blood cells that originate in the bone marrow), which are transformed into plasma cells that produce antibodies capable of destroying a specific organism.
3. *Attack by killer T cells and macrophages:* Alerted by the helper T cells, the *killer T cells* and macrophages can now search out the targeted organisms and kill them.
4. *Memory and suppression of the immune response:* Two other white blood cells, *memory T cells* and *suppressor T cells,* become activated. The memory T cells "remember" the specific antigen, and, if ever that antigen gains entry into the body again, the memory T cells will respond more quickly by alerting the immune system to the presence of the antigen. This is called *acquired immunity,* because the body has developed an antibody system against that specific antigen. Once the battle against any foreign substance is won, the suppressor T cells halt the production of antibodies by B cells, and the body returns to homeostasis.

Acquired immunity also can be conferred through vaccination, in which an injection of killed or weakened pathogens that cause a specific disease stimulates the body to build antibodies specific to it. For example, people are vaccinated against the polio virus with killed pathogens. This approach has nearly eliminated polio. Vaccination programs and their large-scale availability are important in containing and eliminating serious infectious diseases (Weinstein & Rosen, 2003).

SEXUALLY TRANSMITTED INFECTIONS (STIs)

Sexually transmitted infections are transmitted from an infected person to an uninfected person through an exchange of body fluids (blood-to-blood contact and sometimes through the sharing of contaminated needles during intravenous drug use). The organisms that cause STIs all have an affinity for mucous membranes such as those that line the reproductive organs. Transmission usually requires direct contact between genital areas and other areas (including the mouth, eyes, and throat) that have moist, mucoid linings and access to the blood supply. Mucous membranes, such as the lining of the uterus, provide an ideal environment for these organisms to grow and multiply. Some also grow and multiply in the bloodstream.

The incidence of STIs has been increasing steadily, in some cases to epidemic proportions. Common STIs are Candidiasis, trichomoniasis, chlamydia, gonorrhea, syphilis, crabs (pubic lice), genital herpes, hepatitis B, genital warts, and HIV/AIDS. STIs are mostly bacterial or viral: *bacterial*-induced STIs are treatable and curable; *viral*-induced STIs are treatable. Young people who are sexually active are contracting these diseases with great frequency and for many reasons, not the least of which is because they do not believe that they are susceptible.

Once again, educating children about prevention is the first step in giving them control over their health and susceptibility. The second step is their ability to make decisions and choices about behaviors that will keep them healthy. Knowledge about treatments is the third step in the process of protecting children and adults from these diseases.

Some infections of the genitals may or may not be sexually transmitted. For example, yeast and fungal organisms are found naturally in the reproductive tract or genitals. With bacteria, sometimes an imbalance can occur from taking antibiotics destroying the "good" bacteria that can maintain health while leaving the "bad" bacteria to fester. When this imbalance exists, symptoms similar to those of an STI may be present—an abnormal discharge from the vagina or a burning and itching sensation in the genital area, especially when urinating. These "imbalances" are actually infections that can be treated and cured with appropriate medication. However, if one has sexual intercourse or oral sex when a yeast or fungal infection is present, they can be transmitted sexually. Similarly, crabs (pubic lice) and scabies (mites) are also highly contagious and can be transmitted by using the same towel as someone infected as well as from sexual activity.

What follows is a brief description of several of the more common STIs, their symptoms, modes of transmission, and treatment approaches.

Candidiasis (Yeast Infection)

This is a type of *vaginitis*—any inflammation of the vagina—specifically, *Monilia vaginitis,* caused by an overgrowth of *Candida albicans,* a yeast-like fungus. It is not usually sexually transmitted. Symptoms include a thick, curdlike, white discharge associated with vaginal itching and irritation. Diagnosis is made by visualizing yeast buds and hyphae under a low-power microscope. Cultures are not indicated (Feigenbaum & McCarthy, 1987).

There are many ways to treat yeast infections, including vaginal tablets and cream and oral fluconazole (Crooks & Bauer, 2002).

Certain conditions can predispose to yeast infections. These include antibiotic use, pregnancy, oral contraceptives, and diabetes (Feigenbaum & McCarthy, 1987).

MODE OF TRANSMISSION

- Candidiasis is a spontaneous infection, not usually transmitted by sexual activity

Chlamydia

Chlamydia is a sexually transmitted infection caused by a bacteria (*Chlamydia trachmomatis*). Four million new cases are diagnosed per year (King, 2002)—50 percent more than people who contract gonorrhea. Chlamydia is the major cause of mucopurulent cervicitis in the female and nongonoccal urethritis in the male. Left untreated, chlamydia can lead to pelvic inflammatory disease (PID) and possible infertility in men and women. It can also cause epididymitis in males, although this is a much rarer occurrence.

People who are most at risk for chlamydia are under the age of 24, who have multiple sexual partners, who do not use a barrier method of birth control (condom or diaphragm), and/or whose partners have had chlamydia or other STIs during their relationships.

About 70 percent of women infected with chlamydia don't have any symptoms. If they do have symptoms, they may include the following:

- Abnormal vaginal discharge
- Irregular vaginal bleeding
- Bleeding during or after intercourse
- Pelvic pain or discomfort
- Discomfort on urination

Men who have symptoms usually complain of a painful burning sensation when urinating or a clear discharge from the urethra, especially in the morning.

Chlamydia is usually treated with antibiotics such as doxycycline, azithromycin, ofloxacin, or tetracycline, given four times a day for a week. If the person is allergic to tetracycline or pregnant, then the treatment is erythromycin. All medication must be taken as directed and for the full length of the treatment. The person should have a follow-up examination 2 to 3 weeks after treatment to make sure the infection has been eliminated (Feigenbaum & McCarthy, 1987).

MODES OF TRANSMISSION

- The mixing of infected mucous secretions with semen during unprotected anal, oral, and vaginal sex with an infected partner
- Mother to child during the birthing process

Herpes

There are two types of herpes, *Herpes simplex* Type I and Type II, which are both caused by viruses. Type I causes cold sores or fever blisters usually in or around the mouth; Type II, known as *genital herpes,* causes painful sores outside and/or inside the vagina and on the cervix (neck of the womb), and in males, in and around the penis, urethral opening, and the scrotum. Herpes Type I and Type II can be transmitted through direct physical contact, including sex, with a person having active herpes sores. Both types of herpes may also cause an infection of the mouth or throat. Oral sex is a frequent channel for transmitting the herpes virus (HSV-1, HSV-2) from the genitals to the throat (Nevid, 1998). One million new cases are diagnosed every year in the United States (King, 2002).

Genital herpes usually appears anywhere from 2 to 20 days after sexual contact. Often, the first symptoms of herpes may be swollen lymph glands, burning, itching, or a rash in the genital area that develops into blisters with red edges. The blisters burst, bleed, ooze, and eventually scab over. Accompanying symptoms may be pain, fever, vaginal discharge, swollen glands in the groin, and painful urination. Sometimes, however, there may be no symptoms in the early stage, especially if the herpes are located on the cervix. Herpes sores are most contagious from the time they blister until after the sore heals. Recurrent herpes infections may be controlled by a medication known as Zovirax. Although it is not a cure, Zovirax capsules can decrease the severity and frequency of herpes outbreaks.

Currently, there is no known cure for the herpes virus. Healing can take from 1 week to 1 month. Unfortunately, the disappearance of the sores or blisters does not mean that the virus is destroyed. After the sores are healed, the virus remains in one's system in a dormant state. Recurrence of herpes is common and can happen because of a compromised immune system, without further contact with an infected person. Recurrence is most likely to happen if one has vaginitis, gonorrhea, or a fever; is under stress or run-down; and during menstruation, ovulation, and pregnancy.

The long-term effects of genital herpes are unknown. However, it can be dangerous in the following ways:

- While herpes is active and the sores are open, there is a chance that they can become infected. Good personal hygiene can minimize this possibility.
- In pregnant women, herpes can be transmitted to their newborn infants during delivery, causing serious illness or death. It is important to alert the prenatal care provider about past episodes of herpes so that transmission can be avoided.
- Herpes can be prevented from spreading by refraining from sexual contact from the prodrome (beginning of the itching and tingling) until 2 to 3 days after the sores are healed. Sometimes the virus can be transmitted when there are no symptoms. Use of latex condoms is believed to provide some protection against infection during periods with no symptoms. (Feigenbaum & McCarthy, 1987)

MODES OF TRANSMISSION

- Skin to skin during unprotected anal, oral, or vaginal sex with an infected partner
- Kissing (even if no sores are present)

Human Papilloma Virus (HPV)

Genital warts are caused by the human papillomavirus (HPV). This same virus causes all warts, but each type of wart is caused by its own type of HPV virus. Thus, warts that are on the hand don't spread to the genital area or vice versa. Genital warts are sexually transmitted. They can be found on the vulva, inside the vagina, on the cervix, around the anus, and on the urethra in females. They can be found on the penis or in the scrotal area, anus, or the urethra in males.

Genital warts have a long incubation period of up to 2 to 3 months and may be an asymptomatic infection in some people. That is, they have the virus and are contagious, but they don't have any visible warts. Approximately 1 million new cases are diagnosed per year (King, 2002).

External warts are treated by painting the wart with either podophyllin or tricloroacetic acid (TCA). This causes the wart to dry up and fall off. Multiple treatments are generally needed.

Cervical warts are of special concern because they have been found to cause cervical dysplasia, which is thought to be a precancerous condition. Cervical warts require an examination called a *colposcopy,* which is a pelvic examination using a low-power microscope. At the time of the colposcopy, tissue biopsies are taken. If warts are present on the cervix, they are treated using cryosurgery (freezing) or cauterization or a laser beam. Pap smears must be done every 6 months to check for reoccurrence.

Males with *Condyloma* should be seen by a dermatologist or urologist who has knowledge of *Condyloma* treatment. External urethral *Condyloma* can be treated the same way for males as for females. Using a condom can minimize the risk of acquiring or spreading the infection (Feigenbaum & McCarthy, 1987). Anal warts can lead to anal cancer.

MODES OF TRANSMISSION

- Skin-to-skin contact with an infected partner, even when warts are not present
- Sometimes from mother to child during the birthing process

Gonorrhea

Gonorrhea is caused by a bacterium, *Nisseria gonorrhea*. This disease can be spread through all forms of sexual contact. It can affect the cervix, urethra, anus, and throat. This infection is more likely to persist and spread in women than in men. If left untreated, it can lead to epididymitis or a serious pelvic infection (pelvic inflammatory disease [PID]) that can result in infertility. Women who have gonorrhea may not have symptoms, or they will experience minor symptoms:

- Abnormal vaginal discharge
- Irregular vaginal bleeding
- Bleeding during or after intercourse
- Pelvic pain or discomfort
- Painful urination
- Rectal irritation and discharge

Some men will have no symptoms, although most men will complain of the following:

- A thick milky discharge from the penis
- Pain or burning upon urination

As with all STIs, there is an increased risk of gonorrhea with multiple partners, with intercourse without a barrier method of contraception, and/or if a partner has had gonorrhea or other STIs during the relationship.

The incubation time for gonorrhea is short, only about 1 week. There has been an increase in asymptomatic disease, making it more difficult to find and treat people who have gonorrhea. One million new cases per year are diagnosed (King, 2002).

Gonorrhea is usually treated with a large dose of penicillin (ampicillin or amoxicillin) along with probenecid, which helps the penicillin stay in the blood longer. Because gonorrhea and chlamydia often coexist (the presence of one STI makes it likely to be infected by another), a prescription for tetracycline is also given at the same time. Dual therapy consists of a single dose of ceftriaxone, cefixime, ciprofloxacin, or ofloxacin plus doxycycline for 7 days or a single dose of azithromycin (Crooks & Bauer, 2002). Some strains of gonorrhea are resistant to penicillin; in those cases, the treatment is spectinomycin or rocephen (Feigenbaum & McCarthy, 1987).

MODES OF TRANSMISSION

- Mixing of mucoid secretions with semen during unprotected anal, oral, or vaginal sex with an infected partner
- Mother to child during birthing. Infants can contract gonorrhea of the eyes (gonococcal ophthalmia neonatorum) when passing through the birth canals of infected mothers. This disorder may cause blindness but has become rare because the eyes of newborns are treated routinely with antibiotic ointment toxic to gonococcal bacteria (Nevid, 1998).

Hepatitis B and C

Hepatitis B virus (HBV) is transmitted by body fluids and blood. These body fluids include saliva, semen, and vaginal secretions. Sexual intercourse (vaginal and anal) and oral sex are risky activities. The CDC estimated in 1996 that there were 200,000 to 300,000 new cases of hepatitis B each year in the United States. Of these, at least 25 percent and up to perhaps 50 percent are transmitted sexually. In addition, approximately 20,000 babies a year are infected from their mothers. The CDC recommends that all children be vaccinated against hepatitis B.

Hepatitis C virus (HCV) is most often spread through blood-to-blood contact (transfusions) or sharing intravenous (IV) drug needles. It can be spread by sexual activity, but this behavior is much less risky. Only 20 percent of the cases in the United States are related to sexual transmission (CDC, 2002).

There is no vaccine for hepatitis C. It is treated with interferon and ribavirin, which are effective in only 30 to 40 percent of the cases. Cirrhosis of the liver and/or liver cancer will occur if patients do not respond to treatment (King, 2002).

MODES OF TRANSMISSION

- Unprotected anal, vaginal, or oral sex with an infected partner
- Sharing contaminated needles or syringes
- Infected mother to child during birthing or breastfeeding
- Tattoos or blood transfusions

Pubic Lice and Scabies

Pubic lice are parasites that embed themselves in the pubic hair and feed on the blood that they suck from the body. They cause severe itching. They can live for approximately 24 hours away from the human body, but their eggs, which may have dropped or fallen off, can hatch up to 10 days later. Thus, they can be found on sheets, towels, or the clothing of a person who has them and are highly contagious. Kwell lotion, cream, or shampoo can often help to eliminate lice from the pubic hair. Shaving is probably the best cure in the pubic area. All clothing, bedding, towels, and any other material that came in contact with the infected person must be thoroughly washed in very hot water. Having any sexual contact with a person with pubic lice is almost guaranteed transmission.

Scabies are itch mites that burrow under the skin to lay their eggs. They cause pimple-like bumps on the skin that are intensely itchy. Like pubic lice, sexual contact is not essential but would definitely lead to transmission. Special lindane lotion or a single dose of ivernection is highly effective. Also, all clothing, sheets, towels, and other materials must be thoroughly washed in hot water (King, 2002).

MODE OF TRANSMISSION

- Any contact with body, clothing, towels, sheets, and other materials of an infected person

Syphilis

Syphilis is caused by *Treponema pallidum,* a spirochete. Except for HIV, syphilis is the most complex of the STIs because it has four different stages and can go in and out of these stages.

The first stage (primary) usually entails a painless sore called a *chancre* that appears where the spirochete enters the body. This will disappear if left alone, but the bacteria will stay in the body, multiply, and spread.

The second stage develops 6 weeks to 6 months after the onset of the primary stage. By this time the bacteria have spread throughout the body. The symptoms can appear and disappear over several years. They may include a rash that is generalized and affects the hands and feet. One can experience flulike symptoms. These may resolve if left untreated, at which time the latent stage begins; that is, the organism is present without symptoms. There is often a relapse to primary and secondary symptoms during this stage.

The third or tertiary stage can occur 10 to 20 years after initial infection. It is usually evidenced by damage to the heart or brain, as well as other body organs, and is usually fatal.

Diagnosis is by a blood test (VDRL) for syphilis. If this test is positive, a second, more precise test (FTA-ABS) is done to confirm the results. Primary stage syphilis is diagnosed by clinical examination. When a chancre is found, fluid may be drawn from it and examined under a microscope in a procedure called a *dark-field test* that makes the spirochetes more visible to the eye (Nevid, 1998).

Syphilis is treated with the administration of a long-acting penicillin injection. Treatment for syphilis can be administered by a county health department or by a private physician. The treatment may include doxycycline, erythromycin, or ceftriaxone for nonpregnant, penicillin-allergic patients (Nevid, 1998).

MODES OF TRANSMISSION

- Direct contact with sores or rash during unprotected anal, oral, or vaginal sex with an infected partner
- Mother to child during the birthing process
- Infected pregnant women can pass the spirochete to the fetus in utero. Miscarriage, stillbirth, or congenital syphilis may result, causing impaired vision and hearing or deformed bones and teeth. Diagnosis of syphilis in the mother by means of a blood test may help to avoid transmission of the disease to the baby if treatment is administered early in pregnancy. The fetus will probably not be harmed if an infected mother is treated before the 4th month of pregnancy (Nevid, 1998)

Trichomoniasis

Three million new cases of this form of vaginitis occur in the United States every year (King, 2002). Symptoms of trichomoniasis (caused by the organism *Trichomonas vaginalis*) usually begin after menses. They include a greenish-yellow, frothy, malodorous discharge associated with vulvovaginal itching and irritation. Trichomoniasis is sexually transmitted. In the male, *Trichomonas vaginalis* can lead to nongonoccal urethritis (NGU), which may be noticeable by the appearance of a slight penile discharge (usually upon first urination following morning awakening). The urethra may become slightly irritated, leading to sensations of itching or tingling along the urethral tract. However, most men are asymptomatic (Rein & Muller, 1990). The diagnosis is made by visualizing *Trichomonas vaginalis* in a saline wet mount under a low-power microscope.

Treatment is metronidazole twice a day for 1 week for both the male and female. Concurrent treatment of both partners is important. It is important not to drink any alcohol while taking this medication for 2 days after treatment and to avoid the use of mayonnaise and vinegar, which can cause an antabuse effect of vomiting and severe stomach cramping.

Gardnerella (Bacterial Vaginosis)

Gardnerella (*Haemophilus vaginalis*) is thought to be among the normal flora of the vagina. However, at times it can cause symptoms of vaginitis. Among these symptoms are a thin, white-gray discharge sometimes accompanied by a "fishy" odor. Diagnosis is made based on the presence of "clue cells" on a saline wet mount. There is no culture for gardnerella.

Treatment is indicated only if the patient is symptomatic. If treatment is necessary, metronidazole is given twice a day for 7 days. Partner treatment is not necessary unless the infection is recurrent or persistent, especially if the male partner is uncircumcised. Gardnerella occurs only in the female (Feigenbaum & McCarthy, 1987).

MODE OF TRANSMISSION

- Skin-to-skin contact during unprotected anal, oral, or vaginal sex with an infected partner

HIV/AIDS

Of all of the sexually transmitted diseases, teaching about the human immunodeficiency virus (HIV), which causes acquired immune deficiency syndrome (AIDS), has become institutionalized. It is the only area of sexuality education that is mandated for inclusion by most state education departments in K–12 curricula. This approach is due to the fact HIV/AIDS has no realistic cure in the immediate future. Prevention is the first, and probably the only, line of defense in stopping this disease. Although the disease is fatal, armed with information and an ability to make informed decisions about risky behaviors, people can protect themselves from ever becoming infected. Some children are tragically born with HIV, transmitted by infected mothers, but infection of all others can be totally avoided. In other words, an individual must purposely participate in behaviors that pose a risk for infection. However, one cannot always predict a partner's behaviors. It is only the dissemination of accurate information through education, as early and as comprehensively as possible, that we can make an impact on this growing problem, especially among young people.

Half of all new infections of HIV occur in people under the age of 25 and a quarter under the age of 21. With an estimated incubation time between 3 months and 10 years before symptoms of infection occur, the disease is commonly contracted during the teen years. Because the primary sources of transmission involve sexual behaviors, the question is how much to teach students and at what developmental levels. In any case, education must begin in the earliest grades and continue in developmentally appropriate stages throughout a child's education to ensure that young people adopt primary prevention behaviors that eliminate risk (Weinstein & Rosen, 2002).

It should be noted that HIV/AIDS is not distributed evenly among the population. Some subpopulations of ethnic and cultural members seem to have a higher incidence of HIV/AIDS than others. This information is important for service providers and epidemiologists, but it must be used with caution in educational circles. As with other STIs, people practice magical thinking and come to believe that if they are not a member of a "high-risk group," they are unlikely to contract the disease. Hence, they are less likely to take appropriate precautions. Education must stress that it is not the membership in one group or another but rather the behaviors one participates in that put one at risk for infection. Understanding incidence or population rates helps to reach people more effectively with educational messages at their most accessible places and/or create culturally relevant prevention curricula.

THE DISEASE

AIDS is caused by the human immunodeficiency virus (HIV), a virus that breaks down the body's immune system, thereby potentially exposing the infected person to a variety of life-threatening diseases collectively called *opportunistic diseases*. These serious and life-threatening opportunistic diseases, such as Karposi's sarcoma (a form of cancer) and *Pneumocystis carinii* pneumonia, contribute to AIDS. Healthy people with intact immune systems may not contract these diseases even though they are prevalent in the environment. Thus, having both an HIV infection and an opportunistic disease constitute AIDS.

Viruses, in general, are protein-coated packages of genes (DNA) that invade healthy body cells (host cells) and alter the host's normal genetic apparatus, causing them to produce more virus cells. This process often kills the host cell. HIV is one of a group of retroviruses that are unique because (1) their genetic code is carried in the form of RNA instead of the usual DNA, and (2) they attack immune system cells. Retroviruses also carry an enzyme called *reverse transcriptase*. When HIV attacks a cell, it uses this enzyme and the host cell's machinery to manufacture RNA from DNA (new virus particles) within the host cell. This process continues until many new viruses are produced. Then the process may stop for a long time, or it may continue until the viruses rupture the host cell's membrane and escape into the bloodstream, attacking new host cells and thereby continuing to reproduce.

When the HIV virus enters the bloodstream, it targets the body's immune system cells, white blood cells such as macrophages and T4 cells (one type of helper T cell), because these cells have, on their surface, a protein that the virus recognizes. It then bores into these cells and hides there, unrecognized and therefore not targeted for destruction while it repeats the reproductive process described earlier. In an uninfected person, the T4 cells mobilize the immune system to fight infection.

Normally the blood system contains about 1,000 T4 cells per cubic millimeter of blood. The number of T4 cells may remain at about 1,000 per cubic millimeter for several years following infection with HIV, and many people show no symptoms of AIDS while it remains at this level. Then, the number of T4 cells declines (because of viral destruction). But many people may show no symptoms of disease for several more years. People become most vulnerable to diseases when the level of T4 cells falls below 200 cells per cubic millimeter. The result is an immune system deficient in T4 cells and therefore unable to combat other opportunistic infections. The person becomes ill and eventually dies from these infections, which the weakened immune system cannot overcome.

Currently, research suggests that the vast majority of HIV-positive people eventually do develop AIDS. A person whose immune system is compromised in some way before infection with HIV probably will progress from infection with the virus to AIDS more quickly than someone whose immune system is healthy. Also, repeated exposure to HIV and alcohol and drug abuse can accelerate the progression of this disease. A seemingly healthy person, showing no outward symptoms, is as contagious as an infected person who is symptomatic and even severely ill. Therefore, people cannot tell without testing who has the HIV virus and who does not. Although the time frame varies from person to person, the pattern for the course of HIV infection to AIDS generally is as follows:

Stage I: Primary HIV infection. Soon after contracting HIV, some people develop a fever, swollen glands, fatigue, and perhaps a rash. These early symptoms usually disappear within a few weeks.

Stage II: Chronic asymptomatic infection. This stage is marked by a gradual decline in T4 cells but no particular disease symptoms. At the same time, there is often evidence of chronically swollen lymph nodes and an increasing vulnerability to opportunistic infections.

Stage III: Chronic symptomatic infection. At this stage, thrush (a fungus infection in the mouth) may appear. Infections of the skin and moist inner membranes of the body may appear, along with general feelings of discomfort, weakness, night sweats, weight loss, and frequent diarrhea.

Stage IV: Clinical AIDS. This diagnosis is made after one or more of 27 opportunistic diseases have been manifested in an HIV-infected person who also has a T cell count below 200 (Stryker, Coates, De-Carlo, Haynes-Sanstad, Shriver, & Makadon, 1995).

Why HIV infection can take more than 10 years to progress to AIDS is still not entirely clear. In some cases, the person has been exposed and HIV infection is not present. Are these individuals naturally immune? More research is being done on these few cases in an attempt to discover why certain people seem to be protected from getting HIV.

When people are infected with the HIV virus, their bodies combat the infection by activating T cells and producing antibodies. The presence of these antibodies in the blood is what indicates that a person is carrying HIV (is HIV-positive). In most cases, 3 months after exposure to the virus is sufficient time for the antibodies to show up in the commonly used blood test, called ELISA (enzyme-linked immunoabsorbent assay). By 6 months, 95 percent of infected people test positive (Stryker et al., 1995). If insufficient time has elapsed for production of antibodies, the test will be negative even though the person is infected and can infect others. Sometimes the ELISA test is positive even though no antibodies are present (a false positive). Then a second test is done.

When the ELISA test results are positive for both tests another antibody test, the Western blot (immunoblot) test is administered for confirmation. Although it is more accurate than the ELISA, the Western blot is expensive and, therefore, not used as the primary test for HIV. Pharmaceutical companies are continually working on new and better testing methods. In 2003 a new test has become available that pricks the finger for a blood sample, and the results can be attained in 20 minutes. This visually read assay shows a one bar negative/two bar positive result. Additionally, each OraQuick device has an internal procedural control that ensures each result is valid and that the test was run properly. Based on clinical data submitted by OrasSure Technologies, the OraQuick test has been shown to have sensitivity and specificity comparable to laboratory-based tests, 100 percent specific and 99.6 percent sensitive. The test requires no instrument, is portable, and can be stored at room temperature, providing convenience in any setting (Abbot Diagnostics, 2004).

Testing must not create false assurances. It is not uncommon for people to assure partners that they are not infected because they have been tested, when either not enough time has elapsed since exposure or they have participated in risky behavior since being tested. Hence, testing only assures people of HIV-infected status when the appropriate "window of conversion" has been accounted for and no new exposures have occurred.

Contracting HIV is not easy to do. HIV is not circulating in the air or water or living on toilet seats, drinking glasses, combs, or brushes; it is not in foods that infected people touch. Because it is a virus, it does not know a gay person from a straight person, an African American person from a Caucasian person, or a woman from a man, nor does it care. Hence, it can be transmitted from any infected person to any other person without discrimination. The body fluids that best support the transmission of the virus are blood, semen, breast milk, and vaginal fluids. Saliva and tears may contain the virus, but there are no reported cases of transmission from these body fluids (probably because sufficient particles of the disease must be in the fluid, and the fluid must be able to support the life of the virus for transfer to occur). A person must choose to participate in specific high-risk behaviors that give the virus access to the bloodstream or to an unknowing partner's, where it can get into the cells needed to multiply itself.

MODES OF TRANSMISSION

- Having unprotected sexual intercourse, anal or vaginal, with an infected person. The vagina and anus have accessible blood vessels through which the virus, deposited by the semen or vaginal fluid from the infected person, can enter the bloodstream. Although oral sex may be a mode of transmission, the virus must find entrance into the bloodstream through a cut or sore in the mouth or digestive juices will destroy it. Cases of transmission from oral sex are difficult to document because most people who participate in it also participate in other sexual behaviors that could transmit the virus.
- Sharing contaminated drug needles or syringes with an infected person. When people use injected drugs, they often share needles with little concern for sterilization. The blood of the infected person is drawn into the syringe that contains the drug, mixes with it, and then is left as residue that mixes with the next user's drug.

- Women infected with HIV can transmit the virus to their babies during pregnancy, childbirth, or breastfeeding. HIV can be transmitted through the placenta and infect the fetus. Some fetuses, however, receive only antibodies from infected mothers. During childbirth, the blood vessels of mother and baby may rupture, allowing the virus to be transmitted through the blood. However, treatment with AZT during pregnancy can reduce the risk of viral transmission.

Prior to 1985, when blood screening began, some people became infected by receiving blood transfusions. Now that the blood supply is tested, the incidence of transmission through infected blood has virtually been eliminated. Donating blood is not a mode of transmission. The equipment for giving blood is new or sterile for each user. Health care workers including dentists, physicians, and nurses have not been known to transmit the HIV virus in their work. The case of the dentist who treated Kimberly Bergalis in 1991 was the first known case of HIV transmission from a health care worker to a patient. Tests on more than 15,000 patients and physicians had not uncovered one case of health care provider–to–patient transmission (Nevid, 1998).

As of January 1996, according to the CDC, there has not been a documented case of HIV transmission from insect bites of any kind. Also, though the virus is known to appear in saliva and tears, the quantity and the environment do not seem to support its transmission.

With one 15- to 24-year-old becoming infected every 15 seconds around the world, it is apparent that this pandemic will increasingly affect young people. Moreover, 9 out of 10 people do not know they are infected or are living with AIDS. Prevention through educational efforts produces evidence of risk-reducing behaviors among this population, including increased knowledge about STIs and AIDS, delayed sexual activity, decreased number of sexual partners, and greater use of condoms at first coitus (Summers, Kates, & Murphy, 2002). Young people have been brought up in a world where HIV/AIDS always existed. They have become somewhat complacent about prevention. Thus, we must continue our educational efforts that reinforce prevention as our only defense against this devastating disease. Our curricula must be planned so that they are consistent and developmentally appropriate. Education must not only reinforce personal skills but also help young people know where and when to go for services.

PREVENTION

SIECUS (2001) provides a 10-step strategy for helping young people prevent HIV infections. These same strategies can be applied to preventing other STIs, too:

1. End the silence, stigma, and shame assuring that young people will talk freely about related risk behaviors (sexuality, drugs, violence, and so forth).

2. Provide knowledge and information through school and community sources, so that young people know how to protect themselves and others.

3. Provide life skills such as decision making, communication, and conflict resolution that enable young people to put knowledge into practice.

4. Provide youth-friendly health services including access to condoms, medical testing, and treatment in addition to authentic information resources.

5. Promote voluntary, anonymous, or confidential HIV counseling and testing, and let young people know where they can receive these services.

6. Work with young people, and promote participation in the development of relevant activities and presentations. Peer educators not only are effective sources of information to others but are more likely to practice self-prevention.

7. Engage young people living with AIDS who can put a recognizable face on the disease, decreasing the stigma and mythical thinking associated with it.

8. Create safe and supportive environments that have as their mission the condemnation of sexual violence, abuse, and exploitation.

9. Reach out to young people most at risk, including the disenfranchised, refugees, and homeless children.

10. Strengthen partnerships, and monitor progress through collaborative educational programs that are interdisciplinary and include parent groups, community, government, and others.

In addition, always use latex condoms unless there is certainty that both involved are 100 percent infection-free. This certainty may be difficult to ascertain. (Consider the scenario about John and Mary earlier in the chapter. A one-night mistake caused her to unknowingly contract chlamydia, and she infected John.)

Practicing prevention for STIs requires that we

- Become comfortable talking about sex with our partners.
- Never participate in sexual behavior without an effective protective barrier such as a latex condom (skins are porous and allow the virus to penetrate) or dental dam (for oral sex). Only in circumstances where we can be 100 percent positive that our partner is disease-free can we have intercourse without effective protection. Because that is almost 100 percent not possible, *always* use appropriate protection. The degree to which you choose to "trust" your partner is the degree to which you are willing to take a risk of infection.
- Reevaluate your sexual lives. Multiple partners increase the likelihood of exposure and infection.
- Are willing to see abstaining from sex as an option, until a relationship evolves where trust, honest communication, and mutual

medical examinations, including HIV testing, can assure sexually healthy lives.

- Do not use alcohol and/or other drugs before or during sexual activity, recognizing that they cloud good decision making and behavior choices.

Various social attitudes and fears prevent or impede the practice of safer sex. For example, the perception of the need to use a condom can vary. Many high school- and college-age students believe that the longer they are involved in a monogamous relationship, the less they need to use a condom for protection against STIs. (A "long-term" relationship in this age group may be considered a year or less.) In reality, "low perceived need is not based on an actual STI" (Wendt & Soloman, 1992, p. 106). This perception sometimes comes from the social belief, but rather mythical notion, that all marital or committed relationships are monogamous. There is also the perception that if a person looks clean, that person can't possibly have a STI.

This student population also has a sometimes distorted perception of the need to talk about using a condom. High school- and college-age students report that it is much easier to have sex than to talk about having sex. Not only do they feel uncomfortable using the correct language, such as *penis, vulva,* and *vagina,* but they also believe that discussing sex is not "cool," especially for women. They rarely go through a communication process that encourages them to both agree to be sexually active and under what circumstances before the action begins.

Also complicating the practice of safer sex is the perceived role of women versus men in sexual decisions and condom use. Communication between men and women about sexual decisions, and especially condom use, is often hindered by the socially learned double standard that still exists. In many subgroups, it is acceptable for the man to be in a dominant position, playing the role of "actor," while the woman is the "reactor." Thus, if a woman initiates a discussion about sexual history and condom use, she may well be viewed negatively. If she dares to carry a condom, the perception is often that she has "been around" and that she is willing. Obviously, these perceptions inhibit women from being assertive and feeling empowered to initiate honest, open sexual dialogue and condom use. For men, it is often not cool to be worried about diseases.

Finally, the perception of pleasure and condom use can also impede practicing safer sex, as young men may note, "It's like taking a shower with a raincoat." Many young men report that the sensation of orgasm is minimized when they wear a condom. This may be true, but orgasm only lasts a few seconds and takes the least amount of time in the entire human sexual response cycle (see Chapter 3). Furthermore, wearing a condom can significantly protect one from giving or getting an STI, can decrease premature ejaculations, and, in the case of HIV, can actually save one's life. The benefits, therefore, far outweigh the risks. It's time to become "condom-friendly."

EDUCATIONAL CONSIDERATIONS AND DEVELOPMENTAL APPROPRIATENESS

As in other subjects related to human sexuality education, many dilemmas, controversies, and issues exist regarding STIs and AIDS, especially about what is developmentally appropriate to teach. The ability to teach about safer and pleasurable sexual behavior is often replaced by scare tactics and abstinence-only messages, leaving young people without the knowledge or the ability to enrich their sexual lives without risk.

Aggleton (2002) raises some important reflective "educational abuses" to be considered. He believes that the majority of educational curricula proceed from the belief that those who are being educated in schools about STIs and AIDS are not infected, that education often assumes that those who are infected are the problem rather than part of the solution, that there is enormous stigma and discrimination reinforced rather than eliminated, that the inequities of gender-related phenomena continue to affect education and risk, and that the messages that existed initially in the epidemic will continue to be effective today and in the future. Aggleton suggests that pedagogy ought to be designed to include the concerns of individuals rather than social institutions or intervention experts. In other words, rather than telling people what to do and when to do it, one needs to "unleash the power of community to take charge and fight back" (p. 6). He goes on to explain that "ultimately, there are no universal panaceas to discover in prevention science. The approaches we use must be context specific—context is important because of its intimate relationship with what we call vulnerability" (p. 7).

Education about STIs can be included in various units in a human sexuality curriculum. It lends itself especially well to a unit on communicable diseases. A multidisciplinary approach is also useful and can sometimes eliminate the problems associated with overloaded curricula. For example, a team approach might be particularly effective whereby the science teacher teaches about the immune system, organisms, and the like; the social studies teacher teaches about the effects of the epidemic on world populations and other culturally related considerations; and the health teacher teaches about life skills and prevention.

SUMMARY

STIs and AIDS present a serious and long-term health problem for the world community, the U.S. society, and especially youth. They constitute the fastest-growing subgroup of people becoming infected. At this time in the epidemic, the only resourceful defense against infection is education. Education requires that we understand the immediate culture and environment in which young people interact, that we listen to them and meet their needs, and that we provide them with open forums for discussing their concerns. Education considers student's developmental levels and therefore their ability to understand and to incorporate what they learn into their lives.

Characteristics of each disease—its etiology, prevention, mode of transmission, and so forth—have been discussed, as have life skills for optimizing young people's ability to reflect on the implications of infection and for empowering them to assert their beliefs and attitudes even in vulnerable situations. Recognizing that denial about the implications of STIs and knowledge of the myths and misconceptions about them will arm adolescents with a greater ability to recognize worthwhile risks from those that have potentially permanent, health-compromising outcomes. Students can realize that contracting an STI can be virtually avoided by the sexual behavior choices that they make.

WEBSITES

Centers for Disease Control and Prevention, STI information: www.cdc.gov/nch-stp/dstd/diseaseinfo.htm

SIECUS: www.siecus.org

National Institute of Allergies and Infectious Diseases (NIAID), Genital Herpes: www.niaid.nih.gov/factsheets/stdherp.htm

NIAID, Chlamydia: www.niaid.nih.gov/factsheets/stdclam.htm

National HPV and Cervical Cancer Resource Center: www.ashastd.org/hpvccrv

American Social Health Association and CDC, AIDS FAQs: www.ashastd.org/nah/faqs.html

Journal of the American Medical Association HIV/AIDS Information Center: www.ama.assn.org/special/hiv/hivhome.htm

ADDITIONAL RESOURCES

AIDS Hotline: English, (800) 342-2437; Spanish, (800) 344-7432

American Academy of Pediatrics, Publications Department: PO Box 927, Elk Grove Village, IL 60009-0927

Centers for Disease Control and Prevention, National STD Hotline: (800) 227-8922 or (800) 342-2437

National TTY/TDD AIDS: (800) 243-7889 (Monday–Friday, 10:00 A.M.–10:00 P.M. EST)

National Herpes Hotline: (919) 361-8488

National HPV and Cervical Cancer Hotline: (919) 361-4848

SIECUS: 130 W. 42nd Street, Ste. 2500, New York, NY 10036

U.S. Department of Health and Human Services, National AIDS Information Clearing House: PO Box 6003, Rockville, MD 20850

REFERENCES

Abbot Diagnostics. (2004, January 29). *HIV/AIDS*. Available: http://abbotdiagnostics.com/Your_Health/HIV-AIDS/.

Aggleton, P. (2002). HIV/AIDS: Prevention and sexuality education must change to meet their promise. *SIECUS Report, 31*(1), 5–7.

Centers for Disease Control and Prevention. (2002, September 27). Trends in sexual risk behaviors among high school students 1991–2001. *Morbidity & Mortality Weekly Report*. Available online: www.cdc.gov/mmwr.

Cohn, J. A. (1997). HIV Infections. *British Medical Journal, 314*, 487–491.

Crooks, R., & Bauer, K. (2002). *Our sexuality* (8th ed.). Pacific Grove, CA: Wadsworth.

Eng, T. R., & Butler, W. T. (1997). *The hidden epidemic: Confronting sexually transmitted diseases*. Institute of Medicine, Committee on Prevention and Control of Sexually Transmitted Diseases. Washington, DC: National Academy Press.

Feigenbaum, R., & McCarthy V. (1987). *The Teen Advocate Project (TAP) manual*. Hempstead, NY: Planned Parenthood of Nassau County.

Hedgepeth, E., & Helmich, J. (1996). *Teaching about sexuality and HIV*. New York: New York University Press.

King, B. (2002). *Human sexuality today*. Upper Saddle River, NJ: Prentice Hall.

Nevid, J. (1998). *Choices: Sex in the age of STDs*. Needham Heights, MA: Allyn & Bacon.

Powell, E. (1996). *Sex on your terms*. Needham Heights, MA: Allyn & Bacon.

Rein, M. F., & Muller, M. (1990) *Trichomonas vaginalis* and trichomoniasis. In K. K. Holmes, P. Mardh, P. F. Sparling, & P. J. Wiesner (Eds.), *Sexually transmitted diseases* (2nd ed., pp. 481–492). New York: McGraw-Hill.

Sexual Information and Education Council of the United States. (2001). A 10-step strategy to prevent HIV/AIDS among young people. *SIECUS Report, 3*(1), 8–9.

Sexual Information and Education Council of the United States. (2003, March). *Fact sheet*. New York: Author.

Stryker, J., Coates, T. J., DeCarlo, P., Haynes-Sanstad, K., Shriver, M., & Makadon, H. J. (1995). Prevention of HIV infection: Looking back, looking ahead. *Journal of the American Medical Association, 73*,1143–1148.

Summers, T., Kates, J., & Murphy, G. (2002). The global impact of HIV/AIDS on young people. *SIECUS Report, 31*(1), 14–19.

Weinstein, E., & Rosen E. (2003). *Teaching children about health*. Belmont, CA: Wadsworth/Thomson Learning.

Wendt, S., & Soloman L. (1992). Barriers to condom use among heterosexual male and female college students. *Journal of American College Health, 44,* 105–108.

LEARNING EXPERIENCES

Learning about STIs, including HIV, is an interactive experience between students and teachers. Very young students need to begin their learning about the basics of personal hygiene and its relationship to health and the immune system. They will be encouraged to understand the difference between wellness and illness and between communicable and noncommunicable diseases and how people contract diseases. They will recognize how they feel when they are sick and how they feel when they "get better." These personal experiences become the basis for teaching about diseases, what causes them, how to deal with them, and how to prevent them.

The emphasis should be on developing an internal locus of control so students begin to accept the notion that what they do and how they live can affect their health. They can also learn that through sound health practices, they will be less susceptible to disease, and, if they do become ill, they will be more likely to recover more quickly. Even children with chronic diseases can improve if they adopt healthy behaviors within the limitations imposed by their disease.

The following learning experiences provide opportunities for students to practice and develop their decision-making, communication, goal-setting, resource management, relationship management, and stress management skills.

Decision making is important in the prevention of STIs because of its relationship to effectively resolve problems enabling students to make well-thought-out decisions about their sexual behavior, including whether they will be sexually active, what behaviors they will participate in, with whom, where, and when.

Communication skills will help students to share their decisions, feelings, attitudes, values, and knowledge with prospective partners without succumbing to peer pressure. It will also help individuals build self-confidence and establish and maintain relationships. Students will be encouraged to be effective listeners and to recognize and overcome barriers to communication such that they can confidently articulate acceptance of or refuse to participate in behaviors that may put them at risk for an STI.

Goal-setting skills will help students to relate the impact of their present behavior on their future. They are also able to assess which goals are worth achieving and at what cost and benefit.

Resource management skills will help students identify and use the many STI information, treatment, and prevention services available. Managing these resources also means knowing which ones are effective and how and when to contact them.

Stress management skills help students recognize when they are becoming overwhelmed. In high-stress situations, decision making is compromised.

Grades K–2

In these early grades, students should learn about the relationship between disease and modes of prevention—for example, relating germs to cold symptoms such as a sore throat and sneezing. They need to recognize the importance of simple routine behaviors that can keep them healthy, such as how to drink from a water fountain, not to share utensils or to drink from the same cup as another person, to cover their mouth when coughing, to wash their hands before eating and after going to the bathroom, and so on. They also need to learn when and how to report symptoms to a teacher or a parent and when and why they stay home when they are ill. They also should begin to know what to do when they have serious symptoms and who can help them. Hence, by the end of second grade, students will be able to

- Understand the concepts of illness and wellness.
- Explain that some diseases are communicable and others are not.
- Explain what a germ is.
- Recognize that some germs can make people sick.
- Recognize that there are different kinds of germs.
- Describe behaviors that they can practice to prevent themselves from becoming infected.
- Identify people and places in the home, school, and community where they can get information, medical, and other health-related assistance.

Grades 3–4

By third grade, a discussion of immunizations is important. These students are also interested in common childhood diseases such as chicken pox and measles. By the end of fourth grade, children should understand locus of control enough so that they can take responsibility for their health by behaving in ways that promote wellness. They can begin to understand some of the scientific knowledge about the immune system and how certain behaviors are helpful while others are harmful. They can begin to learn elementary concepts about the different types of germs, such as bacteria and viruses.

By the end of fourth grade, in addition to mastering the objectives from grades K–2, students will be able to

- Understand the function of the immune system, types of immunity, and how immunizations prevent disease.
- Recognize that many diseases including HIV/AIDS are caused by bacteria or viruses.
- List the several ways that STIs, including HIV/AIDS, are usually acquired.
- Describe the skills one could practice to prevent STIs.

- Understand that a person cannot become infected with HIV by simply being around or touching someone with HIV.
- Understand how diseases can affect an entire family.
- Explain that some diseases can be controlled or eliminated through medical treatments and others cannot.
- Identify people and places to go to for information and other health services.

Grades 5–6

By now, students are ready to study specific diseases and to discuss their experiences. They are ready to discuss more abstract concepts of disease and the impact of STIs on people's lives. They can begin to relate their behaviors to their risk for infection.

After studying about STIs in grades 5 and 6, students will be able to

- Name the common sexually transmitted diseases, including AIDS, and know how they are transmitted.
- Understand how the immune system functions in relation to STIs.
- Describe the elementary differences between safe and unsafe sexual behaviors.
- Explain the effects of diseases on individuals, family, community, and society.
- Expand their knowledge of community resources that provide services and authentic information about STIs.

Grades 7–9

The data tell us that many of the students we encounter in these grades are beginning to experience sexual activity. They will need to have very specific information and skills in order to keep themselves safe from infection.

Students in Grades 7–9 will be able to

- Compare symptoms of STIs, including HIV infection.
- Explain the stages of the more common diseases.
- Describe the physical consequences of STIs, including HIV infection.
- Explain the potential social effects of STIs on their future health and personal activities.
- Identify and utilize sources for obtaining information, diagnosis, and treatment of STIs.
- Know how to evaluate and trust their sources of information.
- Make decisions about their behavior as it relates to potential infection and communicate them.
- Know what they can and cannot do around people who are infected.

- Recognize the relationship between sex, drugs, violence, and STI and HIV infection.

Grades 10–12

These grade levels probably represent the last opportunity teachers will have to formally educate students about STIs and HIV. It is also a time of greatest challenge because students in these grades often believe that "nothing can happen to them." Their invincibility is the strongest, as is their need to be accepted and to belong. It is also the time when they are most likely to experience their first "love" and intimate relationship. This is an important time to help students develop a concern for their fellow person, a sensitivity for people who are challenged with illness, and other displays of love and empathy.

Students in Grades 10–12 will be able to

- Describe the clinical symptoms associated with STIs and HIV infection.
- Understand the relationship between the human immune system and communicable disease infection, especially how it dysfunctions in cases of HIV infection.
- Understand the significance of infection with an STI and their personal future plans and health.
- Relate sexually risky behaviors and STI infection.
- Understand the relationship between drugs and poor decision making.
- Understand the relationship between multiple partners and increased risk for infection.
- Develop a personal plan of behavior that decreases their risk of contracting an STI.
- Resist peer pressure and advocate for themselves and others.
- Identify their attitudes and behaviors that relate to sexually transmitted infection.
- Identify related resources and evaluate their services.
- Be empathetic to the plight of persons who are infected.
- Understand the impact of STIs to personal health, the community, and society.

LEARNING EXPERIENCE 1

TITLE: Gloves to Keep Me Germ-Free

GRADE LEVELS: K–3

TIME REQUIREMENTS: One session

LEARNING CONTEXT

This learning experience develops communication and decision-making skills. Following this activity, students will be able to

- Define what germs are.
- Describe how germs get into the body.
- Explain how cleanliness helps prevent germs from getting into the body.

NATIONAL LEARNING STANDARDS

1:   Students will comprehend concepts related to health promotion and disease prevention.

3:   Students will demonstrate the ability to practice health-enhancing behaviors and reduce health risks.

5:   Students will demonstrate the ability to use interpersonal communication skills to enhance health.

PROCEDURE

Put on a latex glove and then dip the gloved hand into a dish of sparkles. Show the students the glove, and tell them that you are pretending to be a dentist. The sparkles represent germs that came from a patient's mouth, from saliva or blood. Then touch several students' arms, leaving sparkles on them. Remove the glove and ask the students whether they see any sparkles (germs) on your hand. Explain how germs are spread and how they are not spread.

Questions for Discussion

- Why is wearing a glove important for dentists?
- In what other professions do people wear gloves?
- What are germs?
- How do they get into the body?
- What would happen if the glove was torn and you had a cut on your hand?

RESOURCES

Latex gloves and sparkles

ASSESSMENT PLAN

Assess the students through their participation in group discussion.

LEARNING EXPERIENCE 2

TITLE: Invisible Germs in the Air

GRADE LEVELS: K–3

TIME REQUIREMENTS: One session

LEARNING CONTEXT

After this activity, which develops communication and decision-making skills, students will be able to

- List the important reasons for not spreading germs.
- Describe how to get rid of germs.
- Explain how the first line of defense works.

NATIONAL LEARNING STANDARDS

1: Students will comprehend concepts related to health promotion and disease prevention.

3: Students will demonstrate the ability to practice health-enhancing behaviors and reduce health risks.

PROCEDURE

Use a plastic bottle with a spray nozzle to demonstrate how germs get into the air when we talk, sneeze, and cough. Then cover the nozzle with the tissue. Demonstrate how the tissue blocks the spray and how the germs are invisible. Call on students to discuss these topics:

- Explain why they must practice behaviors that prevent the spreading of germs.
- Describe how to get rid of germs.
- Explain how the body's immune system begins to work.

RESOURCES

Plastic bottle with a spray nozzle and a tissue

ASSESSMENT PLAN

Assess the students through group discussion and observation.

Name: _____

What happens when you catch a cold virus?
You might have a stuffy nose and a sore throat. Maybe you'll get a headache. A few days later, your nose may start to run. A few days after that, you start to feel better.

Your body has been able to fight the cold, thanks to your immune system.
Your immune system fights most of the germs that enter your body before they make you sick. If you do get sick, your immune system works hard to kill the germs so you'll get better faster. Sometimes your immune system is able to remember that virus that caused your cold and will destroy it every time it gets into your body, but there are so many viruses that cause colds, and a new one may cause your next cold.

Complete these sentences:
_____ make the _____ that fight germs such as viruses. Together, they are the key parts of your body's _____.

Just what is your immune system?
Even though your blood looks red because of all its red blood cells, there are many *white blood cells* in it, too. Some white blood cells make *antibodies,* your body's germ-fighting chemicals. Together, white blood cells and antibodies are the key parts of your immune system.

The best we can do is not infect other people while we have the virus. Germs pass through the air when people talk, cough, or sneeze. You can "pick up" some germs by touching door-knobs or telephones, shaking hands, or picking up garbage. Germs will get into your body if you put your fingers, pencils, and other objects in your mouth or if you rub your eyes or nose

Write answers to the following questions:

1. Explain what a germ is and what germs do when they get into the body.

2. Describe ways in which germs enter the body.

3. Describe simple hygiene measures that can prevent people from getting sick.

LEARNING EXPERIENCE 3

TITLE: Understanding Germs

GRADE LEVELS: 4–6

TIME REQUIREMENTS: One session

LEARNING CONTEXT

Communication, decision-making, and goal-setting skills are developed in the following learning experience. After this activity, students will be able to

- Define what germs are.
- Describe how germs get into the body.
- Explain how cleanliness helps prevent germs from getting into the body.

NATIONAL LEARNING STANDARDS

1:   Students will comprehend concepts related to health promotion and disease prevention.
3:   Students will demonstrate the ability to practice health-enhancing behaviors and reduce health risks.
5:   Students will demonstrate the ability to use interpersonal communication skills to enhance health.
6:   Students will demonstrate the ability to use goal-setting and decision-making skills to enhance health.

PROCEDURE

Give instruction index cards to five students in the class, telling two of the students not to take anything from anyone else, not to shake hands with anyone else in the class, and not to tell anyone else what is written on their cards (using good communication to politely refuse). On the other three students' cards is a statement that says they have a bad cold. Instruct all of the students to move around the room and introduce themselves to other people by shaking their hand or offering them their pencil or paper. Then have the students take their seats. Ask the students who had a very bad cold written on their card to stand. Then ask any students who shook their hands to stand, and then ask students who took something from them to stand. Have the three students read what is on their card, and explain that each person who had contact with them and is standing has been exposed to the "germs" that caused the cold. Then have the students sit, and ask the two students who did not have contact with anyone to stand and explain that they were unlikely to have been exposed.

Discuss how easily we can come in contact with some germs. Others do not go from one person to another so easily. Invite students to come up with other ideas for good hygiene that can help prevent germs from spreading. Discuss what personal items can be shared and what should not be shared. Tell students that germs are all around us and that we can't eliminate them, but we can help keep them out of our bodies by practicing good hygiene.

Read the following content aloud with the class: Thousands of germs enter the body every day, but the immune system can fight most of them. You are more likely to get sick, however, if you have not been eating or sleeping well or are under a lot of stress because that can "tire" your immune system and change its efficiency. Fever during illness is a sign that your immune system is working hard; a raised body temperature helps your white blood cells and antibodies fight illness. The body must make a different antibody to fight each type of bacteria or virus that enters. Once a germ invades the body, your immune system "remembers" it and is always ready to make more antibodies, in case that germ enters your body again. That is why we generally get illnesses such as chicken pox just once.

Instruct the students to answer the questions in the following handout (included here). Complete the exercise and discuss the responses in class. The handout can be graded according to a teacher-designed rubric that measures the health content.

RESOURCES
Handout and index cards

ASSESSMENT PLAN
Assess students through the group discussion and their responses on the handout. General answers to the homework questions are as follows:

1. The immune system of a healthy person works like this: If germs get into your body, white blood cells will rush over. They make antibodies to fight the germs. White blood cells that fight germs travel to all parts of the body.

2. Keep your cold germs from spreading to others:
   - Sneeze into a tissue.
   - Turn your head and cover your mouth when you cough.
   - Wash your hands.
   - Throw used tissues in the wastebasket.

3. Keep germs out of your body:
   - Never put your mouth on the spout of a water fountain.
   - Wash hands often with soap and warm water. Dry them on a clean towel.
   - Keep fingers, pencils, and other objects out of your mouth.

LEARNING EXPERIENCE 4

TITLE: Caring about Myself and Others

GRADE LEVELS: 4–6

TIME REQUIREMENTS: Two sessions

LEARNING CONTEXT
The following activity develops skills in communication, decision making, relationship management, and goal setting. Students will be able to

- Identify unhealthy behaviors.
- Identify healthy behaviors.
- Understand how one person's behavior affects another person.

NATIONAL LEARNING STANDARDS
1: Students will comprehend concepts related to health promotion and disease prevention.
2: Students will demonstrate the ability to access valid health information and health-promoting products and services.
3: Students will demonstrate the ability to practice health-enhancing behaviors and reduce health risks.
6: Students will demonstrate the ability to use goal-setting and decision-making skills to enhance health.

PROCEDURE

Session 1

On the chalkboard, write the following three headings: "High Risk," "Low Risk," and "No Risk." Ask the students to list, name, and identify behaviors that fit into each category, relevant to the transmissions of germs. Write the list on the chalkboard or on an overhead; then discuss various risky behaviors as they pertain to communicable infections.

Session 2

Have the students individually respond in writing to the handout (included later). Then, in their groups, have them read their responses to each other and summarize the group responses before sharing one list with the entire class.

RESOURCES
Chalkboard and chalk; handout

ASSESSMENT PLAN

Give a spelling test on any new words introduced in this lesson. Ask students to write in their journals about their individual responses to the handout. Students will be able to

- Spell the new vocabulary words correctly.
- Effectively use writing skills to explain high-risk and low-risk behaviors.
- Effectively use writing skills to describe feelings and behaviors about themselves and others in regard to illness and wellness.
- Differentiate between healthy and unhealthy behaviors.

Some sample answers for the handout are as follows:

- Keep germs away. You can help keep germs out of your body. You can help stop your germs from spreading to other people.
- Use a tissue when you sneeze.
- Cover your mouth when you cough.
- Wash your hands before you eat. Wash your hands after you go to the bathroom. Use soap and warm water.
- Don't drink out of someone's glass. Don't share forks or spoons.

REFERENCE

Adapted, in part, from *HIV/AIDS: Instructional guide, Grades K–12* (Albany: State University of New York, April 1996).

Name: _____

1. I can help myself make healthy decisions when I

   _____

   _____

2. I can help my family, friends, and others make healthy decisions when I

   _____

   _____

3. I show I care about myself when I

   _____

   _____

4. I show I care about others when I

   _____

   _____

LEARNING EXPERIENCE 5

TITLE: Making Healthy Choices

GRADE LEVELS: Can be used with several grade levels by making the choices developmentally appropriate

TIME REQUIREMENTS: Two or three sessions

LEARNING CONTEXT

Students will develop decision-making, problem-solving, and communication skills in this activity. They will be able to

- Understand the concept of making decisions.
- Define the concept of healthy choices.
- Understand the importance of thinking about choices and consequences.

NATIONAL LEARNING STANDARDS

1: Students will comprehend concepts related to health promotion and disease prevention.
2: Students will demonstrate the ability to access valid health information and health-promoting products and services.
3: Students will demonstrate the ability to practice health-enhancing behaviors and reduce health risks.
5: Students will demonstrate the ability to use interpersonal communication skills to enhance health.
6: Students will demonstrate the ability to use goal-setting and decision-making skills to enhance health.

PROCEDURE

Session 1

In small groups, have the students generate a list of at least five things they have to make choices about that could relate to their health. For example: "Would you rather stop your friend's bleeding or call for help?" "Would you rather delay having sex or have sex without a condom?" "Eat potato chips for snack or eat a fruit?" "Go home from the party or stay and drink with everyone else?" The lists generated by the students will be age-appropriate and from their own experiences.

Collect the cards, and then have the students all stand in the center of the room. Read each card individually, and have the students move left for one choice or right for the other. Ask the students to explain why they made that choice, but they must give their own unique reason and not repeat the same reasons that have already been given. After they have made their choices and given their reasons, ask the students to discuss the possible outcomes of their choices on their present goals and on their future goals.

Session 2

Have the students identify in writing at least two short-range goals and two long-range goals for themselves. Using at least three choices they made in Session 1, the students should indicate how their choices would have impacted their stated goals. Then, put the students in groups, and have them share at least one of their choices and outcomes with each other.

As homework, ask the students to respond to the following questions in their journals:

- What did they learn about themselves and what is important to them?
- What did they consider when making their choices?
- Would the choices that they made lead them to their long-range goals?

RESOURCES

Chalkboard and chalk; handout

ASSESSMENT PLAN

Evaluate the students' journals.

REFERENCE

Adapted, in part, from *HIV/AIDS: Instructional guide, Grades K–12* (Albany: State University of New York, April 1996).

LEARNING EXPERIENCE 6

TITLE: AIDS—Facts and Myths

GRADE LEVELS: 7–9 (The list of myths to be used should reflect developmental appropriateness.)

TIME REQUIREMENTS: Two or three sessions

LEARNING CONTEXT

Following this activity, students will be able to understand the differences between HIV and AIDS. They will develop skills in goal setting, communication, resource management, and decision making.

NATIONAL LEARNING STANDARDS

1: Students will comprehend concepts related to health promotion and disease prevention.
2: Students will demonstrate the ability to access valid health information and health-promoting products and services.
4: Students will analyze the influence of culture, media, technology, and other factors on health.
6: Students will demonstrate the ability to use goal-setting and decision-making skills to enhance health.
7: Students will demonstrate the ability to advocate for personal, family, and community health.

PROCEDURE

Session 1

Divide the class into small groups. Provide each group with index cards on which are written common myths and facts about HIV/AIDS. For example:

HIV/AIDS is a disease that primarily affects gay men.

The primary cause of the epidemic is homosexual sex.

HIV/AIDS can be spread by infected people coughing, sneezing, or breathing on another person.

HIV/AIDS can be spread by infected people using the same telephone, water fountain, or bathroom as others.

The spread of AIDS in the United States is part of an evil plot.

The possibility of infection in heterosexuals is very small.

We are falsely being told that HIV and AIDS is a serious problem in this country.

If you feel healthy, you are not infected with HIV.

Mosquitoes and other insects can spread HIV/AIDS.

You can get HIV/AIDS by donating blood.

Individuals under 25 account for most of the cases in the United States.

Most of the people being diagnosed with HIV/AIDS got their disease in their teen years.

The HIV epidemic is decreasing.

Most young people today know about HIV/AIDS and are taking precautions.

HIV can be transmitted through oral sex.

Anal sex is only practiced by homosexual men.

HIV infection can be transmitted by people even though they have no symptoms.

You can tell if a person has HIV/AIDS.

HIV can be transmitted through sharing IV drug needles and sexual intercourse (anal, oral, and vaginal).

HIV cannot be passed from mother to unborn child.

A vaccine is available for AIDS.

AIDS can now be cured with prescriptive drugs known as combination drug therapy.

If you have sex with only one partner you will not get infected.

People who keep themselves clean especially after sex do not get infected.

Session 2

Using the index cards, have each group create a poster without a title. They decide whether their poster is fully depicting myths or fully depicting facts but do not tell their choice to the rest of the class. In the groups, the students with all myths will identify the truths; the groups with all truths will identify corresponding myths. Each group hangs its poster on the wall. The other groups of students must decide whether the poster represents myths or facts, citing reasons. At the end, the groups put a title on their poster. As a class, the students will discuss how they think some of the myths got started.

RESOURCES

Guidelines on myths and facts, poster board, markers, magazines, and index cards

ASSESSMENT PLAN

The students can develop a rubric for evaluating their posters and then use the rubric to evaluate each other. Students should be able to work cooperatively in a group to effectively complete an assignment, produce a creative project (poster) that describes the facts and myths about HIV/AIDS, and differentiate facts and myths about HIV/AIDS.

LEARNING EXPERIENCE 7

TITLE: A Public Service Announcement

GRADE LEVELS: 7–9

TIME REQUIREMENTS: Two 45-minute sessions

LEARNING CONTEXT

Communication, resource management, and decision-making skills are developed in the following learning experience. After this activity, the students will be able to

- Express the importance of advocating for family and community health.
- Describe how HIV is transmitted.
- Identify the behaviors that reduce the risk for HIV infection.
- Identify the risk factors for HIV infection.

NATIONAL LEARNING STANDARDS

1:   Students will comprehend concepts related to health promotion and disease prevention.

2:   Students will demonstrate the ability to access valid health information and health-promoting products and services.

5:   Students will demonstrate the ability to use interpersonal communication skills to enhance health.

7:   Students will demonstrate the ability to advocate for personal, family, and community health.

PROCEDURE

Put the students in small groups of four. Instruct the students to develop a public service announcement that would be used in their school newspaper or their school's radio station. The announcement can be no more than 5 minutes long. Include information about the disease, prevention, and especially where to go for health and medical help. Each group will then present their public service announcement, and the class will choose the best one using the rubric described later. The teacher gets one vote.

RESOURCES

Paper, pencils, class notes, computer access, phone book, and resource materials

ASSESSMENT PLAN

The class uses the following rubric to evaluate the announcements:

A = Does not exceed 5 minutes; all information completely correct; provides information that is appropriate for the age level of the audience; includes information about health services and how to access them; is innovative, creative; and holds interest

B = Does not exceed 5 minutes; most of the information is correct; includes reliable information about health services and how to contact them; is somewhat innovative, creative; and mostly holds interest

C = Does not exceed 5 minutes; several statements of information were incorrect; includes reliable information about health services but no contact information; is interesting but not very innovative or creative

D = Exceed 5 minutes; many statements were incorrect; does not include a reliable source of information and services; is interesting but not very innovative or creative

LEARNING EXPERIENCE 8

TITLE: High-Risk/Low-Risk/No-Risk Behaviors

GRADE LEVELS: 10–12

TIME REQUIREMENTS: 45 minutes

LEARNING CONTEXT

After this learning experience, students will

- Compare symptoms of STIs, including AIDS.
- Describe physical consequences of STIs.
- Identify and use sources for obtaining information, diagnosis, and treatment of STIs.

NATIONAL LEARNING STANDARDS

1: Students will comprehend concepts related to health promotion and disease prevention.

2: Students will demonstrate the ability to access valid health information and health-promoting products and services.

4: Students will analyze the influence of culture, media, technology, and other factors on health.

5: Students will demonstrate the ability to use interpersonal communication skills to enhance health.

PROCEDURE

Put the students in groups of four, and give each group six index cards. Name the groups "High-Risk," "Low-Risk," and "No-Risk." Assign each group with the task of writing at least six behaviors associated with STIs that relate to the assigned group. Collect the cards and shuffle them. For example:

> *High-risk:* poor communication with partner about having sex; sex without a condom
> *Low-risk:* sex with a condom (oral, anal, or vaginal); getting tested for STIs and
> HIV/AIDS; using effective communication about sexual decisions and choices
> *No-risk:* abstinence—no oral, anal, or vaginal sex; masturbation; mutual mastur-
> bation; outercourse; no drug or alcohol use; kissing

On each of four posters, cut in 4 × 8 strips, write "High-Risk," "Low-Risk," "No–Risk," and "Need More Information." Tape them on four different walls in the room.

Holding up one card at a time, ask the students to stand under the poster that best describes their thinking about the risk displayed in the raised card. They will then be asked to explain why they chose the position they took. Then hold up another card and ask the same. They might choose "Need More Information" if, for example, a card said, "Used a condom during intercourse." They might say, "We don't know if it was a latex condom or a skin." The teacher may ask, "What is the difference?"

When the cards are completed, have the students sit in a circle and discuss the following questions:

- Why do people engage in high-risk behaviors? (Sample answers: low self-esteem; peer pressure; sense of adventure; feelings of immortality)

- Aside from intercourse, how can people express physical intimacy? (Sample answers: kissing; petting; "making out"; hugging)
- What are some reasons people decide *not* to have intercourse? (Sample answers: religion; age; no real relationship; do not want to take a risk with their future)

As homework, ask the students to write a journal entry about their personal high-, low-, and no-risk behaviors.

RESOURCES
Index cards, small posters, tape, and chalkboard

ASSESSMENT PLAN
Evaluate journal entries.

LEARNING EXPERIENCE 9

TITLE: What Do They Need To Know?

GRADE LEVELS: 10–12

TIME REQUIREMENTS: Two or three sessions

LEARNING CONTEXT

This activity takes places after a class discussion of the symptoms and consequences of STIs. It develops communication, decision-making, problem-solving, and conflict management skills. Students will be able to

- Identify symptoms and consequences for various STIs.
- Recognize risk factors for infection.
- Describe effective communication skills to use for different STI scenarios.
- Identify appropriate conflict management techniques for different STI scenarios.

NATIONAL LEARNING STANDARDS

1: Students will comprehend concepts related to health promotion and disease prevention.
2: Students will demonstrate the ability to access valid health information and health-promoting products and services.
3: Students will demonstrate the ability to practice health-enhancing behaviors and reduce health risks.
5: Students will demonstrate the ability to use interpersonal communication skills to enhance health.
6: Students will demonstrate the ability to use goal-setting and decision-making skills to enhance health.
7: Students will demonstrate the ability to advocate for personal, family, and community health.

PROCEDURE

Session 1

Distribute a copy of the "STI Case Study" handout (included) to each student. Read each case study aloud. Ask students to identify the symptoms, a diagnosis, and the consequences of each case.

Session 2

Divide the students into groups. Each group will write their own STI case study and present it to the class. The class will identify the symptoms, a diagnosis, and the consequences of each case. (This exercise can be used for reviewing STI concepts.)

RESOURCES

"STI Case Study" handout, index cards, small posters, tape, and chalkboard

ASSESSMENT PLAN

Determine whether the students have the components for reviewing STI and AIDS concepts.

REFERENCE

Adapted from *Preventing sexually related disease: A curriculum for Grades 9–12,* by Betty M. Hubbard, 1989, pp. 80–93 (Santa Cruz, CA: Network Publications).

STI Case Study Handout

Case Study 1: Rosa and Ramon

Even though Ramon and Rosa had been attracted to each other for a long time, they just never seemed to get together. When Ramon was available, Rosa was going steady. When Rosa was available, Ramon was seeing someone else. When they finally began to date, Rosa and Ramon fell in love and decided to begin a sexual relationship. Almost a month after Rosa first had intercourse with Ramon, she developed a fever and headache. Small fluid-filled blisters appeared on her sex organs.

Case Study 2: Jane and Gary

Jane and Gary met at college and dated during their senior year. They made plans to marry after graduation. Two weeks before the wedding, Gary told Jane that he has genital warts.

Case Study 3: Phil

Phil was proud to join the U.S. Navy after high school graduation. While in basic training, he began to visit a local bar on the weekends. One night, Phil had too much to drink and went home with a woman he had just met at the bar. Several weeks after a one-night stand, Phil noticed a sore on his penis. He was concerned at first, but the sore did not hurt and disappeared after a couple of weeks.

Case Study 4: Sunny Brown

Maggie Brown and her husband were filled with joy and excitement when their daughter was born. They named her Sunny. Not long after Sunny's birth, Maggie realized that something was wrong. Sunny developed diarrhea, had no appetite, and did not gain weight. She often cried, even when she was not wet and had just been fed. When Maggie took Sunny for her checkup, she told the doctor about Sunny's problems. The doctor said he would do some tests but not to worry— it was probably just a virus that was going around. A few days later the doctor called Maggie and asked her to bring Sunny back to the clinic for additional tests.

LEARNING EXPERIENCE 10

TITLE: Telling Tomas about His Brother

GRADE LEVELS: 10–12

TIME REQUIREMENTS: Two sessions

LEARNING CONTEXT
After this activity, students will
- Be able to use communication skills to ask difficult questions.
- Develop empathy for persons with HIV/AIDS.
- Recognize personal risk for infection.
- Decrease notions of prejudice about persons with HIV/AIDS.

NATIONAL LEARNING STANDARDS
1: Students will comprehend concepts related to health promotion and disease prevention.
2: Students will demonstrate the ability to access valid health information and health-promoting products and services.
3: Students will demonstrate the ability to practice health-enhancing behaviors and reduce health risks.
5: Students will demonstrate the ability to use interpersonal communication skills to enhance health.
7: Students will demonstrate the ability to advocate for personal, family, and community health.

PROCEDURE
This activity involves role plays. Place the students in a circle with chairs next to one another. In the center of the circle are the chairs to be used by the active role players. While some students will begin in the active role play, each student will be asked to volunteer or be chosen to take a part of one of the role players during the role play in order to add to the dialogue. Thus students must continue to pay attention because they will have to participate at some point or another.

Session 1

Conduct the following role play. Ask the students to write at least four questions that they would ask their parents or their doctor if one of their siblings were diagnosed with HIV or AIDS. Suggest that the students include personal questions about how they would deal with embarrassment, fear, and other emotions.

Role Play

Tomas is a 13-year-old who has many friends and is interested in sports. Although he is interested in girls in his school, the guys he hangs around with make lots of fun of guys who "really like girls." They also make fun of kids whom they label as "gay." They have learned a little about HIV and AIDS in school, but Tomas and his friends are still filled with the common myths. Tomas has been told that his parents want to talk to him about his brother. They will tell him that his brother has been infected with HIV while he is away at college. They will answer all of Tomas's questions with honest and correct answers.

Session 2

After the following role play, ask the students to write down at least four questions that they will ask the brother when he comes home. They are also to be encouraged to ask personal questions.

For homework, ask students to write in their journals about how their lives would change if they were to be diagnosed with HIV/AIDS.

Role Play

Tomas's brother is William, and he is 19 years old. He has been away at college and is in his sophomore year. He took a class in HIV/AIDS and on a fluke decided that since he was sexually active, he would get anonymously tested. When he called in with his number, he found out that he was HIV-positive. Several more tests confirmed it, and he called his parents and told them. They insisted that he come home. He is now having a first conversation with his brother. He is very worried that his brother Tomas will get the same disease someday.

ASSESSMENT PLAN

The teacher will use the role plays to assess whether the information being communicated indicates that the students have correctly grasped the information.

LEARNING EXPERIENCE 11

TITLE: The Community Resource Booklet

GRADE LEVELS: 10–12

TIME REQUIREMENTS: Over the course of several weeks, including several class sessions

LEARNING CONTEXT
After these sessions, the students will be able to
- Recognize authentic sources of information and services.
- Contact various services organization to determine the type of services provided.
- Determine when they need to use STI health- and medical-related services.

NATIONAL LEARNING STANDARDS
2:   Students will demonstrate the ability to access valid health information and health-promoting products and services.

4:   Students will analyze the influence of culture, media, technology, and other factors on health.

5:   Students will demonstrate the ability to use interpersonal communication skills to enhance health.

7:   Students will demonstrate the ability to advocate for personal, family, and community health.

PROCEDURE
The class will collaboratively develop a manual for teens with information and resources related to STIs, including HIV/AIDS. Using the jigsaw classroom strategy, divide the students into groups of four. Each individual in each group will be assigned a task in the process of developing their resource manual as follows:

Person 1: Will be responsible for determining what to look for in an agency or organization that provides health and medical services related to HIV/AIDS. How do you tell whether it is a reliable service?

Person 2: Will research the various types of agencies that provide services and information related to HIV/AIDS

Person 3: Will gather the names and addresses of agencies and organizations in the local area. The group will then select 5 to 10 agencies and organizations they will include in their information booklet

Person 4: Will contact each agency either on the computer if it has a website or by phone or letter, asking the group to send materials about its services

The group will then create and submit their resources in a report to the class. The class will then decide together which services will go into the final booklet. Each group will be assigned a task in putting the final booklet together during a class session. Copies of the booklet can be made available to each student and to other students in the school if desired.

ASSESSMENT PLAN
A rubric will be developed by each student describing his or her grade evaluation. Each group will develop a rubric for evaluating their entire group's final submission.

SEXUAL VIOLENCE

ALANE FAGIN AND PATRICIA CATHERS

OBJECTIVES

After reading this chapter, students will be able to

1. Define different forms of sexual violence, abuse, and assault.
2. Identify indicators of sexual abuse in children.
3. Understand the role of the educator in reporting sexual abuse and assault.
4. Delineate developmental concepts of instruction in personal safety.
5. Understand how classroom teachers can incorporate abuse and violence prevention strategies into classroom learning experiences.

REFLECTIVE QUESTIONS

Elementary School
1. Who are your friends?
2. Complete the sentence: A friend is someone who _____.
3. Can friends be younger than you? Can they be older than you?
4. Do you have family online safety rules?
5. If you were in the mall and needed help, whom could you go to and what would you say?

Middle School
1. What makes a good friend?
2. Is there a difference between an online friend and a school/community friend?
3. How dangerous is this situation?
4. What could a person do to protect him- or herself from an online predator?

5. Would it matter if an online friend were male or female?
6. If you set up a meeting with someone online, would you tell someone?
7. If molestation were to occur as a result of an online friendship, would it be the kid's fault?

High School
1. What are the advantages and disadvantages of online friends?
2. If a friend discloses an incident of sexual abuse, how could you help him or her?
3. What are your personal expectations and boundaries when meeting someone new?
4. List your strengths and vulnerabilities of being a teen and confronting the possibility of sexual exploitation.

─────────────── **SCENARIO** ───────────────

Jessie's uncle takes her to the movies every week. Recently he has started putting his arm around her and touching her private parts while they are watching the movie.

Ever since Anne's mother started working the night shift at the hospital, her stepfather has been coming into her room at night and crawling into bed with her. He has started having sex with her despite her protests.

Judy is a college freshman. She goes back to her date's room following an evening of partying and drinking. Her date pushes her onto the bed, pulls her clothes off, and forces her to have sex with him.

Carla is asked to work overtime by her boss late at night. She is attacked and raped in a desolate office by someone in the building.

Jon has made a friend in an online chat room for teens. He plans to meet this new friend who he thinks is his age at the local mall. Unbeknownst to him, his new friend is a 35-year-old convicted sex offender.

Jason walks to school everyday with his best friend, Tim. These two boys, who are 10 years old, pass a neighborhood park and are approached by a man who suddenly unzips his pants in front of them.

─────────────────────────────────

INTRODUCTION

Hardly a day passes without a case of sexual abuse, sexual assault, or rape headlining the news. Sexual violence, in one form or another, is the topic of television shows and film. It is found in our literature, music, and video games. The statistics around sexual violence are staggering, and its effect on children and adults is long-lasting. In spite of the alarming number of reported cases, school administrators and educators are reluctant to include a discussion of these issues in their health education classes.

How prevalent are these problems? When should these issues be taught in the school? How should we introduce these topics so as not to scare children but to provide them with the tools and strategies enabling them to make healthy decisions and handle difficult situations? The National Victimization Study found that teaching children sexual abuse and victimization prevention could help children cope with real-life situations (Finkelhor, Asdigian, & Dziuba-Leatherman, 1995). Children who participate in these programs are more likely to disclose victimization and victimization attempts.

DEFINING SEXUAL VIOLENCE

Exactly what do we mean by *sexual violence? Sexual assault? Sexual abuse?* Although there is some disagreement in the literature in terminology and definition, for the purposes of this chapter, the terms *sexual violence, sexual assault,* and *sexual abuse* will be used interchangeably. In the broadest sense, sexual violence is based on three concepts—power, sexuality, and control—and is considered a forced sexual act against one's will. It can take the form of a single act or a series of acts. It includes a range of sexually abusive behaviors perpetrated against children and adults, including sexual harassment, molestation, incest, rape, and date rape. The perpetrator can be a family member, a friend, or a stranger. Contrary to what most people might think, most sexual abuse is perpetrated by someone known to the victim. In 50 percent of cases of child sexual abuse, the perpetrator is a family member; in 80 percent of cases, the offender is not a stranger. In more than half of all cases of rape, the perpetrator is an acquaintance.

Child Sexual Abuse

When the abuse is perpetrated against a minor, it is commonly called *child sexual abuse,* and it is illegal. *Child sexual abuse* is defined as any contact or interaction between a child and an adult in which the child is used for the sexual gratification or stimulation of the adult. All states acknowledge that minors are incapable of consent to sexual interactions with adults. Each state defines its own child abuse statutes and age at which an individual can give consent to sexual contact with an adult.

Sexual abuse encompasses a wide range of behaviors or activities, from molestation such as inappropriately touching a child's genitals, buttocks, breast, or other intimate parts; engaging or attempting to engage in sexual activity that is not appropriate to a child's age or development; and using a child in a sexual performance for child pornography or prostitution (Fagin, 2003). When sexual relations occur between relatives, it is called *incest.*

Sexual Harassment

Sexual harassment is defined as any unwelcome behavior of a sexual nature that interferes with a student's ability to learn. For too long, schools have dismissed sexual harassment as an unfortunate part of growing up: "boys will be boys"; "girls will be girls." Sexual harassment is a form of sexual discrimination and is prohibited under Title IX of the Educational Acts of 1972. Title IX protects students from sexual harassment on school grounds as well as on any school-sponsored activity off school grounds. It protects both male and female students regardless of who the harasser is, even if the harasser and target of the harassment are of the same sex. Under Title IX, schools can be held financially responsible for sexual harassment that harms students based on the Supreme Court's 1992 ruling in *Franklin v. Gwinnett*

County Public Schools, a case involving a high school student who was sexually harassed by a teacher (Williams & Brake, 1998, p. 2).

The legal definition of sexual harassment recognizes two types of sexual harassment: *quid pro quo* and *hostile environment. Quid pro quo* in Latin literally means "this for that." It usually involves a person who has power or authority over a student and uses that authority to get the student to submit to sexual advances, requests, or favors or other verbal, nonverbal, or physical conduct of a sexual nature. A teacher who threatens a student with a poor grade unless the student submits to his or her demands constitutes quid pro quo sexual harassment. *Hostile environment* consists of unwelcome behavior of a sexual nature that is sufficiently persistent, pervasive, and severe that the conduct creates an abusive, hostile environment. A group of boys who target a group of girls every week on the playground, making graphic sexual commentaries about the girls' bodies, backing them up against the fence, and attempting to touch them in a sexual way constitutes a hostile environment. This type of sexual harassment may also include criminal misconduct (sexual assault) dependent on the location and type of touching.

Many high school students may already have jobs and may experience or witness sexual harassment in the workplace. Employers must provide an environment free from sexual harassment for their workers, which may include students participating in job training and apprenticeship programs in workplaces or students employed by their school. Title VII of the Federal Civil Rights Act of 1964 prohibits employers from discriminating on the basis of sex (which includes sexual harassment and race). Title VII is enforced by the U.S. Equal Employment Opportunity Commission (EEOC) and applies to workplaces with 15 or more employees.

Stalking

Another form of harassment is stalking. An underlying factor in stalking is the exercise of control and power; stalking does not necessarily have to be sexual in nature. Public policy attention to the crime of stalking has resulted in the enactment of antistalking laws in every state, including the District of Columbia, between 1990 and 1994. In many states, stalking is classified as either a misdemeanor or a felony depending on the specific circumstances. While the specifics of the 50 statutes vary, *stalking* is typically defined as the willful, malicious, repeated following, harassing of another person, or causing credible threat to another individual in an attempt to frighten or cause harm (National Institute of Justice [NIJ], 1993). Stalking behaviors range from hang-up phone calls to more focused, direct threats toward a target (National Victim's Assistance Academy, 2002).

Rape and Acquaintance Rape

Rape has been defined as "sexual intercourse or attempted sexual intercourse with a female against her will by force or threat of force" (Barnett, Miller-Perrin, & Perrin, 1997, p. 1). Depending on an individual state's legal definition, either men and women, or only women, can be victims of rape or sexual assault; in most cases, however, the male is the perpetrator and the female is the victim.

Parrot (1999) defines *acquaintance rape* as forced unwanted sexual intercourse in which the attacker and the victim know each other. Date rape is the most common form of acquaintance rape. Although laws differ from state to state, some states consider only forced sexual intercourse rape, whereas others consider other forced sexual behaviors to be rape as well. Furthermore, facilitating a sexual offense with a controlled substance is considered a federal crime (according to the 1996 Drug-Induced Rape Prevention and Punishment Act).

The use of "date rape" or "predator" drugs that render a victim unconscious or unable to say no is a relatively new rape threat. Although many substances can be used to make a victim incapable of saying no, such as alcohol, marijuana, ecstasy, and other street drugs, generally the term *date rape drug* refers to gamma hydroxy butyrate (GHB), Rohyphnol, and ketamine hydrochloride.

GHB, called the "Mickey Finn of the '90s," is odorless and tasteless, and can be made at home in a chemistry lab. When mixed with alcohol, it results in memory loss, unconsciousness, amnesia, and even death.

Rohyphnol is commonly referred to as "roofies," "roche," "Mexican valium," and "circles." It is popular at fraternity parties, at college gatherings, and in gay bars. Recognized as an antianxiety drug, Rohyphnol is not approved for medical use in the United States, although it is legal in other countries. When Rohyphnol is added to alcohol, serious side effects can occur resulting in decreased blood pressure, drowsiness, confusion, memory impairment, and death.

Ketamine hydrochloride is commonly referred to as "Special K," "Vitamin K," and ketaject. It is considered a "dissociate anesthetic" that makes the person who ingests the drug feel disassociated from reality. This drug is used widely by veterinarians as an anesthetic. A range of side effects can occur, including hallucinations, delirium, respiratory depression, cardiac arrest, and temporary loss of vision.

It is always important to stress prevention strategies when introducing the topic of acquaintance rape and date rape drugs to students. Because these drugs are odorless and tasteless, they can easily be slipped into a drink or food making an unknowing, unaware victim passive, without memory, and without inhibition. Victims of date rape drugs have no memory of what has occurred after the event and therefore might not even be aware that they have been raped. Students should be warned that they should never drink from community punch bowls at parties, that they should never leave a drink unattended, and that they should buy their own drinks or be present when their drinks are served. Keeping an eye on their drink and food is one way of preventing being drugged by a sexual predator and becoming an unwitting victim.

Any discussion of date rape and sexual assault should include both prevention strategies and language for disclosure. Child Abuse Prevention Services (CAPS), a nonprofit organization located in Roslyn, New York, uses a mneumonic—the word *CLEAR*—when teaching date/acquaintance rape prevention to high school students:

C = Communication. Communicate with your partner. Say what you mean. Mean what you say.

L = Listen. Listen to each other. Respect your date's limits. No means no. Listen to yourself— if you have a bad feeling about someone, don't ignore it. Trust your instincts.

E = Equal partners. No one person in a dating relationship should be dominant. An equal relationship means equal partners. No one person should control the other. *E* is also for *economics*—there is no entitlement for sexual favors, regardless of the amount of money spent on a date.

A = Assertive. Be firm. Assert yourself. Don't go along with any behavior that makes you feel uncomfortable. Scream. Kick. Punch if you have to. It's better to be embarrassed than be raped.

R = Responsible. Both men and women share responsibility in dating relationships. Respect each other. *R* is also for *respect*.

HOW PREVALENT IS SEXUAL VIOLENCE?

Because there is no national reporting system that encompasses both intrafamilial and extrafamilial cases of sexual violence for children and adults, the exact incidence is difficult to determine. Furthermore, legal definitions vary from state to state. Wang and Daro (1998), in their study of child sexual abuse trends in 1992, report that 223,650 children were subjects of child protective reports. The National Incident Based Reporting System (NIBRS) calculates that 67 percent of sexual assaults handled by law enforcement agencies are perpetrated against children (Snyder, 2000). The National Victim Center's study "Rape in America" estimates that more than 12 million women and children have been subjected to sexual violence as a child or an adult (Kilpatrick, Edmunds, & Seymour, 1992).

Despite the significant incidence of sexual abuse, most professionals working in the field believe that sexual violence, sexual assault, and sexual abuse are underreported. Experts believe that much abuse goes undetected, and because of the nature of sexual abuse, it is therefore unreported. Some cases are reported long after the incident has occurred; some offenders are convicted on lesser charges, thereby making it difficult to interpret statistics. Our best understanding of the prevalence of sexual abuse comes from retrospective studies and self-report surveys.

Based on extensive research in the 1980s and 1990s, it is believed that one in four girls and one in eight or nine boys will be sexually abused by the time they reach the age of 18. In a telephone survey of adults, 27 percent of women and 16 percent of men reported victimization by age 18 (Finkelhor & Ormond, 1999).

Prevent Child Abuse, in its annual 50-state survey, has demonstrated a decline in identified cases of sexual abuse from approximately 429,000 reports in 1991 to 336,000 reports in 1999. In a survey of state child protection administrators, some respondents have postulated that prevention programs for children in schools and other education campaigns may be responsible for preventing abuse or stopping it in its early stages (Jones, Finkelhor, & Kopiec, 2001).

REPORTING VICTIMIZATION

Educators must be prepared for the possibility of a student making a disclosure during the course of presenting lessons on sexual abuse and victimization. It is advisable to alert the support services within the school community that you will be presenting programs on this topic, and it would be an ideal opportunity to invite the school guidance counselor, psychologist, or social worker into the classroom to introduce him- or herself to the class.

The disclosure of child sexual abuse and victimization may occur at different times in a victim's life. The disclosure may be "indirect"—that is it might be observed through behavioral actions—or it may be purposeful, resulting in a "direct" statement to a friend, adult, or colleague. A child who describes being sexually abused should be reported unless there is clear reason to disbelieve the statement (Besharov, 1990).

Educators should be familiar with state reporting requirements of child sexual abuse and must acquaint themselves with their school's policy and procedure for reporting suspected abuse. School personnel are considered mandated reporters in all 50 states and therefore must report child abuse when they have reasonable cause to suspect that a child has been abused. Failure to report suspected abuse by a mandated reporter is considered a misdemeanor in many states.

Reports of child sexual abuse, where the perpetrator is a parent or regular caretaker and the victim is a minor, should be reported to the child abuse hotline or state central register in the state in which the child resides. In cases of victimization where the offender is not a family member (such as a neighbor, stranger, coach, or date), the incident should be reported to the police. Each state has its own definition of a minor and its own system for reporting and investigating incidents of child sexual abuse and sexual violence.

Reports of sexual harassment must be responded to quickly, fairly, and effectively. Students have a right to go to school feeling safe and to learn in a nondiscriminatory learning environment. It is critical that school officials take action that is responsive to ending the sexual harassment and to prevent its reoccurrence. A student who believes he or she has been sexually harassed should immediately report it to a school official who can take corrective action. Under the law, schools and school districts must have at least one person responsible to respond to sexual harassment complaints. It is important that students, parents, and teachers know who their Title IX coordinator is. Students and parents can file a complaint using the school's grievance procedure. Under Title IX, the rules and procedures for filing complaints must be published in a student handbook and employee manual (Williams & Brake, 1998, p. 15).

Indicators of Victimization

Educators must become familiar with the physical, behavioral, and academic indicators of sexual abuse and victimization prior to teaching lessons on sexual violence or implementing a prevention program. Physical indicators of sexual abuse, such as torn, stained, or bloody underwear, STIs, or pregnancy, may suggest that a child is a victim of sexual abuse or assault. However, it is important to note that physical indicators are not always present in sexual abuse and in fact is only present in less than 50 percent of all reported cases of sexual abuse (Wallace, 1996).

Behavioral and academic indicators serve as "red flags" and should be used to alert the educator or school personnel that a child might be a victim of sexual abuse. Generally it is a pattern of behavioral indicators that would suggest to the professional that the child or adolescent is or has been a victim of sexual abuse or assault.

A range of behavioral indicators have been observed in both young children and adolescents and can include an unwillingness to change for gym, unusual sexual behavior or knowledge, acting out, poor peer relationships, delinquency, and running away. Moreover, younger children may exhibit sexualized play, regression, or school phobias, while older children might present with a sudden drop in academic performance, sexual promiscuity, depression, or suicide attempts. When a child presents with a combination of both sexual and nonsexual indicators, suspicion is heightened, and follow-up should be considered.

When sexual harassment occurs, a student may have trouble learning; experience a loss of self-esteem and confidence; may have physical symptoms associated with stress and anxiety such as stomachaches and headaches; may be frequently absent from school; and may have feelings of fear, humiliation, and a sense of powerlessness. Many times sexual harassment is an openly public event and affects not only the target but the bystanders as well, creating an intimidating environment for all students in the school. Most studies indicate that sexual harassment is a common occurrence in most schools and begins as early as elementary school. Sexual harassment most commonly occurs in school hallways and classrooms. Females are most often the target of sexual harassment. Sexual harassment may very well set the foundation for sexual assault and other forms of sexual violence. It is critical that issues of sexual harassment be addressed because it is against the law and everyone suffers—the victim(s), the harasser(s), the bystanders, the school, and the school district.

Rape victims suffer from a variety of emotional responses including shock, disbelief, fear and anxiety, shame, embarrassment, posttraumatic stress disorder, depression, issues of self-esteem, social maladjustment, sexual dysfunction, and other psychological reactions to rape (Wallace, 1996; Parrot, 1999). Victims of acquaintance rape often feel guilt because they believe that their behavior may have contributed to the rape and therefore they must assume some responsibility for the rape. They often have a difficult time accepting the fact that what they experienced was in fact rape, particularly because rape is often perceived as a violent act by a stranger and not forced sex by someone the victim knows. In all cases of sexual abuse, sexual assault, and sexual violence, it is important to communicate that it is never the victim's fault.

APPLICATION OF SKILLS

Effective communication enhances personal safety and competence and is an overall means of defense in minimizing risk of victimization. Children who learn to communicate effectively are given the message that they have permission to speak on their own behalf. They learn to name and articulate a range of emotions. They widen their vocabulary so they can identify and name specific sexual behaviors and body parts. Learning to communicate effectively enhances a child's vocabulary development and provides them with a dignified language to communicate about a physical violation.

Effective communication incorporates verbal and nonverbal assertiveness training so that children learn to say no assertively to potentially exploitative situations. Children need to learn to express their needs clearly and persistently in order to protect themselves. Effective communication skills assist in promoting safe, respectful communication between genders and in reducing conflict in interpersonal relationships, thereby lessening the chance of victimization and/or of becoming a victimizer of sexual assault. Effective communication skills assist children in advocating for one's self and others. Strengthened communication skills also provide children with the confidence and competence in disclosing issues of sexual abuse and exploitation as well as the tools and language necessary to help a friend who may be victimized or at risk of being so.

Critical decision-making and problem-solving scenarios offer children the opportunity to apply concepts they have learned and turn them into skills. Problem-solving activities may accurately assess a child's handling of a variety of different situations. Children learn to identify behaviors and situations that may be potentially uncomfortable and dangerous that could lead to sexual violence and exploitation and how to effectively respond to them. Development of critical decision-making and problem-solving skills ensures that children are actively participating in decision making that promotes their health, safety, and well-being and minimizes their risk of being sexually abused or assaulted.

Resource identification development skills offer students the opportunity to access health-promoting agencies and services as well as the opportunity to identify the individuals, families, groups, and organizations they can turn to for emotional and informational support and concrete assistance. As the radius of significant others widens as children grow and develop, the ability to utilize and identify different social systems—family members, nonfamily household members, peers, adults in the school system, professional formal organizations as well as informal organizations—becomes critical in assuring and enhancing children's sense of safety and competence and personal empowerment. Specific knowledge of professionals and agencies that have the expertise in dealing with sexual abuse and assault are particularly important in assuring that children get the right help, accurate information, and professional assistance that they need.

SUMMARY

Sexual violence is a pervasive problem that affects many children and adults and can leave lasting emotional scars. In spite of the alarming number of reported cases of sexual violence, from child sexual abuse and incest to forcible rape and date rape, many school administrators and educators remain reluctant to include a discussion of these issues in their health education classes. Research in the field of antivictimization education has demonstrated that children who participate in these programs are more likely to disclose victimization and victimization attempts.

A developmental approach to introducing antivictimization curriculum in the classroom can be started as early as kindergarten and includes recognizing some basic personal safety concepts. In later grades, the concepts take into account the growing maturity of the child as well as the child's increasing independence and broader range of experiences. Underlying any prevention program should be the theme that it is never the victim's fault for abusive behavior and that there are individuals and services in the community that can help. All programs should identify persons in the school and larger community who students can speak with about abuse and assault. Many videos, lesson plans, and curricula are available for educators to use as part of an antivictimization program. However, all materials should be reviewed carefully to determine their appropriateness for the grade level and community.

Given the staggering statistics for child sexual abuse, date/acquaintance rape, and sexual violence, it is quite likely that several children or adolescents in a classroom have been victimized. It is therefore incumbent on the educator to be knowledgeable of school policy and procedures pertaining to reporting sexual abuse before implementation of an antivictimization program. Educators should be informed of state laws and hotlines, as well as resources available in the community that provide intervention and treatment of sexual violence. Sensitivity to the possibility of disclosure as well as identification of behavioral and academic indicators will be helpful in assisting students who may be victims of sexual abuse.

This chapter includes several learning experiences that prospective teachers can use when teaching about sexual violence. Educators should modify the learning experiences so that they are applicable to the particular student population they are teaching.

WEBSITES

American Humane Association: www.americanhumane.org

Childhelp USA: www.childhelpusa.org

U.S. Department of Health and Human Services: www.dhhs.gov

National Center for Child Abuse and Neglect Information: www.calib.com/nccanch

National Center for Missing and Exploited Children (NCMEC): www.missingkids.com

National Clearinghouse on Child Abuse and Neglect Information: www.calib.com/cbexpress

Child Abuse Sexual Abuse Initiatives, Child and Family Canada: www.cfc-efc.ca.

Rape Abuse Incest National Network: www.rainn.org

U.S. Department of Justice, Bureau of Justice Statistics: www.ojp.usdoj.gov/bjs

ADDITIONAL RESOURCES

Rape Abuse Incest National Network: (800) 656–4673

National Clearinghouse on Child Abuse and Neglect Information: 330 C St. SW, Washington, DC 20447; (800) 384–3366

Examples of Comprehensive Child Safety Curricula

Kids and Company: Together for Safety: A personal safety curriculum for Grades K–6, providing children with skills, information, self-confidence, and support that will enhance their self-esteem and help to prevent abduction and abuse. This multimedia curriculum provides engaging activities, puzzles, songs, and games, as well as video-based role playing. Available through the Adam Walsh Children's Fund, (407) 775–7191.

No-Go-Tell: Child Protection Curriculum for Very Young Disabled Children: A personal safety curriculum designed to facilitate the understanding of concepts of sexual abuse as concretely as possible for very young children.

The Safe Child Program: A child abuse prevention curriculum for Grades K–3 that teaches prevention of sexual, emotional, and physical abuse; prevention of child abduction; and safety. This multimedia curriculum introduces concepts and demonstrates skills through videotaped modeling and role-play in age-appropriate segments. Available from Coalition for Children, PO Box 6304, Denver, CO 80206; (800) 320–1717.

Talking about Touching: A Personal Safety Curriculum: A child sexual abuse prevention program with physical abuse and neglect supplement. Photographs and stories serve as the basis for classroom discussion about decision making and personal safety. Individualized for Grades 1–3, 4–5, and 6–8. Available through The Committee for Children, 2203 Airport Way South, Suite 500, Seattle, WA 98134; (800) 634–4449.

Videos for Children, Grades K–6

The following videotapes are a sampling of materials in child abuse prevention, child assault prevention, child abduction prevention, anger management, and violence prevention. All videotapes should be previewed prior to showing to determine suitability for the audience.

Being Safe: A series of videotapes designed to support a developmental elementary school curriculum in child-abuse prevention. Aims to create a sense of self-worth in children. Three videos; 20 minutes each; Grades K–6; available from Altschul Group Corp., (800) 421–2363.

Believe Me: Teaches the difference between good and bad touch; 21 minutes; elementary; Coronet/MTI, (800) 255–0208.

Better Safe Than Sorry: Three simple rules that can help children to prevent or deal with potential sexual abuse: Say No, Get Away, and Tell Someone. 14.5 minutes; primary; available from Altschul Group, (800) 421–2363.

Break the Silence: Kids against Child Abuse: Profiles four courageous children who have survived child abuse. Unique combination of live interviews and animations; 30 minutes; Grades 3–6; available from Aims Multimedia, (800) 367–2467.

Bully No More: Stopping the Abuse: Strategies for dealing with bullying; 20 minutes; Grades 4–5; Aims Multimedia, (800) 367–2467.

Child Sexual Abuse: A Solution: Offers a solution to sexual abuse by giving the message that your body belongs to you and you can control who touches it, using concrete examples of sexual molestation and abuse. Six segments, 10–15 minutes each; Grades K–1, 2–4, 5–6, and parents/teachers; available from James Standifield & Co., (800) 421–6534.

It Happened to Me: Developed for boys 6 to 9 years old, designed to educate them about sexual abuse prevention. 15 minutes; available from Boy Scouts of America, (972) 580–2295.

John Walsh: Talk It Out with Adults You Trust: Talking and listening to an adult when a child needs advice, as part of a safety plan for children; 20 minutes; elementary; available from Coronet/MTI, (800) 255–0208.

Spider-Man: Don't Hide Abuse: Spider-Man helps a young girl solve her problem of how to disclose her father's physical abuse; 11 minutes; elementary; available from Coronet/MTI, (800) 777–2400.

Two Kinds of Touch: Young children learn the difference between "good touching" and "bad touching" and about their right to say no; 14 minutes; primary; available from Altshul Group, (800) 421–2363.

What Tadoo: A combination of original music, live action, and clever puppetry teach fundamental rules to protect young children from hurt and danger; 18 minutes; primary; available from MTITeleprograms, (800) 777–2400.

Who Do You Tell? Young children are encouraged to bring their problems and concerns out into the open and to identify and makes use of support systems available to them; 11 minutes; primary; available from Coronet/MTI, (800) 777–2400.

Yes You Can Say No: One boy's success in stopping his sexual victimization. Demonstrates assertiveness skills for personal safety; 20 minutes; Grades 2–6; available from AIMS Media, (800) 367–2467.

Videos for Adolescents, Grades 7–12

Flirting or Hurting? Students are helped to recognize and respond to sexual harassment. Gives administrators and teachers tools to help students create a safe environment; 57 minutes in three modules; Grades 6–9; available from GPN Film, (800) 228–4630.

Harassment on Trial: A teen accuses three fellow students of sexual harassment and a trial is held in High School Teen Court; 24 minutes; Grades 7–12; available from Intermedia, (800) 553–8336.

La Confianza Perdida: Spanish-language video, open-captioned in English. Offers prevention techniques on date and acquaintance rape in a very realistic manner; 22 minutes; Grades 10–adult; available from Intermedia, (800) 553–8336.

Playing the Game: A Video on Date Rape: Dramatization of a college campus date rape scenario, shows many points of view and clarifies the definition of rape; 15 minutes; high school; available from Intermedia, (800) 553–8336.

Risky Situations: The Reality of Rape: Dramatization of a radio talk show that features calls from teens and two professionals respond to questions about date rape; 34 minutes; high school; available from Intermedia, (800) 553–8336.

Sexual Harassment: It's Hurting People: Demonstrates and defines various forms and serious consequences of sexual harassment in a school setting; 20 minutes; Grades 6–8; available from National Middle School Association, (800) 528–6672 (NMSA).

REFERENCES

Barnett W., Miller-Perrin, C. L., & Perrin R. D. (1997). *Family violence across the lifespan.* Thousand Oaks, CA: Sage.

Besharov, D. (1990). *Recognizing child abuse.* New York: Free Press.

Donahue, A. (2000). *Prevention programs: Cause for concern?* Minneapolis: Center for Early Childhood Development (CEED), College of Education and Human Development, University of Minnesota.

Fagin, A. (2003). Child abuse prevention. In E. Weinstein & E. Rosen (Eds.), *Teaching children about health: A multidisciplinary approach* (2nd ed.). Belmont, CA: Wadsworth/Thomson Learning.

Finkelhor, D., Asdigian, A., & Dziuba-Leatherman, J. (1995). The effectiveness of victimization prevention instruction: An evaluation of children's responses to actual threats and assault. *Child Abuse and Neglect, 19,* 141–153.

Finkelhor, D., Hotaling, G., Lewis, I. A., & Smith, C. (1990). Sexual abuse in a national survey of adult men and women: Prevalence, characteristics and risk factors. *Child Abuse and Neglect, 14,* 19–28.

Finkelhor, D., & Ormond, R. K. (1999). Reporting crimes against juveniles. *Juvenile Justice Bulletin, 14*(8), 799–820.

Jones, L. M., Finkelhor, D., & Kopiec, K. (2001). Why is sexual abuse declining? A survey of state child protection administrators. *Child Abuse and Neglect, 25,* 1139–1158.

Kent, C. (1982). *No easy answers: A sexual abuse prevention curriculum for junior and senior high school students.* Santa Cruz, CA: Network Publishers.

Kilpatrick, D. G., Edmunds, C. N., & Seymour, A. K. (1992). *Rape in America: A report to the Nation.* Arlington, VA: National Victim Center.

Longres, J. F. (1995). *Human behavior in the social environment.* Itasca, IL: Peacock.

National Institute of Justice. (1993). *Project to develop a model anti-stalking code for states.* Washington, DC: Author.

National Victim's Assistance Academy. (2002). *Stalking.* Washington, DC: U.S. Department of Justice, Office of Victims of Crime.

Parrot, A. (1999). *Coping with date rape and acquaintance rape* (rev. ed.). New York: Rosen Publishing Group.

Snyder, H. N. (2000, July). *Sexual assault of young children as reported to law enforcement: Victim, incident and offender characteristics*. National Incident Based Reporting System (NIBRS) Statistical Report 182990. Washington, DC: National Institute of Justice.

Wallace, H. (1996). *Family violence: Legal, medical and social perspectives*. Needham Heights, MA: Simon & Schuster.

Wang, C. T., & Daro, D. (1998). *Current trends in child abuse reporting and fatalities: The results of the 1997 Annual Fifty State Survey*. Chicago: National Center on Child Abuse Prevention Research.

Williams, V., & Brake, D. (1998). *Do the right thing: Understanding, addressing, and preventing sexual harassment in schools*. Washington, DC: National Women's Law Center.

LEARNING EXPERIENCES

Lessons need to be developmentally appropriate, reflecting the uniqueness and specific abilities of the individual children being taught. Lessons should be taught from the child's perspective and be imparted in a way that makes sense to the child and can be readily understood and acted upon. For example, teaching students effective date rape strategies is more appropriate in the 7th through 12th grades than in the K–3 curriculum. Likewise, teaching personal safety rules is more developmentally appropriate for K–3 students, whereas fourth to sixth grade students, who have demonstrated an understanding of personal safety rules, can draw and expand on their knowledge and apply these specific safety rules to assist them in critical decision making in increasingly complex, potentially sexually exploitative situations.

Nonetheless, some developmental tasks and lesson objectives must be taught at every grade level. The complexity of the lessons increase with the child's growing ability to think and solve problems. Learning at all developmental levels should offer students opportunities to explore and assess assertiveness skills, resource identification skills, effective communication skills, and an awareness of self within an ever-changing environment. Throughout lessons on sexual violence, teachers at all times must foster and model interacting with both genders in respectful and appropriate ways. Also, be aware that opportunities will arise to use "teachable moments" throughout the day promoting children's appreciation for their own selves and the rights of others.

Grades K–3

In the early grades, lessons must be specific and concrete and should include role playing, practicing, and rehearsing of specific skills. Children should have the opportunity to discover what works and what does not (Donahue, 2000). It is not enough to tell children to "say no, go, and tell." They need the opportunity to practice it. Children in kindergarten and 1st grade should be taught to use safety rules as the primary decision making tool. Children in second and third grades can begin to use and trust their feelings in distinguishing between nurturing and confusing and exploitative touch. At this age, children's egocentricity often causes them to blame themselves for situations that are out of their control (Donahue, 2000). It is important to reassure them that sexual abuse and exploitation are not their fault and that the responsibility for such acts lies with the perpetrator.

By the end of third grade, students should be able to

- Respect and appreciate their bodies.
- Apply safety rules to potentially dangerous situations.
- Know they have a right to say no to unwanted, unsafe touch.
- Demonstrate assertive responses in potentially exploitative situations.
- Know how to tell.
- Identify adults whom they can go to for help.

- Determine the difference between safe and unsafe touch.
- Understand the difference between a surprise and a secret.
- Know the difference between tattling and reporting a situation that involves safety.
- Recognize and resist potentially unsafe situations.
- Acknowledge and understand their body rights and respect the body rights of others.
- Use a proper and dignified vocabulary and language for learning about their bodies.
- Articulate and name a range of emotions and feelings.

Grades 4–6

At this level, children have substantially grown and matured physically, socially and intellectually. They have mastered the language and have acquired a staggering number of concepts, facts, and premises. It is a time of growing independence, and children at this age want to be considered more responsible; children are given more freedom to play and are achieving more personal independence. They are acquiring more mature social relationships with friends of both sexes. Children are asked to assume more responsibility for themselves. Children at this age are developing moral standards by which they will live. They are learning about gender-specific roles and developing a scale of personal values (Longres, 1995). They can understand relationships and the feelings of others. Their reasoning ability and critical decision-making and problem-solving abilities have heightened as they advance into abstract thought. This is an ideal time for children to apply basic safety concepts and turn them into real skills. It is also a time when children can become confident in trusting their feelings when a touch or action makes them uncomfortable. They can learn to use their critical decision abilities to accurately assess and handle a variety of potential sexually exploitative situations.

At the end of sixth grade, students should be able to

- Trust their feelings, intuitiveness, and internal warning system.
- Identify safe, confusing, and exploitative touch.
- Provide a working definition of *sexual assault* and *molestation*.
- Know how to tell.
- Identify helping resources outside the immediate family.
- Demonstrate strengthened assertiveness skills.
- Understand their right to get help.
- Assess danger and potentially sexually exploitative situations.
- Describe several self-protection strategies to potentially dangerous situations.

Grades 7–9

At this time, children express a continued demand for greater independence from parents, with increased attention to peers, friendships, and group membership. During this explorative and often insecure time, young adolescents push their boundaries and test their limits. Concurrently, an increased sexual drive is a major physiological concomitant of early and mid-adolescence. Students are faced with an increasingly larger world where opportunities for choices are numerous. Peer relationships become paramount. This is an ideal time to assist students in learning how to establish different boundaries for different kinds of relationships including friends, dates, acquaintances, and new people.

At this level, a lot of the information students receive about sexual assault and exploitation is based on rumor, myth, and the popular opinions of their peers. Students need to begin to explore where their ideas about sexual violence originate and understand the myths and facts about sexual violence and exploitation. Rape, assault, sexual harassment, and sexual violence exploitation become increasingly pervasive during the middle and high school years (Longres, 1995). Because students are most likely to tell their friends about an incident it becomes increasingly important to discuss with students how to help a friend who discloses an incident of sexual violence.

At the end of ninth grade, students should be able to

- List their strengths and vulnerabilities of being a teenager in regard to sexual violence (Kent, 1982).
- Define terms related to sexual abuse and sexual violence.
- Demonstrate knowledge of facts regarding the scope of sexual violence.
- Understand the root causes of sexual violence.
- Define their personal boundaries and demonstrate confidence in communicating these boundaries to others.
- Know how to disclose.
- List ways to help a friend who discloses a sexual assault.
- Understand that sexual assault is not the victim's fault.
- Show increased problem-solving skills and responses to exploitative situations.
- Identify specific professionals and community agencies relevant to sexual violence.
- Demonstrate proactive assertive responses to potentially sexually exploitative situations.
- Apply touch continuum concepts to their different relationships.

Grades 10–12

Students at this level are deeply involved in attempts to achieve emotional independence from parents. Peer relationships remain paramount. Relationships with the same and other sex come closer to serving as prototypes for later adult relationships. The need to fit in and respond to peer pressure and social expectations may create potential crises in their lives. Sexual stereotyping and misinformation about young women provoking sexual violence remain prevalent in this age group (Kent, 1982).

Adolescents increase their vulnerability to experiencing sexual violence as victims and/or perpetrators. Teachers at this level must concentrate on teaching skills that will minimize the possibility of victimization while clearly identifying behaviors and situations that place students at risk.

At this level, there is an increase in risk-taking behaviors; students' abilities to analyze potentially sexually exploitative situations need to be honed. Students need practice to evaluate situations and strategize solutions. Students also need time to explore and examine their attitudes, beliefs, and values around different types of sexual violence including incest, rape, and sexual abuse.

At the end of 12th grade, students should be able to

- Understand the underlying causes of sexually violent behavior.
- Demonstrate advanced skills in problem solving in potentially sexually exploitative situations.
- Realize that sexual assault affects both males and females.
- Know how to disclose.
- Demonstrate an understanding of the sexual assault laws.
- Understand the concepts of consent, pressure, and forced assault.
- Describe how gender influences viewpoints and realize that sexual stereotyping is one instrument that perpetuates dominant/subordinate relationships that can lead to sexual violence.
- Define, in depth, sexual assault terms.
- Clearly communicate when communicating messages regarding sexual activity.
- Model interacting with both genders in respectful, appropriate ways.
- List several ways to help a friend who discloses an incident of sexual violence.
- Identify, assess, and utilize sexual assault resources within the community.
- Demonstrate prevention strategies that minimize risk of being victimized.
- Hold perpetrators of sexual violence accountable for their behavior.
- Acknowledge relationship between alcohol/drug use and unwanted sexual behavior.

LEARNING ACTIVITY 1

TITLE: Our Selves, Our Bodies

GRADE LEVELS: K–3

TIME REQUIREMENTS: Two 25-minute sessions

LEARNING CONTEXT
This learning experience develops communication and personal advocacy skills. Following this activity, students will be able to

- Respect and appreciate their bodies.
- Identify body parts.
- Have an accurate vocabulary for learning about their bodies.

NATIONAL LEARNING STANDARDS
5: Students will demonstrate the ability to use interpersonal communication to enhance health.
7: Students will demonstrate the ability to advocate for personal health.

PROCEDURE
This lesson takes place early on in the study unit. Children must have an appreciation and awareness of their bodies and recognize their own uniqueness in order to take control and responsibility over their bodies. Children need to develop clear, recognizable words for body parts in order to communicate effectively with others. An appreciation and respect for one's body as well as a mutually understood language of body parts are important components in the prevention of sexual abuse and exploitation.

Throughout this lesson, encourage body awareness and appreciation of oneself and others. Introduce key learning points: each of us is special and unique, and each part of our body is special. Children identify body parts by playing "Simon Says" with the teacher. Students have the opportunity to engage in physical activity while learning body parts and functions. Introduce the concept of private body parts and, if applicable, offer correct anatomical names for male and female body parts. Summarize the "Simon" lesson, offering clear and positive messages about their bodies and the importance of self-care. Conclude by discussing the concepts of privacy and body rights.

In preparation for this activity, collect a photograph of each student and have a bulletin board strip titled "I Am Special." Have pictures of body parts and their functions animated and demonstrated within a PowerPoint presentation. Prepare a beach or pool scene to be introduced later in the lesson. Begin the activity by stating that human beings have parts that help us in being special. Brainstorm with students on what those parts may be.

Explain the rules for "Simon Says" with students with one exception: that no one sits down if he or she makes a mistake. Students may need to be reminded during the activity not to point out or tease when mistakes are made. Begin the activity slowly, and start with "Everyone stand up." It is likely most children will stand up. Remind students of rules and begin again: "Simon says, stand up!" This activity begins slowly and speeds up as children become more confident in themselves. Be sure to include body parts as well as some simple body part functions—for example: "Simon says touch your feet. Simon says march around the room." Give the directions and change commands back and forth with "Simon says" and commands without that phrase.

Summarize the activity during a PowerPoint presentation, asking questions such as "What part of the body is this and what makes it special?" Following the activity, introduce the concept of private body parts, and, if in a position to do so, provide anatomical names in a very matter-of-fact way. If not in a position to do so, introduce the concept of private parts as those parts of the body that are covered by a bathing suit. Illustrate this point with a picture showing boys and girls and men and women in bathing suits at the beach or at the local pool. Ask students to identify and point out private body parts, reinforcing the message that they own their bodies and introducing the rule that it is never OK for an adult or older child to touch their private parts except to keep them healthy and/or clean.

For an optional homework assignment, ask children to construct a person using magazine photos of different body parts (arms, legs, and so on). Older children may create a more anatomically correct human being, identifying and labeling both inner and outer body parts.

INSTRUCTIONAL/ENVIRONMENTAL MODIFICATIONS

Environmental modification(s) must be made for students with physical disabilities and/or limitations. The teacher may use a digital camera for the student photos. Pictures of body parts and functions can be presented in a PowerPoint presentation. This lesson may be taught concurrently with science curricula.

RESOURCES

Digital camera, computer, photos for a PowerPoint presentation and beach/pool photos, construction paper, glue, markers, and pens

ASSESSMENT PLAN

The teacher will observe and rate each student's participation in the "Simon Says"–type activity:

A = requires no encouragement to actively participate

B = needs only occasional encouragement to actively participate

C = participates only with constant encouragement

REFLECTION

Children can learn to use the correct terms at an early age. They can learn about their bodies through play and activity. Using the correct terms makes explaining what might happen if there is an incident of sexual assault easier. Lacking the words to talk about body parts makes it much harder for children to explain what happened to them. Comfort with words and with their bodies can help children get the help when they need it. It is important to give children the sense that they own their bodies, that they are entitled to privacy, and to assist them in developing a sense of body integrity.

REFERENCE

"Our Selves, Our Bodies," posted by Debra Wrights of the Western Canada Family Child Care Association of British Columbia, April 1998, at www.cfc-efc.ca/menu/childdev. Wrights offers various lessons on this theme.

LEARNING EXPERIENCE 2

TITLE: Safe and Unsafe Touch

GRADE LEVELS: K–3

TIME REQUIREMENT: One 25-minute session

LEARNING CONTEXT

Personal advocacy and decision-making skills are developed in this activity. It immediately follows "Our Selves, Our Bodies." Children have developed a vocabulary for body parts, have identified the private parts of their bodies and have come to understand what is meant by the private parts of the body. They also have been introduced to the personal safety rule that it is never all right for an adult or older child to touch their private parts except for health and safety reasons. Students are now ready to apply the rule to various safe and unsafe situations.

After this activity, students will be able to

- Recite and practice the safety rule about touching private body parts.
- Identify health and safety needs and apply them to the safety rule exception.

NATIONAL LEARNING STANDARDS

6: Students will demonstrate the ability to use goal-setting and decision-making skills to enhance their health.

7: Students will demonstrate the ability to advocate for personal health.

PROCEDURE

Review the personal safety rule with students, and show them picture cards with various situations. Picture cards should include both safe and unsafe touches. Introduce each picture card, and ask directed questions: "What is happening in this picture? Is it all right for the mother to be touching the baby's private parts? Why or why not?" Give children the opportunity to discuss each picture, referring them back to the rule when children need help with decision making. Explain that it is never their fault if an adult touches their private parts and that they should always tell an adult whom they trust about what happened. (It is preferable to identify private parts by name; however, each school community will have its own policy with regard to this discussion.)

In preparation for this activity, collect various picture cards depicting different situations involving safe and unsafe touch, with a written description of the situation on the back of each card. Picture cards should include a wide range of situations where children can practice and discuss applying the personal safety rule. Several pictures should illustrate exceptions to the personal safety rule; they also should include a fair amount of safe touches so children understand that most adults are caring and safe. However, note that the touching rule applies to all adults, even people we know and like.

Students take turns describing situations and answering directed questions for each card. Each student recites the personal safety rule aloud and gives one concrete example of an exception to the safety rule—for example, a parent diapering a baby and a child being examined by the doctor with the parent present. Give students the opportunity to discuss their feelings in relation to any of the situations depicted on the picture cards.

For homework, students may collect pictures showing examples of caring and safe touches between people (adults and children, younger and older children, siblings, and others) for a classroom collage.

INSTRUCTIONAL/ENVIRONMENTAL MODIFICATIONS

Picture cards can be presented within a slide show or PowerPoint presentation. If the class includes students with language limitations, then other communication processes would be enacted, such as sign language.

ASSESSMENT PLAN

> A = Student shows understanding of all concepts taught with practically no errors.
> B = Student shows understanding of most concepts with few errors.
> C = Student shows understanding of some concepts taught with several minor errors or omissions.

REFLECTION

The touching safety rule needs a lot of practice and should be reviewed throughout the year. Children need concrete examples of the exception to the touching safety rule. This lesson can be expanded using puppets, reading stories, and watching and discussing videos on safe and unsafe touch.

REFERENCES

> *Believe Me*—video available from Coronet/MTI, (800) 255–0208.
> *Better Safe Than Sorry II*—video available from Altschul Group Corp., (800) 421–2363.
> Talking about Touching: A Personal Safety Curriculum for Pre-Schoolers and Kindergartners, developed by The Committee for Children, 1998.

LEARNING EXPERIENCE 3

TITLE: Developing a Children's Bill of Rights

GRADE LEVELS: 4–6

TIME REQUIREMENTS: Two 30-minute sessions

LEARNING CONTEXT

This lesson fits in to the social studies or language arts curriculum in a discussion on the Bill of Rights or human rights. It can also be used early on in the school year when creating classroom rules or when discussing "codes of conduct" in the school. Following this activity, which develops communication and advocacy skills, students will be able to

- Identify safe, confusing, and exploitative touch.
- Trust their feelings and intuitions.
- Understand their right to get help.

NATIONAL LEARNING STANDARDS

6: Students will demonstrate the ability to use goal-setting and decision-making skills to enhance health.

7: Students will demonstrate the ability to advocate for personal, family, and community health.

PROCEDURE

Students will create a Children's Bill of Rights based on an understanding of the concepts and liberties of the Bill of Rights. The children will have the opportunity to discuss the meaning and content of the Bill of Rights and the application of key concepts. In small groups, the students will connect the Bill of Rights to their personal experience, discussing the rights that they have.

Duplicate copies of the Bill of Rights, and distribute to the class. Read the Bill of Rights with the students, and go over the basic concepts and liberties. Select a read-aloud book, such as *Nothing but the Truth,* to further illustrate concepts of the Bill of Rights. Discuss why our country needs a Bill of Rights. An additional lesson can be offered to create a Classroom Bill of Rights.

The students will work in small groups to create their own Children's Bill of Rights on poster paper. They will present this "document" to the other students to be displayed in the classroom. Students will give examples of each right they have written. Each student should contribute at least one right to the project. Rights can include relationships with peers, teachers, other adults in the school, older children, and siblings. Children will work at home to create a Family Bill of Rights based on family safety rules that they can share with the other students. A letter should be sent home to the parents to explain the activity and encourage family participation.

INSTRUCTIONAL/ENVIRONMENTAL MODIFICATION
The Bill of Rights may be presented in a PowerPoint presentation.

RESOURCES
Overhead projector or laptop/proxima, copies of the Bill of Rights, poster board or butcher paper, and markers

ASSESSMENT PLAN
The teacher will observe and rate each student's participation in the small-group activity:

A = Student actively participated.

B = Student needed encouragement to participate.

C = Student participated only with constant encouragement.

D = Student neither participated nor contributed to the group.

The Bill of Rights will be assessed on its overall content and the number of rights cited:

A = Content is clear, and bill posts a minimum of five rights.

B = Content is clear, and bill posts three to four rights.

C = Content is unclear, and bill posts two to three rights.

D = Content is inaccurate, and bill posts fewer than two rights.

REFLECTION
It is important for students to know that they have rights; knowing they have these rights is an empowering experience. They now can apply these rights to personal safety rules and situations.

REFERENCES
Avi. (1991). *Nothing but the truth*. New York: Orchard.

Cuiri, P. R. (1998). *The Bill of Rights*. New York: Children's Press.

Stein, R. C. (1992). *The Bill of Rights*. New York: Children's Press.

LEARNING EXPERIENCE 4

TITLE: Brainstorming Personal Safety

GRADE LEVELS: 4–6

TIME REQUIREMENTS: Two 30-minute sessions

LEARNING CONTEXT

This experience is a follow-up to the creation of a Children's Bill of Rights and a discussion of family safety rules. It develops skills in communication, assessment, assertiveness, and problem solving. Following this activity, students will be able to
- Identify safe, confusing, and exploitative touch.
- Trust their feelings and intuitions.
- Understand their right to get help.
- Define and assess situations involving sexual assault and molestation.

NATIONAL LEARNING STANDARDS
6: Students will demonstrate the ability to use goal-setting and decision-making skills to enhance health.
7: Students will demonstrate the ability to advocate for personal, family, and community health.

PROCEDURE

Present students with several situations involving children and issues of personal safety. Students will be given the opportunity to "problem solve" and role-play these situations, referring to their Children's Bill of Rights, classroom bill of rights, and family safety rules. The children will be able to identify dangerous and risky situations and practice assertive and safe responses.

Prepare scenarios with pictures on laminated index cards or paper, and have students read aloud each scenario. Role-play the adult. Students will brainstorm and practice "safe" responses. Scenarios will progress from simple stories to more difficult, dangerous, challenging scenarios. For example:
- Saying no to cross the street without an adult
- Saying no to going over to a friend's house without telling a parent
- Opening the door to a stranger when a parent isn't home
- Feeling uncomfortable when a friend or other person continues to put his/her arm around you
- Responding to a friend's father who wants to take a picture of you without a shirt on

Use books that provide a wide range of "what if" stories. Prepare a vocabulary list of words to define, such as *sexual assault, molestation, fondling,* and *rape.* Model saying no assertively with words and body language, reinforcing verbal and nonverbal body language. If a mirror is available in the classroom, students can practice assertiveness in front of the mirror.

Each student should have the opportunity to role-play a scenario and respond to a challenging situation. Students can pair with each other to practice assertiveness skills, with each student taking a turn at being "assertive" while the other critiques posture, language, and intonation.

For homework, ask students to read a novel on personal safety and write a book report outlining the challenging situation that the protagonist faced and his or her response to it.

INSTRUCTIONAL/ENVIRONMENTAL MODIFICATIONS
Scenarios should be inclusive to reflect the abilities and diversity of students in the classroom. The scenarios can be presented in PowerPoint. A video can be shown to reinforce skills taught.

RESOURCES
Overhead projector or laptop/proxima, laminated index cards, books, videos, mirror, and a copy of each student's family safety rules or the Children's Bill of Rights

ASSESSMENT PLAN
> A = Book report is complete; content is accurate; and message saying "no, go, tell" is clear.
> B = Book report is accurate but incomplete; message is clear.
> C = Book report is accurate but incomplete; message is unclear.
> D = Book report is inaccurate; message is vague.

REFLECTION
All students should have the opportunity to participate, particularly those students who are quiet, shy, and withdrawn. Children need to practice specific skills; it is not enough to tell children to say no. They need the opportunity to practice it. This lesson serves as a kind of rehearsal in the event a child is ever faced with a comparable situation.

REFERENCE
From *It's O.K. to Say No! A Book to Read Aloud Together,* by R. Lenett and B. Crane, 1995 (New York: Doherty Associates).

LEARNING EXPERIENCE 5

TITLE: Who Can I Turn To?

GRADE LEVELS: 4–6

TIME REQUIREMENTS: Two 30-minute sessions

LEARNING CONTEXT

Communication, assertiveness, and advocacy skills are developed in this learning experience. It fits into the social studies or language arts curriculum and is a follow-up lesson to "Brainstorming Personal Safety." Following this activity, students will be able to

- Trust their feelings and intuitions.
- Understand their right to get help.
- Define and assess situations involving sexual assault and molestation.
- Demonstrate strengthened assertiveness skills.

NATIONAL LEARNING STANDARDS

6:   Students will demonstrate the ability to use goal-setting and decision-making skills to enhance health.

7:   Students will demonstrate the ability to advocate for personal, family, and community health.

PROCEDURE

Discuss with the class the different helping professions and services in the community. Students will learn what each professional does and their role in helping children and adults with abuse and sexual violence. The scenarios used in the previous lesson will be discussed again in terms of who would be the appropriate contact in the event of a problem. Students will practice contacting those professionals and will create their own resource list of family, friends, professionals, and school personnel.

Prepare a list of helping professionals, and define their role in the community: social worker, guidance counselor, psychologist, police officer, crossing guard, doctor, nurse, special victims unit staff, hotline counselor, and so forth. Use scenarios from the previous lesson (or create new ones), and ask students to identify the appropriate resource in that particular situation. The class will brainstorm and practice asking for help for themselves and friends.

Follow up by inviting helping professionals into the classroom to talk about what they do and how they respond to certain crisis situations.

Ask students to develop their own personal list of resources with phone numbers and addresses, including family members and local agencies. Pictures of family members and other important trusted adults can be included. Students will be presented with several situations and practice accessing resources by role-playing phone calls.

INSTRUCTIONAL/ENVIRONMENTAL MODIFICATIONS

Scenarios can be presented on an overhead or as a PowerPoint presentation. Students can research different professions and helping agencies on the Internet.

RESOURCES

Overhead projector or laptop/proxima, handouts, pens, pencils, and notebooks

ASSESSMENT PLAN

A = Telephone directory is accurate and complete with more than eight resources.
B = Directory is accurate and complete with five to eight listed resources.
C = Directory is complete with fewer than five resources.
D = Directory is inaccurate and incomplete.

REFLECTION

It is reassuring for children to know that help can be a phone call away. By rehearsing the actual words to say, children gain confidence in their ability to handle emergency situations. In doing so, students will have demonstrated an ability to advocate for their personal health.

REFERENCES

Visit Child Abuse Prevention Services at www.kidsafe-caps.org and the National Center for Missing and Exploited Children at www.missingkids.com.

LEARNING EXPERIENCE 6

TITLE: Helping a Friend

GRADE LEVELS: 7–9

TIME REQUIREMENTS: Two 45-minute sessions

LEARNING CONTEXT

This lesson takes place later in the study unit; it develops communication and personal advocacy skills. Students will have been acquainted with terms related to sexual violence and exploitation and will have demonstrated knowledge of facts regarding the scope of sexual violence. They will have listed their strengths and vulnerabilities of being a teenager and how it relates to sexual violence as well as explore their own attitudes and beliefs around the different types of sexual violence. The students have come to understand that sexual victimization is not the victim's fault.

Following this lesson, students will be able to

- Understand how to help a friend who discloses that he or she was sexually victimized.
- Understand the significance of supporting and believing in a friend who has been sexually victimized rather than blaming the victim.
- List ways to help a friend who has been sexually victimized.

NATIONAL LEARNING STANDARDS

5: Students will demonstrate the ability to use interpersonal communication skills to enhance health and safety.

7: Students will demonstrate the ability to advocate for personal, family, and community health.

PROCEDURE

Introduce sexual assault statistics to students, and point out that statistically there may be a victim of sexual violence, male or female, in the classroom. Have sexual assault statistics readily available (one in four girls and one in six boys will have been sexually assaulted in his or her lifetime). Review with class that sexual assault on males is underreported, and discuss with students why this might be, challenging them to look at the broader social issues as the lesson progresses. Throughout the lesson, remain vigilant and sensitive to students' responses, and realize that the lesson may evoke student disclosures of sexual abuse/violence. Know the reporting responsibilities in the event of a disclosure.

Guide students into a discussion on what they would do if they discovered that one of their friends has been sexually assaulted. The class brainstorms a range of responses that are written on the board. Students have the opportunity to rate which responses are best and why. Challenge them with thought-provoking questions such as these:

- Would you respond differently to your friend if the perpetrator was a friend of yours?
- What if the perpetrator was a member of the victim's immediate family?
- Does your response differ depending on whether the victim is male or female?
- Do our responses differ according to specific circumstances? Why or why not?

Encourage exploration of gender stereotyping as well as the students' beliefs, attitudes, and values regarding sexual victimization.

Distribute short role-play scenarios giving students the opportunity to practice helping a friend who has been sexually victimized. Students have the opportunity to take the perspective of both the victim and the friend. Every student has the opportunity to participate in this lesson either as an actor or active member of the audience. Role-play suggestions include the following:

- A friend discloses that he or she was hitchhiking, picked up, and forced to perform sexual acts with the driver.
- A friend discloses that her stepfather has been abusing her for sometime, and she is planning on running away.
- A friend is infatuated with another friend's older brother, sneaks out of the house to see him, and is subsequently sexually assaulted by him.
- A friend was drinking at the beach and was sexually assaulted in the men's bathroom.
- A friend was coming home from the city, and a man exposed himself to her on the train.

Students should be invited to create their own scenarios that reflect some of their life experiences. Encourage all students to think of alternative responses and endings to the role-play scenarios. After each role play, focus a discussion on how it felt to be the friend and how it felt to be the victim disclosing the abuse and receiving the help. The class evaluates the effectiveness of the skit.

Prepare a handout called "How to Help a Friend," with space available for students to write in their own responses. Suggested responses include these:

- Listen.
- Believe in your friend.
- Help your friend to tell someone.
- Show that you care—don't laugh or tell him or her she's crazy.
- Let your friend know it's not his or her fault.

Students rate what responses might be most effective and why. Encourage exploration of gender stereotyping, and ask provocative questions challenging their attitudes and beliefs about sexual victimization. Suggested questions might include the following:

- Would your response to your friend change if you discovered the offender was a friend of theirs?
- If the offender was the victim's boy- or girlfriend?
- If the offender was a family member of the victim?
- If the victim and victimizer were of the same or other sex?
- If alcohol or drugs were involved?
- If your friend had been someplace he or she was not supposed to be?

For homework, ask students to write a letter to an imaginary friend who has recently experienced a sexual assault. The letter should include an introductory empathic statement, advice on what to do, and what the student can do to help.

INSTRUCTIONAL/ENVIRONMENTAL MODIFICATION
Role plays can be videotaped for evaluation, interpretation, and assessment of learning.

RESOURCES
"How to Help a Friend" handout, video camera recorder (optional), reading materials, pens and pencils, notebook

ASSESSMENT PLAN

Students have the opportunity to assess their peers in role plays, and the teacher observes and rates each student's participation during the lesson:

A = Student requires no encouragement to actively participate in and encourages others participation.

B = Student requires occasional encouragement to participate.

C = Student requires constant encouragement to participate.

D = Student does not participate.

REFLECTION

Many teens experience barriers to disclosing an incident of sexual violence. It is comforting for them to know that their peers are sensitive to the issue and are present for them in case they need help. Students have demonstrated an ability to use interpersonal communication skills to enhance their health and have demonstrated an ability to advocate for themselves and others.

RESOURCES

Visit www.preventchildabuseny.org/pirc.html. Click on "Child Abuse Prevention Materials," and then click on "Helping a Friend." Also see *Gender Violence, Gender Justice: An Interdisciplinary Teaching Guide for Teachers of English, Literature, Social Studies, Psychology, Health, Peer-Counseling, and Family and Consumer Sciences (Grades 7–9),* by Nan Stein and Dominic Capello, 1999 (Wellesley, MA: Wellesley College Center for Research on Women).

LEARNING EXPERIENCE 7

TITLE: Resource Identification

GRADE LEVELS: 7–9

TIME REQUIREMENT: One 40-minute session

LEARNING CONTEXT

This lesson takes place later in the study unit, following the "Helping a Friend" lesson. Students have learned how to help a friend who discloses an incident of sexual violence. It develops resource identification and advocacy skills. Following this lesson, students will be able to

- Identify, assess, and utilize sexual assault resources within the community.

NATIONAL LEARNING STANDARDS

2:   Students will demonstrate the ability to access valid health information and health-promoting products and service.

7:   Students will demonstrate the ability to advocate for personal, family, and community health.

PROCEDURE

Prepare a resource worksheet for students to complete. Lead student teams to brainstorm as many people and places (formal and informal) they can think of to go to or contact for information, referral, and support. Arrange for a guest speaker from a local community sexual assault agency (for example, a rape crisis center, child protective services, or the police department's special victim's unit).

Students will work together as teams in order to successfully complete the resource worksheet. They will select a spokesperson from each team to share the results with the rest of the class, and they will have prepared a minimum of two questions for the guest speaker.

For homework, ask students to create a laminated personal bookmark illustrating a minimum of five identified helping resources on it.

INSTRUCTIONAL/ENVIRONMENTAL MODIFICATIONS

Students may use the Internet to identify sexual violence resources. Students are also encouraged to access information from traditional sources such as phone books, community resource books, and newspapers. The teacher and students may research culture specific agencies (faith based, multilingual agencies, and so on) that accommodate students' cultural, faith, and ethnic needs. If requested, an overhead projector and/or VCR and monitor will be made available to enhance the guest speaker's presentation.

RESOURCES

Resource worksheets, speaker, audiovisual equipment, computers with Internet access, local resource books, pens and pencils, and notebooks

ASSESSMENT PLAN

The teacher will observe and rate each student's participation during the lesson. Bookmarks will be graded based on content and design:

> A = Student has listed five or more relevant agencies, and the content is complete and accurate. Bookmark is neatly done.
>
> B = Student has listed four relevant agencies, and the content is accurate but not complete. Bookmark is neatly done.
>
> C = Student has listed three agencies, content is not complete, and work is not neat.
>
> F = Student has not handed in the assignment.

REFLECTION

Students find it empowering and comforting to know that resources exist within the community to help them with their questions and concerns. It is important that teens be reassured that they do not have to solve everything on their own and be granted permission to ask for help.

REFERENCES

Visit www.preventchildabuseny.org/pirc.html; click on "More Helplines." Also see http://education.indiana.edu/cas/adol/risk.html: Center for Adolescent and Family Studies School of Education Indiana University Bloomington. This site is a collection of electronic resources intended for parents, educators, researchers, health practitioners, and teens and also notes general sources for adolescent health information.

Under Megan's Law, each state now has a directory of convicted sex offenders. Depending on state law and category of sex offense, access to the directory may be available to the public through the police department.

LEARNING EXPERIENCE 8

TITLE: Preventing Sexual Assault

GRADE LEVELS: 10–12

TIME REQUIREMENT: One 45-minute session

LEARNING CONTEXT

This lesson fits into the health education, social studies, or language arts curriculum and is a follow-up to lessons on healthy relationships, abuse prevention, communication, and peer pressure. It develops skills in communication, assertiveness, and advocacy. Following this activity, students will be able to

- Set standards for what are sexually violent behaviors.
- Demonstrate advanced skills in problem-solving exploitative situations.
- Understand concepts of consent, pressure, and forced assault.
- Define in depth sexual assault terms.
- Demonstrate prevention strategies that minimize risk of being victimized.

NATIONAL LEARNING STANDARDS

6: Students will demonstrate the ability to use goal-setting and decision-making skills to enhance health.

7: Students will demonstrate the ability to advocate for personal, family, and community health.

PROCEDURE

Define with the students sexual assault terms including *date rape, acquaintance rape,* and *sexual abuse,* and review the state's penal code for sexual assaults. Show the video *Playing the Game;* if it is not available, break the class down into small groups, and distribute scenarios depicting different forms of sexual violence with discussion questions. Each group will brainstorm responses, and the class will reconvene to discuss and reach consensus.

As homework, ask students to research organizations that work in the field of sexual violence prevention and treatment (for example, rape crisis centers and date rape prevention organizations). Students will create a resource list of phone numbers, hotlines, and websites with information on sexual violence prevention.

INSTRUCTIONAL/ENVIRONMENTAL MODIFICATIONS

Scenarios can be presented on an overhead projector or as a PowerPoint presentation.

RESOURCES

Overhead projector or laptop/proxima, scenario handouts, guest speakers, video, pens, pencils, and notebooks

ASSESSMENT PLAN

The teacher will observe and rate each student's participation during the lesson:

A = Group demonstrates understanding of scenario, forms of sexual violence, ways to prevent it, and several resources necessary for intervention.

B = Group demonstrates understanding of scenario and forms of sexual violence, and can identify limited resources for intervention.

C = Student demonstrates limited understanding of scenario and resources necessary for intervention.

D or F = No participation in exercise.

REFLECTION

It is important for students to problem-solve various situations, clarifying the basic problem and identifying a range of solutions. Problem solving, particularly in the area of sexual abuse and sexual violence, can be emotionally charged, especially when the problem is not clear-cut. Students need time and practice to explore, identify, and solve complex issues.

REFERENCES

Parrot, A. (1991). *Acquaintance rape and sexual assault: A prevention manual.* Holmes Beach, FL: Learning Publications.

Playing the game: Date rape. Video (15:30 minutes) (Seattle: Intermedia).

LEARNING EXPERIENCE 9

TITLE: Creating a Dating Bill of Rights

GRADE LEVELS: 10–12

TIME REQUIREMENTS: One 45-minute session

LEARNING CONTEXT

This lesson fits into the health education, social studies, or language arts curriculum and can be used as a follow-up to lessons on preventing sexual assault. It develops skills in communication, assertiveness, and advocacy. Adolescents need to understand that acquaintance/date rape is no different than stranger rape and is not considered a lesser offense. It only defines the relationship between victim and offender.

Following this activity, students will be able to

- Set standards for what are sexually violent behaviors.
- Demonstrate advanced skills in problem-solving exploitative situations.
- Understand concepts of consent, pressure, and forced assault.
- Define in depth sexual assault terms.
- Demonstrate prevention strategies that minimize risk of being victimized.

NATIONAL LEARNING STANDARDS

6:   Students will demonstrate the ability to use goal-setting and decision-making skills to enhance health.

7:   Students will demonstrate the ability to advocate for personal, family, and community health.

PROCEDURE

Refer to the video *Playing the Game* and the "Preventing Sexual Assault" lesson in which sexual assault terms were defined and discussed. Introduce the concepts of consent, communication, and alcohol and drugs, and their relationship to dating. Split the class into small groups, equally distributing male and female students. Each group will develop their own list of Dating Rights, from the perspective of the female and the male students. They will brainstorm individual dating rights, based on concepts that they have learned pertaining to communication, consent, and alcohol and drug use. Input from both male and female students will be required. The class will reconvene to discuss each right and to reach consensus. Develop, with the students' input, a document called a "Dating Bill of Rights" on poster paper or the overhead projector.

For homework, ask the students to research relevant penal code sex offenses for their state. Another assignment could ask students to research date rape drugs in newspaper and magazine articles and report to the class on the effects of these drugs.

INSTRUCTIONAL/ENVIRONMENTAL MODIFICATIONS

The Dating Bill of Rights can be created as a PowerPoint presentation or using an overhead projector.

RESOURCES

Overhead projector or laptop/proxima, handouts, speakers, pens, paper or butcher paper, and markers; and the video *Playing the game: Date rape* (15:30 minutes) (Seattle: Intermedia)

ASSESSMENT PLAN

The teacher will observe and assess each student's participation during the lesson and will grade group and student participation:

> A = Group demonstrates understanding of communication, consent, and drugs and alcohol in relation to date rape prevention and contributes seven rights.
>
> B = Group demonstrates understanding of communication, consent, and drugs and alcohol in date rape prevention and presents five rights.
>
> C = Group demonstrates limited understanding of date rape prevention and offers three rights.
>
> D = Student participates minimally in exercise.
>
> F = Student does not contribute to Dating Bill of Rights.

REFLECTION

Acquaintance rape is one of the most common forms of sexual abuse among adolescents, yet it is often misunderstood and underreported. It is important to emphasize that the victim is often manipulated or blamed; however, it is never the victim's fault. The responsibility lies with the offender.

REFERENCES

For additional information for this lesson, contact the National Coalition against Sexual Assault at (717) 728-9764 and the Rape, Abuse, and Incest National Network at (800) 656-HOPE.

LEARNING EXPERIENCE 10

TITLE: Risky Business: Identifying Dangerous Situations

GRADE LEVELS: 10–12

TIME REQUIREMENTS: One 45-minute session

LEARNING CONTEXT

This lesson fits into the health education, social studies, or language arts curriculum and is a follow-up to lessons on creating a Dating Bill of Rights. It develops skills in communication, assertiveness, and advocacy. Following this activity, students will be able to

- Set standards for what are sexually violent behaviors.
- Demonstrate advanced skills in problem-solving exploitative situations.
- Understand concepts of consent, pressure, and forced assault.
- Define in depth sexual assault terms.
- Demonstrate prevention strategies that minimize risk of being victimized.

NATIONAL LEARNING STANDARDS

6: Students will demonstrate the ability to use goal-setting and decision-making skills to enhance health.

7: Students will demonstrate the ability to advocate for personal, family, and community health.

PROCEDURE

Have students "visualize" what a stereotypical rapist and victim look like, and ask them to share these visions with the class. Use these descriptions, and provide facts to dispel some of the myths that are associated with rape and sexual assault. Some examples of myths include the following:

Most sexual assault victims do not know their assailant.

If a woman goes out alone after dark, she is asking to be raped.

The way some women dress is an invitation to rape.

If a person is drunk, he or she can still consent to sex.

If a guy is drunk, he really can't be responsible for his actions.

You can't be raped by a friend or someone you are in a relationship with.

Distribute a true/false test on sexual assault. Answers will be discussed in class to consider myths and facts with students.

As homework, ask students to identify five different situations that might put them in danger or at risk for sexual coercion and how they might handle the situation. The focus should be on dating and peer relationships.

INSTRUCTIONAL/ENVIRONMENTAL MODIFICATIONS

The list of offender and victim images, as well as the true/false test, can be created on an overhead or as a PowerPoint presentation.

RESOURCES

Overhead projector or laptop/proxima, handouts, speakers, pen, and paper

ASSESSMENT PLAN

The teacher will observe and assess each student's participation during the lesson using the following rubric:

A = Student demonstrates understanding of sexual assault by participation in myths and scores 90 percent correct on true/false.

B = Student demonstrates understanding of sexual assault by participation in myths and scores 80 percent correct on true/false.

C = Student demonstrates limited understanding of sexual assault with limited participation and scores 70 percent correct on true/false.

D = Student has minimal participation in exercise and 60 percent on true/false.

F = Student does not contribute.

REFLECTION

Adolescents are bombarded by media coverage of sexual assault and sexual imagery. It is important for students to figure out what is true and what is false in the area of sexual abuse and sexual violence. It is important for students to differentiate between sexuality and sexual abuse. Students need to think about the types of messages they receive about sexuality and sexual violence.

REFERENCE

See *Without Consent: Peer Education Training for Secondary Schools: Preventing Sexual Abuse,* a video of activities for those working with children and adolescents (Wayne County, NC: The Lighthouse, n.d.).

LEARNING EXPERIENCE 11

TITLE: Sexual Harassment Scenarios: What's Wrong with This Picture?

GRADE LEVELS: 10–12

TIME REQUIREMENTS: Two 45-minute periods

LEARNING CONTEXT

This experience is an important discussion builder for the topic of sexual abuse. It encourages students to think critically about incidents of sexual harassment that happen daily in school life but that are coded as "normal."

This activity could introduce a unit on school sexual harassment or be a part of a unit on gender issues. It helps to develop personal life skills through communication, stress management, relationship management, and conflict resolution. It is advised that respectful, open communication requires active listening and that the goal of this learning experience is to establish or review a procedure for responding to school life incidents that are sexually harassing.

NATIONAL LEARNING STANDARD

3: Students will demonstrate the ability to practice health-enhancing behaviors and reduce health risks.

PROCEDURE

Students work in groups of four. Give each group a handout with one of the scenarios (listed later). Ask them to respond to the following questions, as a group:

Is this typical behavior in school life? Why or why not?

Have you ever encountered a similar situation that you can discuss?

What is wrong with this picture? Where is the sexual abuse?

Is this just a case of annoying behavior? Why or why not?

There is a lot of confusion about what sexual harassment is. Can you come up with your own definition?

What procedure, if any, could you follow to report these incidents?

RESOURCE

Scenario handout, cut so that one scenario is on a slip of paper for each group

ASSESSMENT PLAN

Students respond to these questions, individually and in writing:

1. Which of these scenarios, if any, reminded you of an incident that you experienced or observed?
2. Which gender do you think is more victimized by sexual harassment? Why?
3. What should a student do if she or he observes or experiences sexual harassment?
4. Which case of sexual harassment do you believe to be more prevalent? Peer abuse or teacher–student abuse? Please state your reasons.

REFLECTION

Sexual harassment is often not well understood. Under the guidelines established by the Office for Civil Rights (OCR), sexual harassment is a form of sex discrimination prohibited by Title IX of the Education Amendments of 1972. The regulation implementing Title IX, Section 106.31 outlaws sexual harassment as a form of disparate treatment that impedes access to an equitable education. OCR identifies two types of sexual harassment in schools: quid pro quo and hostile environment. *Quid pro quo sexual harassment* occurs when a school employee causes a student to believe that he or she must submit to unwelcome sexual conduct to participate in a school program or activity. It can also occur when a teacher suggests to a student that an educational decision such as grades will be based on whether or not the student submits to unwelcome sexual conduct. *Hostile environment harassment* occurs when unwelcome verbal or physical conduct is sufficiently severe, persistent, or pervasive that it creates an abusive or hostile environment for the affected student.

Scenarios

1. Mr. M. is a fourth grade teacher who rubs the backs of his students when they get upset. Sometimes he touches their shoulders and legs when administering back-rubs. The students say they feel uncomfortable with the rubbing, but other than this, they like Mr. M.

2. Mr. R. is a geometry teacher who has worked hard to develop math materials that will keep his students' interest. He accompanies his lectures with pictures of women in sexually suggestive positions to demonstrate angles. He also tells students jokes about his sexual exploits to keep his students interested.

3. Ms. L, a high school English teacher, calls the girls "honey" and puts her arms around them. Ms. L. also puts her arms around the boys and calls them "studs."

4. Mr. F. is a middle school teacher and football coach who calls his players "pussy," "fag," or "girls" when they do not meet his expectations. In his social studies class, a student calls a classmate who doesn't play football a "pussy."

5. The students walk into chemistry class and one of the boys calls a girl a "slut" as they stream into the classroom. Ms. S., the science teacher, says nothing, although she is in earshot of the remark.

SEXUALITY IN SOCIETY AND CULTURE

MICHAEL LUDWIG AND JEAN L. HARRIS

OBJECTIVES

After reading this chapter, students will be able to

1. Describe a variety of ways that society and culture interact to affect a person's understanding of sexuality.
2. Demonstrate respect for people with different sexual values.
3. Promote the rights of all people to accurate sexuality information.
4. Reject stereotypes about the sexuality of diverse populations.
5. Identify legal issues related to sexuality and sexuality education.
6. Identify how religious affiliation influences one's understanding of sexuality.
7. Describe the impact of race and ethnicity on sexuality.
8. Examine how literature has treated sexuality.
9. Demonstrate strategies for developing media literacy, particularly related to sexuality and sexuality education.
10. Evaluate the validity of the Internet as a source of information on sexuality.
11. Describe a variety of ways that the arts use sexuality.
12. Examine the impact of sexually explicit images on students across all developmental ages.
13. Describe our society's complex relationship with prostitution.

REFLECTIVE QUESTIONS

Elementary School
1. What is a law, and where does one come from?
2. What are the different kinds of media you are familiar with?
3. How do commercials try to get us to buy things?
4. What are some of the holidays your family celebrates, and what do they do to celebrate them?

Middle School
1. Why is it necessary to have laws?
2. How does each of the different media try to influence us?
3. What are the strategies used by commercials to promote their products?
4. How do your family's values influence the types of movies you can go to?
5. What are the roles played by culture in relationships?
6. How does religion affect relationships?
7. How does religion affect your family's beliefs and values?

High School
1. How are laws made?
2. What laws regarding sexuality affect teens the most?
3. How does religion affect relationships when both partners belong to the same religion? What about when they belong to different religions?
4. How do race and ethnicity affect relationships when both partners belong to the same race/ethnicity? What about when they belong to different races/ethnicities?
5. What effect do the media have on our understanding of gender roles?
6. What effect do the media have on our understanding of different racial and ethnic groups?
7. What is the purpose of marriage?
8. How has marriage changed over the last 100 years?
9. How do different cultures (religions) view marriage?

─────── **SCENARIO** ───────

Jonathan and Iris have been seeing each other for a few months. They knew each other in high school and now attend the same community college. The community college is located in a large urban-suburban area with a diverse population. Jonathan's ethnic background is Eastern European and is Jewish; Iris is of Latin background and is Catholic. Each of their parents is concerned about the differences in ethnicity and religious background and has made their views known to their child. Jonathan and Iris think their parents are being old-fashioned and that things like ethnic background and religion don't matter as much as they used to.

Jonathan and Iris enjoy going to the movies together. Iris is taking a film studies class at her community college, and Jonathan is studying business. In the film class, students explore the portrayal of gender, religious, and ethnic background, and as a result, Iris has developed a more critical eye when it comes to the films she sees. After seeing a film, Jonathan and Iris frequently go to a coffee shop to talk about the movie. Recently, these discussions have become more animated as Iris enjoys pointing out what she sees as biases in the movies. Jonathan generally dismisses her concerns and counters by saying, "You're reading too much into the films—they're just entertainment." Iris agrees that they are entertainment but suggests they are also much more—they are cultural phenomena that instruct and that frequently support a particular set of beliefs and values. For example, she says, "Many Disney animated features depict women as subservient to men and suggest that a woman is defined by her relationships to men rather than on who she is." Jonathan believes she has gone too far as he grew up watching Disney's animated features and thinks Iris is mistaken and that the films are fun entertainment and harmless for children to watch. Iris is hurt by Jonathan's blatant rejection of her ideas. She says that she cannot continue to see someone who denigrates her ideas. She gets up and leaves the coffee shop.

In what other ways could Jonathan have voiced his opinion to Iris?
What role do each person's parents' beliefs and values play in this
  scenario?
How does gender influence communication?
How does ethnicity influence communication?
How does religious background influence communication?
How else could Iris have made her points?
What would you do if you were Jonathan?
How valid is Jonathan's point of view?
How valid is Iris's point of view?
How can Jonathan and Iris resolve this dispute?
What specific types of communication did you notice in the scenario?

INTRODUCTION

Society and culture are complex phenomena that influence how people view themselves, the values they hold, and behaviors they exhibit. This is particularly true of sexuality. If there is a universal truth regarding sexuality, it is that the diversity of its understanding and expression both within a particular society and culture and in comparison with different societies and cultures is broad and varied. Although social and cultural beliefs, values, and behaviors related to sexuality share many commonalities, it is also important to recognize and respect differences. In pluralistic societies such as the United States, where people of many backgrounds and beliefs come together, it is especially important for educators, students, and the community at large to recognize this.

The functional knowledge regarding the social and cultural aspects of sexuality should be integrated into the K–12 curriculum using a skills-based approach. Both the functional knowledge and the skills will be operationalized in the Learning Experiences section of this chapter. As you read through the material, think of how to integrate the functional knowledge with the skills-based curricular design outlined in the introduction to this text.

LEGAL ISSUES

Most Americans would be surprised to learn that many states have laws on the books regulating sexual behavior. Most of these laws are old and difficult to enforce. In a recent landmark decision, the U.S. Supreme Court ruled that sodomy laws are unconstitutional (*Lawrence & Garner v. State of Texas,* June 23, 2003). At the time of the ruling, 13 states still had sodomy laws on their books. Some of the sodomy laws apply only to same-sex contact and some apply to both same-sex and male-female sexual contact. The *American Heritage Dictionary* (1993) defines *sodomy* in three ways: anal sexual contact between two males; anal or oral sexual contact between a male and female; sexual contact with an animal. Another definition of sodomy states that it is any sexual contact, other than vaginal-penile intercourse. In the Texas case cited, laws regulating male-to-male sexual contact were deemed unconstitutional.

Another example of the law's impact on sexuality and decision making is abortion. Again, this precedent was set because of a Supreme Court decision (*Roe v. Wade,* January 22, 1973). The Court (the decision was based on a case that originated in Texas) held that a woman's right to an abortion fell within the right to privacy protected by the Fourteenth Amendment. Since the initial decision, several other Supreme Court decisions are related to federal financing for abortion and the age at which a person may obtain an abortion. Although a state-level issue, the Supreme Court has upheld a state's right to limit access to abortion in certain cases.

Sexual harassment can happen anywhere: in the workplace, in schools, among friends, in the community. Since the passage of Title VII in 1964 (banning workplace discrimination of any kind), reports of sexual harassment have grown tremendously. It is not a new phenomenon; rather, the recognition of sexual harassment, particularly as related to the workplace where it is most often experienced, has raised awareness of this problem and given its victims legal recourse. Sexual harassment is typically defined as consisting of two distinct types: quid pro quo and the hostile work environment. *Quid pro quo* sexual harassment is the more obvious condition that occurs when a benefit results from submission to sexual advances or a benefit is denied as a result of the denial of sexual advances. A *hostile work environment* can include such things as jokes, suggestive remarks, pictures, cartoons, or sexually derogatory comments that affect the character of the workplace. In general, one or more of the items enumerated under the hostile work environment must be repeated or continual to constitute sexual harassment. The law has dealt with sexual harassment by rulings in a series of court cases. Employers and schools need to be aware of sexual harassment and take steps to prevent it. Recent publications have highlighted the issue of sexual harassment in schools, providing evidence of extremely high rates of occurrence (Stein, 1999).

The law has a broad influence over a minor's sexuality. This includes the age of consent and access to contraception and other reproductive health services. The age of consent is the age at which the law says a young person can agree to have sex. Before people reach the age of consent, they are not allowed to have sex with anyone, whatever the age of their partner. The law states both partners must be over the age of consent to legally engage in sexual behaviors. In the United States, the age of consent is set by each state. The most common age of consent in the United States (a particular state may be different) is 16 years. This is a difficult law to enforce, and it presents an example of how culture influences the enforcement of the law. For example, while an adult having sex with a child clearly presents a legal violation of the age of consent, many would view the situation differently where one partner is 30 years old and the other 15 years old depending on the gender of both the older and younger participant.

States also regulate minors' access to contraceptive services. According to the Alan Guttmacher Institute (2003), 27 states and Washington, DC, allow minors access to contraceptive services, 7 states allow access under certain circumstances (such as the minor's health and status as married, a parent, or pregnant), and 16 states have no explicit policy. All 50 states and Washington, DC, allow minors to access testing and treatment for sexually transmitted diseases. A majority of states have laws requiring parental involvement (either consent or notification) in a minor's decision to have an abortion (Alan Guttmacher Institute, 2003).

RELIGIOUS CONSIDERATIONS

Religion and religious institutions are another group of factors influencing sexuality within a society and across different cultures. Religion can mean many things. It can include a belief in and respect for supernatural powers, membership in a particular institutionalized system, a set of values and be-liefs, the following of a spiritual leader, a combination of part or all of the above, and more. Religious teaching about sexuality will reflect the par-ticular values of particular religious institutions. In the United States, al-though the majority of the population would self-identify as Christian, one of the founding tenets of the United States is religious freedom.

Christianity, in all its various denominations, grew out of Judaism, hence the Judeo-Christian tradition. The Judeo-Christian tradition repre-sents a wide variety of religious institutions with a wide array of beliefs and values related to sexuality. Traditionally, the Judeo-Christian tradition em-phasizes the creation of men and women by *God* who intended them to marry and "be fruitful and multiply and replenish the earth." This view suggests, by omission, that the main goal of sexuality is procreation.

Although nothing in the Bible specifically mentions such things as mas-turbation, oral sex, or contraception, theologians and other Christian writ-ers have addressed these issues. It is important to remember, then, that much of the Judeo-Christian tradition is based on the views and interpre-tations of post-Bible religious writers, many of whom had negative views of sex (Bullough, 1995). The Old Testament has many passages with sex-ual themes. It is also the place where some proscriptions are made—for ex-ample, same-sex relations and intercourse during menstruation. The New Testament reinforces the Old Testament and also prohibits prostitution and same-sex behavior. Adultery is condemned throughout the Bible, as are sexual fantasies involving someone other than one's spouse.

In general, both the Old and New Testaments are male centered and view sexual expression as a procreative activity only. To use Catholicism as an example, the official teachings of the church ban the use of contraceptive devices, prohibit divorce and abortion, and teach that marriage is only be-tween a man and a woman. Many practicing Catholics ignore these teach-ings as is evidenced by data from the National Survey of Family Growth (NSFG) that reports 96 percent of all Catholic women who have ever had sex have used contraceptive methods and devices at some point in their lives. Furthermore, the NSFG data show that 75 percent of Catholic women of childbearing age who are currently sexually active use a contraceptive method forbidden by the church (Amba, Chandra, Mosher, Peterson, & Piccinino, 1997).

Judaism, though part of the Judeo-Christian tradition, has its own set of attitudes and teaching regarding sexuality. Its holy book is known as the Torah, which is what Christians refer to as the Old Testament of the Bible. It is important to recognize that within Judaism there is a diversity of sex-ual understanding and expression related to the particular institution to which one belongs. Orthodox Judaism and Reformed Judaism represent two different institutions among many that have different approaches to sexuality. Sexual expression is not viewed solely as a procreative function in Judaism, but according to Jewish teachings, it is only permissible within the context of marriage. Sex is viewed as the woman's right, not the man's— it is one of the wife's three basic rights along with food and clothing. In Or-thodox Judaism, the laws of separation are strictly adhered to. The laws of separation forbid sexual intercourse during and after menstruation and last a minimum of 12 days. Judaism does not ban the use of contraceptives; however, the condom is forbidden because it blocks or destroys the seed. Abortion is viewed within the context of the mother's life being most important; therefore, there is no notion of prohibition, but it is not something to be done casually. Lastly, homosexuality, particularly homosexual acts, are clearly forbidden by the Torah.

Islam, a growing religious tradition in the United States and the major religion in most Middle Eastern cultures, is experiencing profound shifts related to sexuality. Islam's sacred text is known as the Koran, and one of the tenets of the Islamic faith is that premarital sex is forbidden. However, Foster (1993) reports that in Tunisia, women's age at marriage has been rising, while the average age of women's first sexual experience has been falling. Assuming this dissonance is present in an Islamic country, it is safe to assume that this trend is present in the United States among those who are part of the Islamic religion.

Islam is a patriarchal religion, and "overwhelming social pressure against premarital sexual intercourse remains" (Foster, 1993, p. 102). This pressure can be openly hostile to women in some Islamic states. With the rise of fundamentalism, women are expected to be covered from head to toe in order to maintain decorum and purity. Even though Islam allows polygamy and men can have concubines, it is not the norm in the Muslim world and certainly not in the United States. Sexual intercourse is seen as a pleasurable activity that is both a privilege and an obligation and is to be practiced only in marriage. "To be attentive to one's own body, to assume it in its totality, to take one's own fantasies seriously, to make the quest for orgasm an essential aim of earthly life and even of the life to come, are some of the aims of Islam" (Bouhdiba, 1985, p. 159).

Hinduism, most commonly associated with India and other Eastern cultures, reflects a range of beliefs. There is no central text as in Christianity and Islam. Hinduism views love and sex as having divine origin, and the pursuit of sexual pleasure is a form of worship. As evidence, one needs to look no further than the *Kama Sutra*, an early Indian treatise on politics, social customs, love, and intimacy written in the 4th century by Vatsyayana. The *Kama Sutra*, while much more than a collection of sexual positions, is viewed by many as an early edition of books such as Alex Comfort's *Joy of Sex.*

Buddhism is an offshoot of Hinduism and has a branch that promotes self-discipline and one that is more liberal in that sexuality and love are seen as positive expressions. Buddhist monks practice a celibate lifestyle, suppressing sexual desire and channeling it into intellectual and spiritual growth.

These brief snapshots of various religions are not meant to be definitive descriptions but merely outlines of their major tenets and the conflicts that often arise between official teachings and everyday practices of members of each religious institution. Despite this tension, there is no argument that religion and religious teachings have a profound impact on sexual attitudes and sexual behavior.

ETHNIC ISSUES

The United States is a diverse society of approximately 281 million people. Gross numbers do not reflect the degree of diversity in the United States. The data on race/ethnicity in the United States identify the population as 69 percent white, 12 percent black, 13 percent Hispanic, and 5 percent other. "Other" includes Asian Americans, Pacific Islanders, American Indians, Aleutians, and Eskimos (Henry J. Kaiser Family Foundation, 2003b).

One of the biggest issues, as it relates to health generally and sexual health specifically, is poverty. The poverty rate of the U.S. population is 11 percent white, 30 percent black, 29 percent Hispanic, and 19 percent other (Henry J. Kaiser Family Foundation, 2003b). Persons in poverty are defined as those who make less than 100 percent of the Federal Poverty Level (FPL), referred to as the *poverty threshold*. The federal poverty threshold for a family of three was $14,128 in 2001.

These levels of poverty affect the sexual health of the populations represented here. For example, the July 2001–June 2002 data on new adult/adolescent AIDS cases show 49 percent black, 30 percent white, 19 percent Hispanic, and 1 percent Asian/Pacific Islander (Henry J. Kaiser Family Foundation, 2003b). The teen birthrate in the United States shows the following distribution: 42 percent white, 25 percent black, 29 percent Hispanic, 2 percent Asian/Pacific Islander, and 2 percent American Indian (Henry J. Kaiser Family Foundation, 2003a). These data are better understood using classic epidemiological rates. The rate of teen births per 1,000 population (in 1999) is 34 for whites, 81 for blacks, 93 for Hispanics, 22 for Asians/Pacific Islanders, and 68 for American Indians (Ventura, Mathews, & Hamilton, 2001). Although there are disproportionate numbers of the black and Hispanic population living in poverty, the role of culture cannot be denied. That is, there is much less stigma attached to teenage childbearing in black and Hispanic cultures than there is in others.

On the other hand, some evidence indicates that the health care gap in some areas is nonexistent. For example, the overall rate of women ages 18 to 64 who report having had a Pap smear within the last 3 years in 2000 shows 87 percent white, 88 percent black, and 82 percent Hispanic (Henry J. Kaiser Family Foundation, 2003b). Clearly, the message of the value of having a Pap smear as well as ways to provide access for those who do not have health care has been heard. There is similar data on the rates of women who report having had a mammogram in the last 2 years.

When dealing with as sensitive a topic as human sexuality can be, the issue of cultural competence becomes of paramount concern. Cross, Bazron, Dennis, and Isaacs (1989) describe *cultural competence* as a set of congruent behaviors, attitudes, and policies that come together in a system or agency or among professionals that enable effective interactions in a cross-cultural framework. Diversity in public schools is a fact of life in much of the United States. As such, culturally competent sexuality educators must be able to not only promote awareness and tolerance but also must be able to help their students build skills so that they can also be culturally competent.

Advocates for Youth (1994) outlines a four-step model for teachers to build cultural competence:

1. Learn about culture and important cultural components.
2. Learn about your own culture through a process of self-assessment that includes examining your culture's assumptions and values and your perspectives on them.
3. Learn about the individual young people in your program.
4. Learn as much as possible about important aspects of their cultural backgrounds, with a focus on sexuality-related issues.

It is beyond the scope of this chapter to provide training in cultural competence, but a list of important cultural components is a starting point to understanding the complexity of this issue. Important cultural components include language and communication style, health beliefs, family relationships, sexuality (including sensuality, sexual intimacy, sexual identity, reproductive and sexual health, and sexualization), gender roles, religion, level of acculturation, immigration status, political power, racism, poverty and economic concerns, and history of oppression.

The impact of culture on the expression of love and sexual desire is an area where researchers have begun to chart differences and similarities among cultures from around the world. There is "clear evidence that passionate love and sexual desire are cultural universals" (Hatfield & Rapson, 1996, p. 4). Often, much is made of the differences between Western and Eastern cultures, particularly the more individualist focus of the West and the collectivist focus of the East. However, Yamaguchi (1994) suggests that self-interest may underlie both individualist and collectivist sentiments. Hatfield and Rapson (1996), while acknowledging differences based on culture, state that major cultural groups are more similar in their views of love and sex than stereotypes suggest, that the rate of assimilation affects cultural influences, that personality may be more powerful than culture, and that truth trumps ideology concerning relative advantages or disadvantages of various cultures.

Many differences regarding love and sex are evident across cultures. Buss (1989) found that the degree of sexual experience upon marriage varies widely. In China, India, Indonesia, Iran, Israel (the Palestinian Arabs), and Taiwan, young people were insistent that their mate be chaste (never engaged in sex before marriage). In Finland, France, Norway, the Netherlands, Sweden, and West Germany, most thought chastity was unimportant. The anthropological research demonstrates great variety in sexual attitudes and behavior. Mead's (1935) pioneering work demonstrated wide differences in gender role standards among three cultures in the South Pacific. Geertz's (1960) study of the Batak in northern Sumatra noted the differences in sexual initiation based on gender: boys were isolated and instructed in both talk and practice by older men, whereas the girls were also isolated but were limited to talk because virginity was prized.

There are numerous other examples regarding cultural expectations about dating, relationships, love, sexual activity, and marriage. When teaching sexuality, it is vitally important to know who your students are and to give them the opportunity to share their cultural background and beliefs as well as to provide them with a safe environment to learn about other's cultural background, beliefs, and practices.

THE MEDIA

The media encompass both the familiar and the new: newspapers and other print media, radio, television, films, music, music videos, computer programs, video games, and the Internet. An analysis of each medium is beyond the scope of this text, but there *is* a set of media literacy principles that can be applied to each medium named here as well as any other new media that may be created in the future.

Media literacy comes from a commitment to critical thinking with students actively involved in their own learning. This becomes a particular challenge in the area of human sexuality since it is such a powerfully charged emotional issue to many. However, in survey after survey, a majority of Americans support sexuality education in the schools (Alan Guttmacher Institute, 2003). Furthermore, it is evident that sexuality is used as a powerful motivator and marketing tool in much of what the media produce. It is the intersection of the media and sexuality that demonstrates how widespread the need is for students to not only understand sexuality but also how the media uses it to entice, to motivate, and to sell. As Considine and Haley (1999) state, "questions about ideology, power, social relations, and the way knowledge is constructed, carried, and conveyed by media representations necessitate a commitment to both critical thinking and a critical pedagogy" (p. 8).

In addition, the concept of media literacy, embraced by this text, is based on three notions: preparation, protection, and pleasure. That is, while many are concerned about the content of the media, it is often viewed in monolithic terms as a negative entity. That is not to deny the negative aspects of the media but rather to acknowledge that, in addition to preparing students to decode and deconstruct the various media they interact with, it is sometimes necessary to protect students from either the effects or the actual media while, at the same time, acknowledging the fact that the media are a source of pleasure and entertainment.

The "Principles of Media Literacy" (Considine & Haley, 1999) follow, with a brief explanation:

- *Media are constructions.* This concept addresses the fact that regardless of the medium, it has been built with a particular purpose in mind and reflects the decisions of its makers/designers. In other words, each medium has a particular point of view.
- *Media representations construct reality.* This concept deals with the difference between the real and perception. For example, if the media constantly produce stories about anorexia, we may begin to believe it is a very common disorder. That is not to say

it is not a serious and possibly life-threatening condition that warrants attention but rather that the constant portrayal of it by the media may cause the public to believe it is a bigger problem than is based on actual epidemiological data.

- *Media constructions have commercial purposes.* This point may seem obvious, but many do not make the connection. Every media product is a commodity that must sell in order to survive. Programming is based on market research. Another aspect of this principle is the issue of media ownership and how who owns the media affects what is produced/shown.

- *Audiences negotiate meaning.* The media attempt to constrain the meaning consumers take away from interacting with the product. However, each person has a different background and a different set of lenses with which to "view" the media. Therefore, potentially endless interpretations to what a particular product means are possible. The most important notion is that this concept rejects the idea of a passive consumer of the media. Each person interacts with the products that he or she consumes and produces his or her own meaning. While admitting to a potentially endless stream of meanings, each product is designed to limit interpretation so that a common message is understood.

- *Each medium has its own conventions and forms.* This concept illuminates the various forms and properties of each medium. Even within a particular medium, such as television, there are conventions and forms for particular genres. For example, most television shows follow somewhat traditional narrative conventions.

- *The media contain and convey values and ideologies.* This concept recognizes that, while there is a surface message, each media text attempts to deliver that underneath this message (such as to entertain or inform) are certain values or ideologies being promoted. Examples of the types of values being promoted include such ideas as patriotism, individualism, and stereotypical views of masculinity and femininity. Disney animated features, though undeniably high-quality entertainment with superb voiceovers, animation, and music, have frequently been cited as promoting a view of femininity that suggests women and young girls only find fulfillment via relationships with men.

- *Media messages may have social consequences.* This last concept attempts to understand how the media influence knowledge, attitudes, and behavior. Using the Disney example, one could argue that its animated features influence how young women understand their place in the social order. That is not to say that Disney animated features cause young women to select only traditional identities but that it is one factor among many present in the culture. A similar argument could be made about the normalization of alcohol and tobacco use. By seeing thousands of depictions of alcohol and tobacco use in the media, often without consequences, children grow up believing that these are desirable activities.

These principles can be used with any medium or media product. For example, advertising is produced in every format: print, audio, visual, telecommunication, e-mail, and the Internet. Therefore, teachers and students should look for a common thread for each product.

Marketing and advertising have become ubiquitous in Western culture. It is nearly impossible to find advertising-free zones. Advertising revenue is what supports all media and it often includes both direct and indirect references to sex and sexuality. Going back to the notion that media literacy has three goals—preparation, protection, and pleasure—one can demonstrate how these goals apply to advertising. Preparation enables students to become aware of the environment in which they live so that they can better understand how advertising seeks to influence their choices. In the realm of sexuality, it can help students to understand that the images of men and women they see in advertisements represent a minute portion of the population. That is, the mostly white, young, fit, and beautiful models that appear in the advertisements are not the norm. Even the models' pictures have often been enhanced so that they are at least partially digital creations.

Second, protection is an area where more attention is being paid. For example, tobacco advertisements have been regulated by the Food and Drug Administration to prevent young people from adopting a smoking habit due to the images of attractive young people engaged in fun activities. The "Joe Camel" campaign (by the R. J. Reynolds Company) used a cartoon character to promote smoking in youth and was one of the primary motivators in the policy to reduce youth access to tobacco advertisements.

Lastly, it would be remiss not to acknowledge the creativity that goes into advertising. As a creative endeavor, albeit with a product or lifestyle to promote, advertising is a source of pleasure for many.

Today, an estimated 30 percent of all video rentals are X-rated tapes. The adult video industry is a multibillion-dollar business (Winks & Semans, 2002). (The issue of sexually explicit materials and attempts to promote or censor it is addressed later.) Whatever one's point of view on sexually explicit materials, the messages and values related to sex and sexuality, as they appear in the mainstream media, are the focus of the reason for developing media literacy skills. Students, teachers, parents, and other community members must be cognizant of the skills needed to deconstruct the messages we receive about sexuality in the media. This in no way equates the representations of sex and sexuality in the media as an unmitigated evil. Rather, it is to promote the three-pronged approach of preparation, protection, and pleasure and to recognize the role each plays in media literacy.

The Arts

The intersection of sexuality and art, like other cultural phenomenon, has been a subject of controversy and discussion throughout history. To suggest that the arts are somehow outside the media is a false distinction. The arts—literature, theater, dance, music, painting—exhibit a complex relationship with the societies in which they are produced. Art both reflects and creates culture. The dictionary definition (*American Heritage Dictionary,* 1993) states that *art* is the human effort to imitate, supplement, alter, or counteract the work of nature.

Both the visual and performing arts have been subjected to various forms of censorship. It is beyond the scope of this chapter to present the history of censorship as it relates to the arts as each form of artistic expression has been subjected to censorship. Perhaps the form most familiar is censorship of literature. In the United States today, many schools have banned books because of what is often called inappropriate content. *Inappropriate content* is often a euphemistic term for content with a sexual theme. Censored authors include Shakespeare, Kurt Vonnegut, J. D. Salinger, Chaucer, D. H. Lawrence, Mark Twain, Alduous Huxley, Henry Miller, Judy Blume, and scores of other well-known and highly acclaimed writers. The working assumption in banning the works of these authors suggests that reading work with sexual content will lead to increased levels of teen sexual activity. This belief has never been demonstrated empirically but rather reflects a generalized fear of teenage sexuality. In fact, the banning of books—a practice that is ethically questionable—can lead to increased attention as the forbidden often becomes more attractive to the very audiences being targeted. Although a case can be made for limiting access to certain materials on the basis of developmental readiness, there is no logic in preventing generally agreed-on valuable works of literature from being read by adolescents.

Pornography

What is pornography? Many may fall back on the often quoted statement by Supreme Court Justice Potter Stewart when he wrote (in *Jacobellis v. Ohio,* 1964), "I imply no criticism of the Court, which in those cases [previous pornography cases] was faced with the task of trying to define what may be indefinable but I know it when I see it." The notion that pornography is knowable may be specific to the time when the verdict was reached.

Miller v. California (1973) sets out the "modern" test for obscenity. The way to judge obscenity (according to the ruling in this case) is based on (1) the proscribed material must depict or describe sexual conduct in a patently offensive way; (2) the conduct must be specifically described in the law; and (3) the work must, taken as a whole, lack serious value and must appeal to a prurient interest in sex. What is patently offensive is to be determined by applying community values, but any jury decision in these cases is subject to independent constitutional review. The Supreme Court has upheld that states may proscribe sexual material involving minors.

What is apparent in this brief legal discussion is the difficulty involved in defining pornography. *Pornography* is derived from the Greek word meaning "the writing of [or about] prostitutes." The word *pornography* is a morally laden term with negative connotations. It is associated with the words *obscenity* and *prurient.* A more positive term is *erotica,* which suggests that whatever is being discussed has artistic value. A more neutral term is *sexually explicit material,* which more accurately describes the phenomenon without judging its merit.

With the advent of personal viewing products (such as the VCR, DVD, and the computer), the use and consumption of sexually explicit material has become much more of a private behavior. Before the advent of these technologies, sexually explicit material was limited to photographs or films shown in movie theaters, typically in cities that had "red light" districts. With the advent of the videocassette recorder, persons wishing to view sexually explicit films only had to go to their neighborhood video rental outlet and discreetly rent a video.

The last 20 years have witnessed an explosion of sexually explicit materials, what is often referred to as the adult entertainment market. The sale and transmission of sexually explicit materials over the Internet have become one of the most profitable business applications of the Internet and the World Wide Web. The production, distribution, and sale of sexually explicit videocassettes and DVDs is also highly profitable. The renting of sexually explicit videocassettes and DVDs is often the most profitable component of the rental business. Clearly, there is a market for these materials. Rich (2003), writing in the *New York Times,* states, "Taboos are falling so quickly that the word *taboo* itself increasingly has an archaic ring. . . . Few bemoan the 'porning' of America these days. Except for the usual fire-and-brimstone sermonizers in the pulpits and on the Supreme Court, most conservatives have joined most liberals in giving up the fight against all but the scourge of child pornography" (pp. 1, 15).

One of the reasons for this view is that, with the media giants' increasing monopoly powers, sexually explicit material is a highly profitable product, and the corporate powers that be are very influential in the political arena. In short, the media corporations do not want a substantial part of their bottom line to be regulated by the government, especially in light of the widespread acceptance of sexually explicit materials by the majority of the American public.

Rich (2003) outlines the latest trend in sexually explicit material:

> The cliché has it that when formerly contraband becomes accepted, it loses its cachet. With sex, that is not really an option. What does seem to be happening is a digitalization of sex—and not only in the sense that porn is distributed digitally, whether by Internet or DVD or television or spam. In a more profound sense, the erotic is being figuratively and literally dismembered as it is broken down into its various discrete bytes. . . . The newest trend in hard-core porn movies is the "eschewing of plot"; each body part or type, sexual taste, fetish, whatever, boasts dedicated videos catering exclusively to that particular niche as clinically and single-mindedly as possible. (p. 15)

Without doubt many regard this view of sexuality, as observed in the sexually explicit materials currently being produced and distributed, as limiting if not degrading. However, from a strictly economic point of view, it is merely with the development of many niche markets in sexuality now that sexually explicit materials seem not to be as shocking or outside the mainstream as they were just 10 years ago. Menon (2003) has found evidence of corporate sponsorship, stating that "through subsidiaries and other partnership agreements, companies such as General Motors, EchoStar Communications, AT&T, Liberty Media, On Command, Hilton, and Marriott, to name a few, are making money from adult entertainment, even though few publicly discuss this branch of their business" (p. H01). The oft-quoted remark (made in 1953) by General Motors president Charles E. Wilson, "We at General Motors have always felt that what was good for the country was good for General Motors, and vice versa" (cited on www .Bartleby.com), becomes either ironic or prophetic depending on one's point of view regarding sexually explicit materials (Rich, 2003).

PROSTITUTION

When sex is viewed solely as a commodity and as a way of earning a living, it is called *prostitution*. Although often viewed in terms of women providing sexual service to men, prostitution also includes men providing sexual services to other men. Much more rarely do male prostitutes provide sexual services to women, and even more rarely do female prostitutes service other females.

"In clichéd terms, prostitution is often referred to as 'the oldest profession.' It is a controversial practice while at the same time being a part of most cultures worldwide. However, historians increasingly recognize that the sale of sexual services is hardly an essential feature of all societies in all historical eras" (Gilfoyle, 1999, p. 119). In the United States, it is illegal in 49 out of 50 states with only a few counties in Nevada legalizing prostitution. It is legal in other countries, most notably Argentina and the Netherlands (Amsterdam in particular), and tolerated in many others (McAnulty & Burnette, 2003).

Evidence indicates that, in open and tolerant societies with greater freedom and opportunity for both genders, prostitution is less prevalent than in economically depressed countries (Goode, 1990). This seems to hold true in the United States if one compares the reported rates from the 1940s to more recent surveys. Kinsey, Pomeroy, and Martin (1948) reported that two-thirds of white males surveyed admitted visiting a prostitute at least once. In a later survey (Janus & Janus, 1993), only 20 percent of men reported visiting a prostitute. This holds true for sexual initiation as well. Kinsey et al. (1948) reported approximately 54 percent of male high school graduates and 20 percent of male college graduates had their first sexual experience with a prostitute. Compared with data in a more recent survey, Laumann, Gagnon, Michael, and Michaels (1994) found only 1.5 percent of 18- to 24-year olds males reported having had their first sexual experience with a prostitute.

Evidence of prostitution around the globe demonstrates its existence dating to the beginnings of recorded history, which is not to say that it is ubiquitous or that it is common to all societies and cultures. Even in the current-day United States, where multiple notions of sexuality and sexual practices are accepted, prostitution continues to engender heated debate.

Gilfoyle (1999) outlines the parameters of the debate through a series of questions: "Is prostitution a recognizable profession or a form of proletarian exploitation? Is prostitution the ultimate form of sexual enslavement or a profound rejection of male domination? Is it symbolic of capitalist domination or a rejection of the monotony of the capitalist workplace? Do prostitutes embody a form of self-destruction or an expressed desire for an eroticized lifestyle?" (p. 139)

SUMMARY

Human sexuality is heavily influenced by social and cultural environments. This is not to discount genetics or biology but to acknowledge the significant role played by social institutions and cultural traditions. The legal system is a powerful social institution that affects sexuality in many ways: by defining who can and cannot get married, by attempting to regulate sexual behavior even though this has recently been challenged, and by regulating who has access to reproductive services including abortion. The legal system also deals with sexual harassment and sexual assault by prosecuting alleged offenders and punishing those convicted of sex-related crimes. Religious traditions form the foundation of moral systems relating to the expression of human sexuality. In a pluralistic society such as the United States, diversity in religious expression and practice are the norm. It is important to understand how various religions understand and view human sexuality so that tolerance can be advanced. Ethnicity also exerts a powerful influence on human sexuality. The United States is a racially and ethnically diverse nation and, as a result, has a wide divergence of views related to sexuality.

The media are ubiquitous. Some people use this fact to suggest that all problems related to sexuality can be traced back to the media. Although there is no denying the media's power, a more productive approach is to promote media literacy to help facilitate both understanding and critical thinking. The arts, by definition, are an area of human expression where meanings and accepted wisdom can be challenged. As such, it is not unusual for the arts to use sexuality as a means of expression and as a way to challenge the status quo. Censorship of the media and the arts constitutes an ongoing site of struggle, particularly as it relates to children's consumption of both media products and works of art.

Pornography and prostitution represent two areas often regulated by the state using the legal system. However, with the advent of all the electronic media and forms of communication, both of these practices have discovered new ways to market their products. If looking only at what is and what has been labeled pornographic, it is possible to gain an appreciation of the impact that social institutions and culture have on human sexuality.

Human sexuality is both an ever-constant and ever-evolving realm of human expression that, when viewed through the dual lenses of society and culture, presents a diverse and rapidly changing picture.

WEBSITES

Alan Guttmacher Institute:
   www.guttmacher.org
Kinsey Institute for Research in Sex, Gender,
   and Reproduction: www.indiana.edu/
   ~kinsey
University of Washington's Society for Human
   Sexuality: www.sexuality.org
Planned Parenthood Federation of America:
   www.plannedparenthood.org
Society for the Scientific Study of Sexuality:
   www.sexscience.org
International Foundation for Gender Educa-
   tion: www.ifge.org
Office of the U.S. Surgeon General:
   www.surgeongeneral.gov/sgoffice.htm
Surgeon General's Call to Action to Promote
   Sexual Health and Responsible Sexual
   Behavior: www.surgeongeneral.gov/
   library/sexualhealth/default.htm

U.S. Department of Health and Human Ser-
   vices, Office of Population Affairs:
   http://opa.osophs.dhhs.gov
Advocates for Youth:
   www.advocatesforyouth.org/teens
Kids Health: www.kidshealth.org
National Campaign to Prevent Teen Preg-
   nancy: www.teenpregnancy.org
Center for Sexuality and Religion:
   www.ctrsr.org
Center for Reproductive Law and Policy:
   www.crlp.org
Population Council: www.popcouncil.org
It's Your (Sex) Life: www.itsyoursexlife.com
Circumcision Information and Resource Pages:
   www.cirp.org

REFERENCES

Advocates for Youth. (1994). *A youth leader's guide to building cultural competence.* Washington, DC: Author. Available online: www.advocatesforyouth.org.

Alan Guttmacher Institute. (2003). *State policies in brief.* Available online: www.agi-usa.org/pubs/spib.html.

Amba, J., Chandra, A., Mosher, L., Peterson, L., & Piccinino, L. (1997). Fertility, family planning and women's health: New data from the 1995 National Survey of Family Growth. *Vital and Health Statistics,* Series 23, No. 19.

American heritage dictionary. (1993). Boston: Houghton Mifflin.

Bartleby.com. Charles E. Wilson, confirmation hearing, January 15, 1953. *Nominations,* hearings before the Committee on Armed Services, United States Senate, 83d Congress, 1st session, p. 26 (1953).

Bouhdiba, A. (1985). *Sexuality in Islam.* London: Routledge & Kegan Paul.

Bullough, V. L. (1995). Sexuality and religion. In L. Diamant & R. D. McAnulty (Eds.), *The psychology of sexual orientation, behavior, and identity: A handbook* (pp. 444–456). Westport, CT: Greenwood.

Buss, D. M. (1989). Sex differences in human mate preferences: Evolutionary hypotheses tested in 37 cultures. *Behavioral and Brain Sciences, 12,* 1–49.

Considine, D. M., & Haley, G. E. (1999). *Visual messages: Integrating imagery into instruction.* Englewood, CO: Teacher Ideas Press.

Cross T., Bazron, B., Dennis, K., & Isaacs, M. (1989). *Toward a culturally competent system of care* (Vol. 1). Washington, DC: Georgetown University Press.

Foster, A. (1993). Young women's sexuality in Tunisia: The health consequences of misinformation among university students. In D. L. Brown & E. A. Early (Eds.), *Everyday life in the Muslim Middle East.* Bloomington: Indiana University Press.

Geertz, C. (1960). *The religion of Java.* Chicago: University of Chicago Press.

Gilfoyle, T. J. (1999). Prostitutes in history: From parables of pornography to metaphors of modernity. *American Historical Review, 104*(1), 117–141.

Goode, E. (1990). *Deviant behavior* (3rd ed.). Englewood Cliffs, NJ: Prentice Hall.

Hatfield, E., & Rapson, R. L. (1996). *Love and sex: Cross-cultural perspectives.* Boston: Allyn & Bacon.

Henry J. Kaiser Family Foundation. (2003a). *State health facts online, Centers for Disease Control and Prevention of HIV/AIDS Prevention—Surveillance and epidemiology.* Available online: www.statehealthfacts.kff.org.

Henry J. Kaiser Family Foundation. (2003b). *State health facts online, Division of Vital Statistics, National Center for Health Statistics, Centers for Disease Control and Prevention.* Available online: www.statehealthfacts.kff.org

Janus, S. S., & Janus, C. L. (1993). *The Janus report on sexual behavior.* New York: Wiley.

Kinsey, A. C., Pomeroy, W. B., & Martin, C. E. (1948). *Sexual behavior in the human male.* Philadelphia: Saunders.

Laumann, E. O., Gagnon, J. H., Michael, R. T., & Michaels, S. (1994). *The social organization of sexuality: Sexual practices in the United States.* Chicago: University of Chicago Press.

McAnulty, R. D., & Burnette, M. M. (2003). *Fundamentals of human sexuality: Making healthy decisions.* Boston: Allyn & Bacon.

Mead, M. (1935). *Sex and temperament in three primitive societies.* New York: Dell.

Menon, V. (2003, August 3). Pornography unscrambled: For better or worse, porn has become so mainstream it's losing its smut appeal. *Toronto Star.* Available online: www.thestar.com.

Rich, F. (2003, July 27). Finally, porn does prime time. *New York Times.* Available online: www.nytimes.com/2003/07/27/arts/27RICH.html.

Sexuality Information and Education Council of the United States, National Guidelines Task Force. (1996). *Guidelines for comprehensive sexuality education: Kindergarten, 12th grade* (2nd ed.). Washington, DC: Author. Available online: www.siecus.org/school/sex_ed/guidelines/guide0000.html.

Stein, N. (1999). *Classrooms and courtrooms: Facing sexual harassment in K–12 schools.* New York: Teachers College Press.

Ventura, S. J., Mathews, T. J., & Hamilton, B. E. (2001). Births to teenagers in the United States, 1940–2000. *Division of Vital Statistics Report, 49*(10). Hyattsville, MD: National Center for Health Statistics.

Winks, C., & Semans, A. (2002). *The Good Vibrations guide to sex.* San Francisco: Cleis.

Yamaguchi, S. (1994). Collectivism among the Japanese: A perspective from the self. In U. Kim, H. C. Triandis, C. Kagitcibasi, S. C. Choi, & G. Yoon (Eds.), *Individualism and collectivism: Theory, method, and applications: Cross cultural research and methodology* (Vol. 8, pp. 175–189). London: Sage.

LEARNING EXPERIENCES

These activities represent the content for society and culture at each of the developmental levels discussed in this book; main points within that content are listed here. The learning experiences were originally published by the Sexuality Information and Education Council of the United States (1996, pp. 40–44) and are part of the *Guidelines for Comprehensive Sexuality Education, Kindergarten–12th Grade* (second edition).

Grades K–3

- Religions teach people how to love each other, how to behave, not to hurt others, and what is right or wrong.
- Some families go to a church, a mosque, or synagogue to worship; some families do not.
- Different religions may teach similar or different values.
- Individuals differ in the way they think, act, look, and live.
- Talking about differences helps people to improve their understanding of each other.
- A stereotype generalizes the behavior of all members of a group.
- Stereotypes hurt people.
- All people should receive fair and equal treatment.
- People who are different are often treated negatively or unequally.
- Some of the material on television, in the movies, in books and magazines, on radio, and on the Internet is true, and some is not.
- Some commercials try to make people and things look different and better than they really are.
- Some television programs, movies, and computer forums are not appropriate for young children.

Grade 4–6

- Many religions teach that sexual intercourse should occur only in marriage.
- People are sometimes discriminated against because of race, culture, ethnicity, language, socioeconomic class, and disability.
- People are sometimes discriminated against because of sexuality factors such as gender, appearance, sexual orientation, family, and living arrangements.
- Discrimination can lead to lower self-esteem, unequal opportunities, and physical and emotional problems.
- Discrimination limits a society's ability to use the full capabilities of its members.
- Discrimination has negative consequences for the individual, family, group, and society.

- People can refuse to watch, read, and/or listen to anything that offends them.
- Parents have the right to determine what is appropriate viewing material for their own children.
- No one really looks as perfect in real life as certain actors and actresses appear in the media.
- The media often present an unrealistic image of what it means to be male or female, what it means to be in love, and what parenthood and marriages are like.
- The media sometimes negatively portray certain cultural groups.
- The media can influence the way people think and behave.
- A parent or trusted adult can help when media messages are confusing.

Grades 7–9

- Every culture communicates norms and taboos about sexuality.
- In the United States, people from many different cultural backgrounds have a wide range of views about sexuality.
- In a pluralistic society, the individual's right to hold different opinions is valued.
- American societal messages about sexuality are often confusing and contradictory.
- Messages received about sexuality from one's home and culture may be different from the general societal messages.
- In most schools, there are unwritten norms about sexuality for teenagers.
- Individuals need to examine messages received from different sources and establish guidelines for their own behavior.
- The Supreme Court has determined that people have the right to make personal decisions concerning abortion, sterilization, contraception, and other reproductive matters.
- Some states have passed laws that restrict abortion, in that they require parental notification and/or consent for a minor to have an abortion.
- There are state laws concerning the age of consent for sexual behavior.
- Incest is illegal in all states.
- Laws prohibit sexual harassment.
- Views about sexuality and sexual behavior are culturally determined.
- All world religions have views about sexuality and its place in the human experience.
- Many religions today acknowledge that human beings were created as sexual beings and that their sexuality is good.
- Conflicts may result in teenagers and adults who have been raised in a religion that does not fully accept human sexuality.

- One's religious values can play an important role in sexual decision making.
- People have the right to speak up when they encounter discrimination and when they see others being discriminated against.
- Laws, policies, and procedures can help someone to fight discrimination.
- People's lives are enriched when they understand and celebrate diversity.
- Sexual images are often depicted in the arts, such as music, films, drama, and literature.
- The media usually do not portray sexuality realistically.
- The media sometimes depict stereotypes about the sexuality of certain cultural groups.
- The media sometimes portray stereotypes about men and women.
- Some television shows and movies provide positive models of relationships and sexuality.
- Soap operas and talk shows may give inaccurate and unrealistic information and portrayals of sexuality.
- Real relationships require more effort than is often portrayed in the media.
- Teens and adults have a responsibility to help younger children avoid or deal effectively with negative media influences.
- Communicating one's reactions about the portrayal of sexual issues is important.

Grades 10–12

- Understanding the diversity of views about sexuality is important.
- Because of the wide range of sexual values and beliefs, people need to communicate their views to their friends and partners in order to negotiate behaviors that are acceptable.
- About half of the states have laws that protect sexual behaviors between consenting adults.
- About half of the states have laws that restrict some types of sexual behaviors.
- Public nuisance behavior such as exhibitionism and voyeurism are viewed as unlawful acts in most states.
- Prostitution is illegal in all states except Nevada.
- Court cases have provided guidelines for determining what is obscene, including whether the material portrays sexual conduct in an offensive way and is without value, and if a "reasonable" person finds the work possessing no social value.
- People have different views on what is obscene.
- Child pornography is illegal.
- Laws are currently being developed to govern new reproductive technologies.

- Some states and cities have passed laws banning discrimination on the basis of sexual orientation.
- Many states have laws requiring HIV and sexuality education.
- Some people continue to respect their religious teachings and traditions but believe that some views are not personally relevant.
- Partners with very different religious backgrounds may have difficulty reaching an agreement about their sexual relationship.
- Contemporary religions struggle with many issues related to sexuality and reproduction.
- A growing number of congregations welcome openly gay men and lesbians.
- Examining one's views about diversity occurs throughout life.
- Workplaces benefit from having employees from diverse backgrounds.
- Confronting one's biases and prejudices can be difficult.
- The nature of sexual images in art has changed through time.
- Erotica images in art reflect society's views about sexuality and help people understand sexuality.
- Art with sexual images that reflect a culture's norms may be considered obscene in another culture.
- Some people try to regulate or eliminate sexual images in art.
- No evidence exists that erotic images in the arts cause inappropriate sexual behavior.

LEARNING EXPERIENCE 1

TITLE: Different Religions, Similar Lessons

GRADE LEVELS: K–3

TIME REQUIREMENT: One session

LEARNING CONTEXT

Students will demonstrate knowledge of the main areas of agreement among different religions and develop communication and advocacy skills.

NATIONAL LEARNING STANDARD

4: Students will analyze the influence of culture, media, technology, and other factors on health.

PROCEDURE

Describe different religions (Judaism, Islam, Christianity, Catholicism, Hinduism, Buddhism, and so on), noting that although they are all different in some way, in many ways they are the same. Have students interview parents about the religion practiced by the family. If a child's family does not participate in a particular religion or religious activities, have him or her interview parents about how the family treats each other, how to behave toward others, and what is right or wrong. Ask the same questions regarding a particular religion that is practiced in each child's home. Use the information to create a series of pictures drawn by each student to illustrate what the religion/family structure suggests about love for family and others, how to behave, how *not* to hurt others, and what is right and wrong. Students will hang their artwork around the room and describe what the pictures represent.

INSTRUCTIONAL/ENVIRONMENTAL MODIFICATIONS

Recognize that not all children live in a home where religion is discussed or practiced, and adapt by talking about family approaches to the same issues.

RESOURCES

Paper; crayons; basic information on different religions

ASSESSMENT PLAN

The teacher will assess the presentation of artwork and students' ability to recognize common aspects of all religions.

REFLECTION

- Why is religion important in people's lives?
- Does one have to practice a particular religion to be considered a spiritual person?
- What are other ways to express spirituality?

LEARNING EXPERIENCE 2

TITLE: The Internet and How It Works

GRADE LEVELS: K–3

TIME REQUIREMENTS: Two sessions

LEARNING CONTEXT
This activity develops decision-making, self-management, and communication skills. Students will be able to

- Describe the Internet as a series of computers all over the world that are all linked to one another.
- Identify safe practices for surfing the World Wide Web.
- Describe how hypertext linking works.
- Recognize the anonymous nature of the Internet.

NATIONAL LEARNING STANDARD
4: Students will analyze the influence of culture, media, technology, and other factors on health.

PROCEDURE

Session 1

Photocopy pictures of computers so that each student will have one. Color-code each picture with colored construction paper or colored markers. The colors should include red, blue, purple, green, brown, black, orange, pink—depending on the size of the group, there may be more than one of each color. Each picture should also have the name of a different part of the city, state, country, or world on it so that there is no overlap.

Divide the class into four teams and select a team leader. Have each team come up with a name (such as Net Adventurers, Cybersurfers, Computer Commanders, and the like). You may also do a brief team-building exercise if time allows.

Have all the students, except the team leaders, go back to their color-coded "computer." Explain how on the Internet, all computers are linked to all other computers. Ask students for examples of the type of messages they would send to a good friend. Ask students for examples of the type of messages they would send to every member of the class. Describe how a hyperlink, or underlined text, on a web page can take you to another place on a particular computer or to another computer.

Tell the students that the different colors on each computer represent a hyperlink to that computer and that when you hear your team leader call out a particular color, you are to find a computer with the same color and physically go to that computer. Have no more than three students at any computer at the same time (make sure there are enough computers of each color to accommodate all the students of the class).

Have the team leaders come to the front of the class or wherever they can be seen by all in the class. Provide them with a list of colors they are to call out so that their team members can then go to the computer that matches that color. Each team leader should have a different list of colors. Each round will start by having each team leader call out the first color on his or her list.

Once all members of the team have found the right colored computer, the leader then calls out the next color on the list.

After finishing the list of colors each leader had, discuss how hypertext links allow Internet users to go to different places all over the world. Many new ideas and facts are located on computers that can be anywhere in the world. As part of the processing for this activity, ask students whether they ever found a computer of the right color that was full and what they did (wait; find another computer of that color; go back to their own computer). Use a real computer displayed for the class to demonstrate what a hypertext link is and how a hypertext link takes the user to a different place on the Internet. If you have computers in the class or access to a computer lab, have teams go to preselected sites and explore the hypertext links on that web page.

Assign partners for each member of all groups. Ask the students to write a message describing hypertext links in their own words and include something about themselves they would be willing to share with their partner.

Give each student four envelopes. Have students put their partner's name on each of the four envelopes. Before beginning the next part, be sure to remind the students *not* to close the envelope, then ask the students to cut the message in four parts and put one part of the message in each envelope.

Hand the envelopes in so they can be used tomorrow when this experience continues. Take the envelopes the children made and insert a sticker in at least one of the envelopes addressed to each child. Depending on your tolerance for mess, insert baby powder, confetti, a picture of a mean character such as a "Big Bad Wolf," a spring, or a bell in other envelopes selected at random. Seal all the envelopes. This is for tomorrow's class.

Session 2

Recall yesterday's hypertext linking exercise by asking for descriptions of what a hypertext link is. Reinforce the fact that clicking on a hypertext link can take you to unexpected places. While it is a way to explore, ask about students exploring in the real world. How do kids know where it's safe to go? What rules do they use to "play safe"? Introduce the need to surf safely when using the Internet. Outline how the Internet is different from the real world (ask students first to describe how it is the same and how it is different).

Review "Online Rules" (included at end of activity). These should be posted somewhere in the room and reviewed periodically.

Distribute four envelopes randomly to each student, and have them "deliver" the envelopes to the child whose name is on the cover in the following manner. (Tell them "no peeking" until they have received the envelopes that have their names on it.)

Have each student return to their "computer." They must send the message over the web, by handing each envelope, one at a time to the nearest child along the web, who then hands it to another child along the web, who then hands it to another child, until all four envelopes reach the addressee. Once everyone has their four envelopes, have the children open the envelopes and reconstruct the message.

Talk about the "surprise" messages, and reinforce the need for personal safety skills. What might some of these surprises be on the real World Wide Web? (This might include an e-mail message from a stranger, electronic spam from a marketer, a link to an inappropriate website, a nasty or threatening message, a computer virus, and so forth).

Reinforce to students that people never know when they are going to receive an electronic "surprise," so they always have to be careful. Using the "Online Rules" handout as a starting point, have them brainstorm ways in which they can minimize their chances of encountering nasty stuff on the Internet.

For homework, have students create posters of a highway complete with road signs describing safe surfing rules. The posters can be titled "Safe Driving on the Information Highway." Hang the posters in the hallway, the computer classroom, or the library for other students to see.

INSTRUCTIONAL/ENVIRONMENTAL MODIFICATIONS
Teachers will have a wide variety of skill levels depending on each child's familiarity with computers and the Internet. When forming groups and pairs, be sure to include those with higher and lower computer and Internet skills.

RESOURCES
Colored construction paper or markers; copies of pictures of computers—one for each student; "Online Rules" as a handout; enlarged copy of "Online Rules" for display; envelopes; other materials to put in the envelopes; pencils and paper

ASSESSMENT PLAN
Ask students to write a brief journal entry or verbal reflection on what they learned in each activity. Review their journal entries as well as their participation in the classroom activities.

REFLECTION
- How well did the learning experience meet the stated objectives?
- Did the students have adequate practice time to work on the skills?
- How might you modify the learning experience in the future?
- How did the various skill levels of the students affect the learning experience?

REFERENCE
Adapted from the Media Awareness Network (www.media-awareness.ca).

Online Rules (from the Media Awareness Network)

- I will not give out any personal information online without my parents' permission. This includes my name, phone number, address, e-mail, location of my school, my parents' work address/telephone numbers, credit card number information, and my picture.

- When using the Internet, I will always use a pretend name or nickname that doesn't reveal anything about me.

- When creating a password, I will make one up that is hard to guess but easy for me to remember. To avoid having it stolen, I will never reveal it to anyone (except my parents)—not even my best friend. I will not respond to any message that makes me uncomfortable. I will show an adult right away.

- I will *not* arrange to meet a friend I have made on the Internet unless one of my parents has been informed and will be present. I will not open e-mail, files, links, pictures, or games from people that I don't know or trust. I will always ask an adult first.

- I will practice responsible online behavior.

- I will not post or send insulting or rude messages or threats to anyone online.

- I will not take words, pictures, or sounds from someone else's website without their permission.

- I will not disable any filtering software that my parents have put on the computer.

- I will not make any online purchases without my parents' permission.

- I will not believe everything I read on the Internet. When doing online research, I will always check the source of the information and confirm it with a parent, teacher, or librarian.

LEARNING EXPERIENCE 3

TITLE: Discrimination

GRADE LEVELS: 4–6

TIME REQUIREMENTS: Two to three sessions

LEARNING CONTEXT

This lesson develops communication and advocacy skills. Students will be able to
- Describe different forms of discrimination.
- Recognize discrimination.
- Display behaviors that can challenge discrimination at school and in the media.

NATIONAL LEARNING STANDARD

4: Students will analyze the influence of culture, media, technology, and other factors on health.

PROCEDURE

Ask students whether they have ever felt discriminated against (treated differently) only because they are children. Put answers on the board. Decide as a class whether any of the ways individuals feel they were discriminated against were justified or not justified. For example, children are not allowed to drive, cannot walk to school alone (depending on age), and do not set their own bedtime. Next brainstorm ways the students are aware of regarding how adults are discriminated against (based on things such as race, culture, ethnicity, language, socioeconomic class, or disability).

Working in groups, have the students pick a category of discrimination. Using computers with Internet access, research a particular kind of discrimination. Design a campaign to raise awareness and to inform others that discrimination is illegal and harmful. A campaign item can be a poster, a public service announcement, the script for a radio commercial, or a brochure.

RESOURCES

Access to computers and other art materials

ASSESSMENT PLAN

The teacher will evaluate the product of group work using a rubric for group work (evaluating collaboration and cooperation).

REFLECTION

- How does discrimination affect those discriminated against?
- How does discrimination affect those who discriminate?
- Where does discrimination originate and what is it based on?

LEARNING EXPERIENCE 4

TITLE: Prejudice and Body Image

GRADE LEVELS: 4–6

TIME REQUIREMENTS: This learning experience can take up to four to five class periods to complete all activities. However, one may select one or more of the activities to do in one or two class periods.

LEARNING CONTEXT

This learning experience develops skills in decision making, self-management, stress management, and advocacy. Students will be able to

- Recognize the media's role in dictating standards of attractiveness to society.
- Understand how media images can affect their own feelings toward their own bodies and toward others.
- Understand how unattainable these standards can be for much of the population.

NATIONAL LEARNING STANDARD

4: Students will analyze the influence of culture, media, technology, and other factors on health.

PROCEDURE

Background Information for the Teacher

It is important for students to realize that over time, different societies have had diverse notions about beauty. Prior to the 20th century, Europeans and North Americans admired larger women because they seemed stronger and healthier. Being larger, smaller, taller, shorter, darker, lighter, older, or younger has been admired in various societies, for reasons particular to that culture.

Today, we live in a society where thinness is among the more admired traits, where most of us want to be thin (including 80 percent of 11-year-olds) and where fat and fat people are often stigmatized. It has been noted by some that obesity is one of the last socially condoned prejudices in North American culture. In fact, by the age of 6, most children have already learned to regard the obese as ugly, lazy, stupid, or unworthy.

Pictures portraying images of beauty in other cultures and in other historical periods are useful in demonstrating how ideals are socially constructed. For example, pictures of Victorian women can be used to demonstrate the popularity of the curved figure, achieved through wearing a corset. Pictures of Chinese foot binding can also be used to show how small feet, a sign of beauty in Imperial China, were achieved.

Pressures to Be Thin

A study of women who were *Playboy* centerfolds and Miss America pageant contestants has shown that their body weights and shapes progressively diminished between 1959 and 1979. Over these same 20 years, however, the average weight has increased for women in the general population, particularly those in young adulthood. Thus, there is a growing disparity between the ideal and reality. One good way of demonstrating this is by collecting and discussing images of women in fashion magazines.

Women respond to pressures to be thin by dieting. A 1978 Neilson survey reported that 56 percent of females aged 24 to 54 dieted periodically, 76 percent of whom dieted for appearance rather than health reasons. The Canadian Weight Gallup Poll conducted in 1984 showed only 17 percent of women in Canada "eat what they want." More than 80 percent of women dislike their bodies, and dieting is becoming a concern of women of all ages, from 9-year-olds to the very old.

This situation is not surprising given that women are constantly told to diet and are made to feel guilty for eating. A survey of women's magazines during the period from 1970 to 1978 found the number of diet articles had doubled from the previous decade. And it's important to note that health is not the primary goal of diet and exercise in our culture: beauty is; health only legitimates it.

Men are not immune to these messages. The result of years of being bombarded by images of buff young men with "six pack" stomachs in magazines, film, music videos, and television is a generation of teenage boys who are flocking to gyms in record numbers in an attempt to achieve that "ideal look." Body image disturbance is the term used to describe the condition where young boys and men go to any lengths, from overexercising to abusing steroids, in order to reach their goal of a perfect body.

Advertisers, movies, and television programs use deeper societal pressures to be thin to sell their products. Having thin, attractive women and men model expensive products and play glamorous characters works to link thinness with wealth, success, and happiness. Hip, muscular, young men and thin, scantily clad women in music videos link attractiveness and sexuality with being cool. Using fat women or men to demonstrate "before" pictures in diet ads and play poor or unhealthy characters reinforces the myth that fat people are poor, unsuccessful, lazy, unhappy, and unhealthy.

Ironically, at the same time, marketers are spreading the gospel of thinness. They have been identified by health practitioners as a significant contributor to what has been termed an "epidemic" in childhood obesity, through their relentless promotion of junk food, soft drinks, and fast food. Children need to become aware of these conflicting messages in order to use their own judgment in determining what a healthy body looks like, and to feel more comfortable with their own self-image.

Some Myths about Obesity

Obesity is one of the few remaining socially sanctioned prejudices. There are four widely shared, inaccurate stereotypes about obesity that perpetuate the prejudice against fat people.

- *The obese eat more than the nonobese.* In 19 out of the 20 studies conducted before 1979, obese people were shown to eat the same or less than the nonobese, disproving the view that obese people are heavy because they eat more.
- *The obese are more emotionally disturbed than the nonobese.* Several studies have shown that obese people have no more or fewer emotional problems than the nonobese. Personality and level of adjustment also appear to be similar for both groups, despite the fact that the obese must deal with tremendous social pressure against them.
- *Moderate obesity is associated with increased sickness and death.* Some studies have extrapolated the health risks associated with extreme obesity affecting those who are moderately obese as well. But the Framingham study showed that "over"weight women had a lower mortality risk than "under"weight women. The highest mortality (death) rate for women was for those who were "under"weight. The lowest mortality rates were for women 10 percent and 20 percent over

average weight. Although it may be true that increased blood pressure and deaths due to heart disease may be associated with being "over"weight, there is some speculation that it may be the yo-yo effect of dieting and then regaining the weight that accounts for the increase in blood pressure.

- *Long-term treatment through dieting is successful.* Several long-term follow-up studies have shown that the success rate of diets, over time, is dismal at best. In fact, it is estimated that approximately 95 percent of diets simply do not work over the long term. Dr. Susan Wooley (the executive director of the American School Health Association) suggests that the diagnosis of obesity should be eliminated. She believes that you can't treat something you can't diagnose and that obese individuals should instead be helped to improve their sense of self-esteem.

In any given class, there are probably heavier children who are discriminated against because of body size. In light of this, the challenge for educators is to present information on overweight in a highly sensitive and supportive manner.

Class Discussion

Begin the class by explaining that billions of people live on Earth, each one unique in their color, size, features, and personality. Each one of us has traits that make us unique. Some of us are small, some of us are big; some are fair, some are dark; some are girls; some are boys. Tell students to look around the room and their classmates, saying, "Look at all the differences between just the people in this one room!"

The people that we see in the media represent only a small percentage of the different types of people that live in the real world, and this is a problem. When we see the same type of people each time we turn on our TVs or open a magazine, or when we are told in advertisements that it is better to look like one type of person than another, it can make us dissatisfied with the way we look—with our body image. Use these questions to guide a class discussion:

- What makes a body healthy? (Balanced diet, exercise, lots of sleep, and so on.)
- Do you have to be thin to be healthy?
- How might wanting to look like the people we see on television and magazines be a negative thing? (People who desperately want to be thin may develop eating disorders, exercise obsessively, or turn to smoking or drugs as a way to control appetite. They may develop low self-esteem and become depressed if they can't change the way they look.)

Think about the people whom you see on TV and in advertisements.

- What are some words that you would use to describe the women?
- What are some words that you would use to describe the men?
- What is the message that these images tell us about how people should look?
- Think of your own family and friends—do they look like the people you see in the media?

The truth is that very few of us look like the people you see in the media. In fact, if you met a celebrity in real life, he or she probably wouldn't look anything like his or her media image. This is because the images of people that we see in ads or on TV are carefully constructed—photographs are touched up to make them look more attractive, or the people are filmed using lots of makeup and special lighting. They even have special software that can alter a picture of someone and give them longer legs or even make them thinner. Nevertheless, many of us are influenced by these images, both in our feelings toward others and in our feelings about ourselves.

Activity 1

Pretend that you are an alien traveling through space. One day you come across a deserted space station from earth. In the space station you find all sorts of magazines (those astronauts got pretty bored just floating through space!). Because you've never seen a human before, this is very exciting, so you put together a report on humans based on the magazines that you've found.

In small groups, go through the magazines that you've brought to class. From the images that you see in those magazines, create a description of what a "typical" earthling looks like based on what you've found. (Students might like to create a composite man and a composite woman using bits and pieces of the people they've found in various ads and photos.) As well as physically describing earthlings, what would our aliens say about people based on these magazines? (For example, humans are always smiling and happy, humans live on beaches, and humans wear cool clothes). Present your reports to the class.

Activity 2

Review the story starter (included at the end of the learning experience) with students. Distribute this material directly to students, or provide verbal prompts and work through the story section by section.

After students have finished their stories, discuss how they felt in their "alien worlds." Try to transfer their alien experience to the pressures within our own world to conform to a certain look.

Activity 3

Compare the story the groups put together in Activity 1 with the story starter from Activity 2.

- What are the similarities?
- What are the differences?

Activity 4

Write a letter to one of the magazine editors, corporate sponsors of an ad, or TV show producers asking that they use actors that look more like average people.

RESOURCES
Magazines and story starter handouts

ASSESSMENT PLAN
The teacher will evaluate alien stories (Activity 1), completed stories (Activity 2), comparison reports (Activity 3), and letters (Activity 4).

REFLECTION

This experience lets students take a good look at pressures to conform to standards of beauty—particularly current pressures to be thin and the related prejudice against being overweight. Through class discussion and activities, students begin to recognize how the media pressure people to achieve a certain look and how media images may lead to prejudice against those who don't conform to their standards of attractiveness. Consider the following questions:

- How well did the learning experience meet the stated objectives?
- Did the students have adequate practice time to work on the skills?
- Do students demonstrate more sensitivity to those in class who are overweight?
- How did overweight/obese students react to the activities and discussion?
- How might you modify the learning experience in the future?
- How did the various skill levels of the students affect the learning experience?

REFERENCES

Adapted from the Media Awareness Network (www.media-awareness.ca). The background information is adapted with permission from Teacher's Resource Kit: A Teacher's Lesson Plan Kit for the Prevention of Eating Disorders, National Eating Disorders Information Centre, © 1989. © 2003 Media Awareness Network.

Story Starter (Media Awareness Network, 2002)

This is a story about a strange vacation you took to another planet in a distant solar system. It tells of the day you were discovered by a spacecraft of aliens and taken away to a strange world. These aliens were really huge; they weighed about 400 pounds and were 7 feet tall. At first you thought they were ugly. Yet when you arrived at their planet you found that all the aliens were huge, and the largest were considered the most beautiful by this society. When you opened a magazine or turned on a television, all you saw were enormous aliens. You also saw advertisements and commercials promising to help the aliens become even bigger! Please write an account of this vacation.

_____ (Story Title)

Describe exactly where and how the aliens found you. Did you apply for an ad in the newspaper to go to a strange world? Were you at an amusement park and picked up by aliens who thought you were their friends in disguise?

- What did they look like? What was your reaction to them? What was their reaction to you?
- What was the inside of their spaceship like? Were you afraid? How long did the trip take you? How far away was their planet from the Earth?
- Did you meet any creatures your own age when you arrived? How big were they? What was your reaction to them? Did they view you as a strange creature? Did they ask you questions? Did you see a product that promises to make its customers larger? What is the product that they are selling? A green slime bath that will make their bodies expand? A reverse exercise machine that will add on pounds instead of taking them off? And what does the commercial promise will happen when they become bigger? Will they be more popular and get invited to the Galaxy Space Dance? Will they be more successful and become presidents of their own spaceship companies? Will their lives suddenly become more exciting than the lives that they have now?
- Why were the most famous and admired creatures also the largest? How did the smaller aliens who were short or thin feel about their bodies?
- Describe the feelings you had after being on this planet for a few months. Did you start liking the way the aliens looked? Did it make you feel worse or better about your own body size?
- When and how did you leave? What did your experience tell you about social pressures to be a certain size or shape? If you could give one important message to the people on earth about body size and shape, what would it be?

When you have finished, reread your paragraphs. Add details where you think they are missing. Rewrite the paragraphs with connecting sentences so that they make a continuous story. Read what you have written. Change anything that needs changing. Read and change until you are pleased with your story.

Now try drawing a picture to illustrate your story!

LEARNING EXPERIENCE 5

TITLE: Learning Gender Stereotypes

GRADE LEVELS: 7–9

TIME REQUIREMENTS: This learning experience needs to be completed over a three session time frame.

LEARNING CONTEXT

The objective of this learning experience is to encourage students to develop their own critical intelligence with regard to culturally inherited stereotypes, and to the images presented in the media—film and television, rock music, newspapers and magazines.

The learning experience begins with a review of stereotypes that are associated with men and women and their possible sources—including the role of the media. Students deconstruct a series of advertisements based on gender representation and answer questions about gender stereotyping about articles they have read.

Students will

- Understand the importance of distinguishing between fantasy (what happens on television, in the movies, and in ads) and reality (what really goes on in their lives).
- Understand that stereotypical perfection is illusory and unreal.
- Recognize the futility and the harmful effects of striving to attain stereotypical perfection.
- Appreciate the benefits of celebrating who they really are.

NATIONAL LEARNING STANDARD

4:   Students will analyze the influence of culture, media, technology, and other factors on health.

SKILLS

Decision-making
Self management
Stress management
Advocacy

PROCEDURE

Background

From infancy, our culture teaches what it means to be a boy or a girl. From the colour of clothes to the toys we play with, the messages begin at a very early age. Young people are influenced by a barrage of messages to conform to a variety of expectations, to buy this widget, and to preserve a rigid set of values that stress the differences between genders.

The world of make believe as it is presented on TV and in the movies—from thriller films to soap operas on television—has a big effect on the viewer. Even though the plot and characters are fictitious, the underlying attitudes and messages are not. They communicate cultural values, which shape the way we think and the way we interact. Understanding this, it is important to begin to unmask a double standard that is pervasive in our culture. The dichotomy is that we buy into the stereotypes that reinforce abuse, while trying to "root out" violence in our community.

In order to combat this destructive hypocrisy, students must begin to ask questions, rather than passively accepting whatever they see and hear. Recognizing media myths for what they are is a good first step. The objective here is to draw a thick line between the stereotypical behavior of TV, film, and video heroes, on the one hand, and our own lives, on the other.

Activity: Messages from Magazine Ads

Facilitator's Introduction: Last time we exposed the gender stereotypes in the Act Like a Man/Be Ladylike Box, and what it meant to be outside them. We concluded by naming some of the influences in our lives that can teach us or pressure us to fit into these stereotyped ideas of what it means to be a man or a woman. In today's activity, we're going to explore how the media helps to build these stereotypes.

- display the flip chart sheets from Act Like a Man/Be Ladylike, in the lesson Exposing Gender Stereotypes, for reference.

Ask your students:

- How can parents pressure us to act like a man? (Preference for the color blue, as opposed to pink, "don't cry," "be strong," go out for sports, etc.)
- What about being pressured at home to be ladylike? ("Don't get your hands dirty," "have good manners," develop the right interests like cooking, decorating, tidying up the house, etc.)

It's easy to see that our parents encourage us to do certain things, like going out for sports if we're boys and paying more attention to our wardrobe if we're girls. The way the media influences us is not always so obvious.

- What do we mean by "media"? (Write students' definitions on the chalkboard and list examples under the areas of television, films, videos, newspapers, magazines, and radio.)

Discussion

The media, in whatever form, is a business that sells information and reaches millions of people. The partnership between advertisers and the media dates back to the eighteenth century when the first advertisement appeared in a newspaper (a slave owner requesting the return of his lost "property").

Advertisers have since developed a multi-billion dollar industry to convince consumers (like us) that we need to buy their products. The Pepsi/Coke wars are a recent example of how marketers rally for the buying public's attention and loyalty. Statistics tell us that we see 350,000 ads by the time we graduate from high school. How this influences our attitudes is rich material for social scientists. One thing is for sure: ads do influence our choices when we go to buy something. But the influence of advertisements is tricky to deal with because they affect us subliminally.

Activity One

We often see ads that feature superficially beautiful or "desirable" models, so it comes as no surprise that sexual imagery is used to sell products. But depicting people this way can also contribute to gender stereotypes. Today, we're going to take a look at some media messages that tell us how to be a man, and how to be a woman.

- Display on an overhead: *The Insult that Made a Man out of 'Mac'* and *Pick a Fight After School* comic book ads.

Ask students:

- Do you think the message to act like a man has changed in the twenty years between the publication of these two comic book ads?
- Organize students into working groups of four to six. Distribute the Activity Sheet Media Messages and the magazine ads they brought.

Instructions

These ads were taken from popular women's and men's magazines. Answer the questions, bearing in mind there are no right or wrong answers—just write down what the picture means to you. Don't spend much time on each question; just write your first impressions, and go on to the next one. (Note: For **question 6**, ask students to refer to the stereotype boxes on the board.)

Question 7 may be difficult for students to answer. It may be necessary to point out that, by association, advertisers depict people who look like they have it together so that their products will look desirable to the consumer.

Procedure options

- Have students come forward one group at a time to relate how the ad portrays the stereotypes in the box.
- Ask a student from each group to read answers to questions and record their responses on the board or flip chart for comparisons.
- Hand out flip chart paper to each group.
- Have students draw the outline of a female and a male, and fill in the outline with the expectations or stereotypes projected by the ad.
- Present and display their results for the class to see.

Closure

Ask students:

- What common themes are present in all of these ads?
- What are these ads saying about roles for men and women?
- How do you think these ads can affect our attitudes and our expectations for gender roles?

Activity Two

Homework assignment: Provide additional copies of the Media Messages activity sheet and ask students to find, and bring in, magazine ads that portray sex role stereotypes to share with the class.

Hand out news articles: "Sex, Violence and Advertising" and "Women's Magazines Send Us a Strange, Confusing Message" for discussion.

Process this activity the following day by asking students to present the ads they chose and the reasons they believe it to be an example of a gender stereotype.

INSTRUCTIONAL/ENVIRONMENTAL MODIFICATIONS

Preparation and Materials

- Have students bring in magazine ads depicting men and women together.
- *Act Like a Man/Be Ladylike* flip charts (from the lesson Exposing Gender Stereotypes)
- Overhead transparencies or copies of comic book ads
- Copies of activity sheet Media Messages for each group
- Overheads *The Insult that Made a Man out of 'Mac'* and *Pick a Fight After School*
- Handouts "Sex, Violence and Advertising," "Analyzing an Ad," and "Women's Magazines Send Us a Strange, Confusing Message" for extension activities

RESOURCES

Provide magazines for students who may not have access to them at home.

A print-friendly version of the five handouts/overheads (listed above) can be found at: http://www.media-awareness.ca/english/resources/educational/lessons/secondary/gender_portrayal/gender_stereotypes.cfm

ASSESSMENT PLAN

Completion of handouts
Participation in discussion

REFLECTION

- How does the media influence your own perception of gender?
- What evidence of gender stereotyping do you observe in your students before, during, and after this learning experience?
- How can we better help students see the limitations of gender stereotyping?
- What are the cultural dimensions of gender stereotyping? That is, can any conclusions be made about gender stereotyping based on cultural heritage?

REFERENCES

This lesson was adapted to meet the NY State Health Education Learning Standards and National Health Education Learning Standards from the Media Awareness Network (www.media-awareness.ca)

LEARNING EXPERIENCE 6

TITLE: Individuality versus Conformity

GRADE LEVELS: 10–12

TIME REQUIREMENTS: One session, but part of a 3-day experience

LEARNING CONTEXT

This experience is designed to introduce students to the concept of popular culture and the role that it plays in their lives. It develops skills in decision making, self-management, planning and goal setting, and advocacy. Students examine the pressures that exist to conform to popular culture and its effect on their lives. They will have the ability to

- Understand the prevalence of popular culture in their daily lives.
- Be aware of the pressures within popular culture to conform to its ideals.
- Appreciate the argumentative essay as a means of expressing an opinion.

NATIONAL LEARNING STANDARD

4:   Students will analyze the influence of culture, media, technology, and other factors on health.

PROCEDURE

In a class discussion, have the students identify fads or trends that are popular within their own school. Topics should ideally be those that are somewhat controversial within the school, such as these:

- Body piercing
- Skateboarding
- Tattooing
- Smoking
- Clothing (for example, skimpy clothing for girls, bandanas for boys that may be prohibited because of gang-related connotations)

Once several topics have been suggested, divide your students into small groups. Assign each group one of the topics for discussion.

Explain to your students that they have 20 minutes to discuss answers to the following questions. Remind students that each group member is responsible for recording the group's discussion.

1. With respect to your assigned topic, why do (or don't) you conform or participate in this activity?
2. Are you pressured to participate in this activity? If your answer is yes, how are you pressured? Where does the pressure come from?
3. Do you feel that popular culture emphasizes individuality, or does it ask you to conform?
4. Does popular culture lead trends or follow them?

Using their assigned topics and group discussion notes, students are to write a brief argumentative essay on individuality and conformity in popular culture.

Additional Activities

- Have students trace the origins of current fads or trends in popular culture.
- Debate a controversial fad or trend in popular culture. The chosen topic should be relevant to the lives of your students.
- Have students decide which current trend is the most controversial. Through a show of hands, see how many of your students are in favor of this trend and how many are opposed. Divide your class in half on the basis of those who support and those who oppose this trend (if these groups are lopsided, ask some students to play devil's advocate and join the other side).Give each side 10 minutes to form their debate. Remind students to select an individual to present the opening statement, and a second student to present the closing statement.
- Ask students to design a poster, public service announcement, or brief educational lesson to educate their peers about the risks involved with various fads or trends.
- Ask students to write a letter or start an e-mail campaign to reach elected representatives about better regulation for fads that are illegal (such as access to tobacco and stricter enforcement of age requirements for tattoos).

INSTRUCTIONAL/ENVIRONMENTAL MODIFICATIONS

Prepare materials that address both the risks and the benefits of the fads and trends discussed. For example, the Centers for Disease Control and Prevention website (www.cdc.gov) is an excellent source of health information on smoking, body piercing, and tattooing.

RESOURCES

Internet materials promoting or condemning various fads and trends; poster board

ASSESSMENT PLAN

The teacher will evaluate the following items, depending on the activity:
- Group or individual student projects from selected activities.
- Poster or public service announcement on fads or trends.
- Letter to elected representatives on illegal fads and trends with suggestions on how to better regulate.

REFLECTION

- What trends and fads were popular when you were in high school?
- What pressures did you feel to conform to any of these fads or trends?
- How can your experience translate to the pressures high school students are feeling today?
- What effect does cultural background have on the adoption of fads and trends?

INDEX